READING AND STUDY
Strategies for
Nursing Students

READING AND STUDY Strategies for Nursing Students

Marilyn Meltzer, M.A.

Hunter College
New York, New York

Susan Marcus Palau, M.A.

Learning Specialist
Formerly, Phillips Beth Israel School of Nursing
New York, New York

W.B. SAUNDERS COMPANY

A Division of
Harcourt Brace & Company

Philadelphia London Toronto Montreal Sydney Tokyo

W. B. SAUNDERS COMPANY
A Division of
Harcourt Brace & Company
The Curtis Center
Independence Square West
Philadelphia, PA 19106

Library of Congress Cataloging-in-Publication Data

Meltzer, Marilyn
    Reading and study strategies for nursing students / Marilyn
Meltzer, Susan Marcus Palau.—1st ed.
      p.   cm.
    ISBN 0–7216–4483–X
    1. Nursing—Study and teaching. 2. Study, Method of.   I. Palau,
Susan Marcus. II. Title.
    [DNLM: 1. Education, Nursing. 2. Learning—nurses' instruction.
3. Reading—nurses' instruction.   WY 18 M528r]
RT73.M396 1993
610.73'07—dc20
DNLM/DLC   92–48190

READING AND STUDY STRATEGIES FOR NURSING STUDENTS

Last digit is the print number: 9 8 7 6 5 4 3 2 1

To Joe, Serena, Pepy, and Clowe
S.M.P.

To Sheldon, Sara, and Michael
M.M.

Preface

Reading and Study Strategies for Nursing Students is intended for those nursing students who need to improve their reading and study skills. The purpose of this text is to teach students the strategies necessary for reading the assigned texts in their courses. This book is designed to have nursing students practice basic concentration, vocabulary, and reading and study skills on materials in their own area of study. The exercise materials are taken exclusively from recent nursing texts so that the skills are not presented in isolation but are practically applied within the nursing field.

ORGANIZATION

Unit 1, Improving Concentration, helps students to become organized and focused. These techniques transform students from passive to active readers and provide a foundation for improving comprehension.

Unit 2, Vocabulary Development, gives nursing students specific ways for learning the specialized vocabulary in nursing texts, which is often a hurdle for students. They can learn and retain new words through a variety of approaches including word structure, context clues, and using inferences and index cards.

Unit 3, Reading Comprehension, shows students how to recognize the main ideas, details, and organizational plans of textbook materials. These strategies help students better comprehend and retain what they are reading.

Unit 4, Study Skills, provides nursing students with the necessary tools for better understanding their textbooks and classroom lectures. Test-taking techniques are included to help students learn how to prepare for and get better results on examinations.

Unit 5, Reading Selections, includes 15 readings from nursing textbooks, which will allow the nursing students to apply comprehensively all the skills learned in the previous units.

Each chapter in Units 1 through 4 includes the following:
- objectives
- key words
- skills presentations
- examples
- practice exercises
- vocabulary check
- chapter summary

Unit 5, the reading selections, gives students the opportunity to apply the following skills to 15 selections from nursing textbooks:

- prereading
- identifying key vocabulary
- summarizing
- answering multiple choice questions

USING THE TEXTBOOK

Reading and Study Strategies for Nursing Students is designed to be used in one semester; the 15 chapters can be completed weekly. The reading selections in Unit V can be used in conjunction with Chapters 1 through 15 or done after the student has completed Chapter 15.

This text can be used in a traditional classroom setting or can be used by the nursing student for self-study on an individual basis or in consultation with an instructor. The pages are perforated for maximum flexibility. The answer key at the back can be removed by the instructor to allow graded assignments or used by the student for self-evaluation.

SETTING UP THE COURSE

Participants for the reading and study strategies course can be any student who scores below the 12th grade level on the nursing school entrance examination or on standardized adult reading tests. Nursing programs may want to consider making this course a requirement for prefreshman or freshman students. In any case, the course would be especially helpful for returning adult students who need special learning strategies to get back to academic work. Instructors who teach bridge courses for licensed practical/vocational nurses who are entering registered nursing courses will find the book useful to introduce students to the higher expected level of academic work.

If this textbook is to be used in a classroom setting, the instructor should provide guided practice: working closely with the students at the beginning of the exercises in each chapter, then allowing the students to practice the exercises independently toward the end of the chapter. If the students are working independently in the text, they are encouraged to work through the chapters sequentially. But since the text is divided into four independent units, they can be used in any order. The instructor can assess the students' work in class, or students can evaluate their own work using the answer key individually or in small groups. Finally, the classroom can be structured so that the students are working together in small groups (collaborative learning) or the students can work individually at their own pace.

MOTIVATING THE STUDENTS

When doing the lessons in this textbook, students will have strategies to help them concentrate and comprehend and retain textbook information that will help them do well in nursing school. These strategies are concrete, providing plans for organizing study time and the information the nursing students need to learn to feel more in control of the time and academic pressures they face. Once the students see the positive results gained from using this text, motivation problems will be solved.

ACKNOWLEDGMENTS

We would like to thank our word processors *extraordinaire*, Robin Levine, Sandra Bella, and Michael Martin; the following people at W. B. Saunders who helped in preparation of the manuscript: Michael Brown, Cass Stamato, Marilyn Marsella, Ilze Rader, and Marie Thomas; and Mary Espenschied and Jeanne Gulledge of CRACOM Corporation who helped us in the production process.

Also a special thanks to the Phillips Beth Israel School of Nursing faculty and students for providing the inspiration for this book and to our colleagues and students at Hunter College for their encouragement and support.

Marilyn Meltzer
Susan Marcus Palau

Contents

UNIT I **IMPROVING CONCENTRATION** 1

   1 Time Management 3

   2 Prereading Strategies 12

   3 Monitoring Your Comprehension 24

UNIT II **VOCABULARY DEVELOPMENT** 35

   4 Affixes 37

   5 Using Context Clues 45

   6 Dictionary, Glossary, and Thesaurus 61

   7 Word Bank 78

UNIT III **READING COMPREHENSION** 83

   8 Topics and Main Ideas 85

   9 Details 102

   10 Paragraph Organization 113

UNIT IV **STUDY SKILLS** 127

   11 Reading the Textbook 129

   12 Graphic Aids 154

   13 Active Listening 173

   14 Note Taking in the Classroom 179

   15 Test-Taking Strategies 197

UNIT V **READING SELECTIONS** 219

   References 287

   Glossary 288

   Answer Key 293

   Index 315

• U N I T •

I

IMPROVING CONCENTRATION

As nursing students, you are probably finding yourself in a bewildering new world of facts, theories, and words. Every day the classroom and clinic offer new challenges to your intellect.

Your nursing textbooks present a vast array of facts in intimidating volumes. This may be the first time in your academic career that you are expected to read so much material in so little time. Therefore you need to read your nursing textbooks as efficiently as possible. To be an efficient reader you must concentrate.

Many nursing students find it difficult to concentrate on their textbook assignments. Their minds wander, they do not connect ideas, and when they are finished, they do not retain the information.

Tested strategies can increase your reading concentration. Concentration is the first step to improving reading comprehension and retention.

Unit 1 introduces the technique of improving concentration. Chapter One, "Time Management," helps you to set priorities, schedule your study time, and work in a focused, purposeful style. Chapter Two, "Prereading Strategies," introduces techniques for becoming actively involved with the author's ideas. Chapter Three, "Monitoring Comprehension," helps you keep track of your comprehension as you read and introduces five strategies for getting back on track when your concentration falters.

A vocabulary check is included at the end of each chapter in Units 1 through 4. This vocabulary exercise reinforces the words that are essential to understanding the information in each chapter.

Reading textbooks with concentration requires your active participation. Unit 1 gives you the strategies needed to learn how to concentrate on your nursing studies.

• Chapter 1 •

Time Management

OBJECTIVE

KEY WORDS

QUESTIONS TO THINK ABOUT
BEFORE READING

USING TIME MANAGEMENT
    Getting Organized
    Setting and Prioritizing Goals
    Using Calendars
    Identifying Time Wasters

VOCABULARY CHECK

SUMMARY

• OBJECTIVE

To organize your time so that you will improve your study habits.

• KEY WORDS

Pay attention to the key words, which are listed below. They are underscored the first time they appear in this chapter. Try to determine the meanings of these words from the surrounding words in the passage. If you need further help, use your dictionary or the glossary in the back of this book.

As you read the exercises in this chapter, write additional words you need to learn in the space provided.

GENERAL VOCABULARY

anxiety	internal
avoidance	priority
concrete	procrastination
consistency	_____
excessive	_____
external	_____
extracurricular	_____

• QUESTIONS TO THINK ABOUT BEFORE READING

When you are doing assignments, do you:

1 Fall behind?   Yes _____   No _____

2 Procrastinate?   Yes _____   No _____

3 Save difficult assignments for last?   Yes _____   No _____

4 Waste time?   Yes _____   No _____

5 Find it difficult to get started?   Yes _____   No _____

• USING TIME MANAGEMENT

If you've answered yes to these questions, you have to learn about time management. Time management helps you to get organized and focused. You will learn to control your time rather than letting time control you. The most successful students have learned time management.

• Getting Organized

There are different ways to manage your study time more efficiently. Following a few simple steps will enable you to set goals so that you can successfully complete your assignments.

The most anxiety-producing situation for any student is to fall behind in completing assignments. Establishing goals will help you to solve this problem. You will learn how to set goals so that you can keep up with all your nursing studies and eliminate the anxiety that comes with procrastination.

• Setting and Prioritizing Goals

To manage your time most efficiently during the course of the semester, you should think about the goals you want to achieve by the end of the semester and place these goals in the order of importance to you (prioritizing). When setting semester goals, you must think about how you need to have your life structured. Are you required to take three or four courses? Do you want a part-time job? Are there home and family responsibilities that you must meet? Are you allowing time for hobbies and other recreational interests? List on notebook paper everything you want to accomplish for the semester. Make sure that your goals are *balanced*. You will not be happy with just studying and working; give yourself the opportunity to relax.

When you prioritize these goals, you will notice that some activities have greater urgency than others. In nursing school, studying for your major, or your nursing course, should have priority over some lesser activity. When you order your goals, some priorities will limit other goals. For example, studying for a nursing exam may not allow you to go to the gym that week. However, keep in mind that in prioritizing the most important goals should be met first. Be realistic about what you expect to accomplish in a semester. If you overextend yourself, you may have difficulty meet-

TABLE 1–1   One Student's Semester Goals

Setting Semester Goals	Prioritizing Goals
• Taking full-time schedule at nursing school	1 Taking full-time schedule at nursing school
• Working part-time 10 hours a week	2 Preparing family meals
• Practicing in choir	3 Working part-time 10 hours a week
• Exercising in gym	4 Practicing in choir
• Preparing family meals	5 Exercising in gym

ing any of your goals. Determine what is most important to you and focus on achieving these chosen goals. Table 1–1 is an example of how one student set and prioritized semester goals.

• Using Calendars

Once you have set and prioritized your goals, calendars can help you organize your time efficiently. By using monthly, weekly, and daily calendars, you will be able to follow any schedule you establish to meet your goals.

Each of these calendars has its own function:
• Monthly calendar—to plan long-range assignments
• Weekly calendar—to learn consistency
• Daily calendar—to help you set priorities

MONTHLY CALENDAR

Some helpful information to place on your monthly calendar (Fig. 1–1):
• Exam dates
• Due dates of papers
• Special projects

• EXERCISE 1–1 •

Directions.   Fill in the monthly calendar (Fig. 1–1). What other information might you add to the monthly calendar?

_____

_____

_____

_____

_____

WEEKLY CALENDAR

The weekly calendar (Fig. 1–2) helps you to organize your time and think about consistency. Consistency is staying with a regular schedule. Successful students do

JANUARY

SUN	MON	TUE	WED	THURS	FRI	SAT
	1	2	3	4	5	6
7	8	9	10	11 med-surg exam	12	13
14	15	16	17	18	19	20
21	22	23	24	25	26	27
28	29	30	31			

FIGURE 1–1 Monthly calendar.

assignments at scheduled times. They are not haphazard. They establish a study time and place.

How to Use the Weekly Calendar

Fill in the hours you sleep, have meals, work at part-time employment, and attend classes. Look at the hours left. Circle the hours each day that are free for study. Be realistic. Allow time for extracurricular activities and recreation. Circle the hours you intend to use for study each day with a red pen. Now decide where you will study. Many students find that they are less distracted when they study in a school or neighborhood library than when they work at home. It doesn't matter where you choose to study, but your study area should be quiet, well lit, and free from distractions.

Once you have decided when and where you will study each day, you are beginning to get organized. The next step is sticking to the schedule you planned on your weekly calendar. Learning consistency will help you to manage time.

TIME	SUN	MON	TUES	WED	THURS	FRI	SAT
7–8 AM							
8–9							
9–10							
10–11							
11–12							
12–1 PM							
1–2							
2–3							
3–4							
4–5							
5–6							
6–7							
7–8							
8–9							

FIGURE 1–2 Weekly calendar.

• **EXERCISE 1–2** •

Directions. Fill in the weekly calendar. As you go through the week, make a checkmark (√) next to each task you complete. You'll see at a glance whether you're accomplishing your goals.

Write out a weekly calendar each Sunday. You may have to make changes, but at least you will have a <u>concrete</u> plan for scheduling your time.

Self-Monitoring

At this point in your time management, you must evaluate whether your schedule is allowing you to meet your established goals. One good way of doing this is to monitor your activities as they relate to your weekly schedule. Ask yourself the following questions:

• Are my nonscheduled activities interfering with my school activities?

- Does my study schedule accurately reflect my prioritized goals?
- Am I allowing myself enough time to study?
- Is my weekly schedule flexible enough to allow for the unexpected?
- Does my weekly schedule show that I am wasting time?
- Did I establish a good balance between work and recreation in my schedule?

When you have answered these questions, you may need to rethink your weekly schedule. Keep monitoring and evaluating your weekly calendar to determine whether it is helping you to organize your time efficiently.

DAILY CALENDAR

The daily calender helps you learn to set priorities. Each evening, think about what you want to accomplish the next day. Start by writing a "to-do" list.

To-Do List

A to-do list is an informal listing of all the activities you need to do for the following day. This "to-do" list encompasses both academic and nonacademic tasks. Each night as you think about the next day's activities, write down everything you need to do on a piece of paper. Then number these activities in the order you want to accomplish them. Make sure that you write down specific activities and assignments. Do not be vague. Then transfer this information to the time slots in your daily calendar.

Table 1–2 is an example of a nursing student's to-do list. In step 1 the student wrote down all necessary activities. In step 2 he prioritized the activities according to when he wanted to do them. Note how specific the student was when listing school assignments.

TABLE 1–2 To-do List

Step 1	Step 2	
• Do grocery shopping	2	Do grocery shopping
• Read Chapter 5 in *Anatomy and Physiology*	1	Read Chapter 5 in *Anatomy and Physiology*
• Pick up shirts at cleaner	3	Pick up shirts at cleaner
• Pay phone bill	7	Pay phone bill
• Review clinical notes	4	Review clinical notes
• Write first draft of English essay	5	Write first draft of English essay
• Make dental appointment	6	Make dental appointment

• EXERCISE 1–3 •

Directions. Fill in the daily calendar (Fig. 1–3). Again, be realistic when you set your goals. Make a checkmark (√) next to each assignment that you complete. You will then monitor what you are accomplishing each day. Set your priorities. Decide which tasks are the most important to complete.

(✔)   When   Completed

Time	
9:00 - 9:30	
9:30 - 10:00	
10:00 - 10:30	
10:30 - 11:00	
11:00 - 11:30	
11:30 - 12:00	
12:00 - 12:30	
12:30 - 1:00	
1:00 - 1:30	
1:30 - 2:00	
2:00 - 2:30	
2:30 - 3:00	
3:00 - 3:30	
3:30 - 4:00	
4:00 - 4:30	
4:30 - 5:00	
5:00 - 5:30	
5:30 - 6:00	
6:00 - 6:30	
6:30 - 7:00	
7:00 - 7:30	
7:30 - 8:00	
8:00 - 8:30	
8:30 - 9:00	

FIGURE 1–3 Daily calendar.

- **Identifying Time Wasters**

   Using calendars helps you to avoid wasting time. Some common time wasters are:
   - Procrastination: "I'll do it later." Procrastination, or delaying what needs to be done, is the greatest source of anxiety for students. Do it now—not later. Your grades will improve and you'll be more relaxed. Do not save difficult assignments for last. Do them first when concentration is best. Avoidance only increases anxiety.
   - Excessive socializing: Students can allow socializing to get in the way of completing assignments if they don't stick to a schedule. In your weekly and daily

calendars leave some realistic time for socializing. Staying on schedule eliminates the tendency to allow socializing to take up too much of your time.
- Distractions: Students are often distracted. Both <u>external</u> and <u>internal</u> distractions get in the way of efficient studying.

EXTERNAL DISTRACTIONS

External distractions are elements in your surroundings that prevent you from paying attention to your studies.

Learning consistency, establishing a study place and time, helps to eliminate external distractions. You should plan to study away from the telephone, television, and other distractions.

INTERNAL DISTRACTIONS

Internal distractions are your thoughts and feelings that prevent you from concentrating on your schoolwork.

Using the daily calendar to establish priorities helps to eliminate internal distractions. Instead of worrying about the things you can't control, you can focus on managing your time and completing the tasks on your daily calendar. Sticking to a schedule keeps you organized and improves your concentration.

Remember, if you set and prioritize goals and use monthly, weekly, and daily calendars, you will learn to manage time. Time management is an essential skill for nursing school students.

• VOCABULARY CHECK

Directions.   Below are 10 words taken from the key words section of this chapter. Circle the letter of the best definition from the four choices.

1 Consistency
  a instability
  b contentment
  c disorder
  d regularity

2 Priority
  a goal placed in order of importance
  b activity done beforehand
  c task left uncompleted
  d action done previously

3 Extracurricular
  a an assignment for extra credit
  b additional course information
  c outside the regular course of work
  d illogical circular reasoning

4 Concrete
  a abstract
  b hard
  c false
  d definite

5 Procrastination
  a delaying what needs to be done
  b rearranging events
  c failing to establish goals
  d forgetting crucial assignments

6 Anxiety
  a bodily pain
  b chronic pain
  c emotional pain
  d pain reduction

7 Avoidance
  a reaching out to something
  b withdrawing from something
  c rejecting the truth
  d answering a complaint

8 Internal
  a outside the body
  b inside the body
  c away from the body
  d damaging to the body

9 External
  a outside the body
  b inside the body
  c away from the body
  d damaging to the body

10 Excessive
  a too regular
  b too few
  c too much
  d too little

• SUMMARY

Time management helps you to become a successful nursing student. The first step in time management is setting and prioritizing goals. The use of calendars will help to manage your time most efficiently. Monthly calendars are useful for long-range planning. Weekly calendars help you to learn to be consistent and follow a regular study routine. Daily calendars allow you to set priorities and focus on completing everyday activities in order of importance. You will eliminate the time wasters of procrastination, excessive socializing, and distractions. Time management will help you to become an accomplished nursing student.

• Chapter 2 •

Prereading Strategies

OBJECTIVE

KEY WORDS

QUESTIONS TO THINK ABOUT BEFORE READING

USING PREREADING STRATEGIES

FIVE PREREADING STRATEGIES
   Read the Chapter Title
   Read the Introduction and
   Summary
   Read All Headings
   Look at Key Words
   Examine All Graphic Aids

VOCABULARY CHECK

SUMMARY

• OBJECTIVE

To learn to use prereading strategies to improve reading concentration and comprehension.

• KEY WORDS

Pay attention to the key words, which are listed on the following page. They are underscored the first time they appear in this chapter. Try to determine the meanings of these words from the surrounding words in the passage. If you need further help, use your dictionary or the glossary in the back of this book.

Look up the medical terminology in your medical dictionary or the glossary. As you read the exercises in this chapter, write additional words you need to learn in the space provided.

MEDICAL TERMINOLOGY	GENERAL VOCABULARY
analgesia	credence
dressing	delegate
gastrointestinal	document
inflammatory	extraneous
interventions	impending
irrigate	inherent
ostomy	lifestyle
regimen	locus
sterile	motivated
trauma	protocol
_____	_____
_____	_____
_____	_____

• QUESTIONS TO THINK ABOUT BEFORE READING

When you are assigned chapters in your nursing textbook, do you:

1 Find it hard to get started? Yes _____ No _____

2 Find it difficult to identify the main idea? Yes _____ No _____

3 Have trouble concentrating? Yes _____ No _____

4 Have difficulty understanding what you are reading? Yes _____ No _____

5 Have trouble connecting ideas in the chapter? Yes _____ No _____

• USING PREREADING STRATEGIES

If you've answered yes to these questions, you will find that prereading strategies will help you to tackle assignments in your nursing textbooks.

Many students open a text and just begin reading. They then find it difficult to get involved with the chapter information and complain that the assignment is boring. Instead of giving up before you begin, use prereading strategies as a way to become actively involved with the reading material.

Prereading strategies enable you to concentrate and comprehend textbook assignments by helping you to:

• Get started.
• See how the parts fit into the whole.
• Organize information into main ideas and supporting details.
• Become familiar with the subject matter.
• Read your assignments more efficiently.

• FIVE PREREADING STRATEGIES

The following five prereading strategies will help you to stay involved with the material and actively read with a purpose.

• Read the Chapter Title

The title gives you the topic of the chapter. It tells you who or what the chapter is about. Write the title of this chapter. _____

• Read the Introduction and Summary

The beginning paragraph or paragraphs will usually indicate the contents of the chapter. Carefully reading the introduction gives you a focus. You will know what to concentrate on as you read the rest of the chapter. In a phrase write what the introduction is about.

_____

_____

The summary is usually found in the last paragraph or paragraphs. The summary concisely restates the main ideas of the chapter.

Read the summary of this chapter. List the important ideas.

_____

_____

_____

_____

• Read All Headings

Headings are the titles that are in larger or darker print for emphasis. These are the main topics of the chapter. When done properly, these headings are the outline of the chapter. The largest headings should indicate the most important divisions of the chapter. List all the boldface headings in this chapter.

_____

_____

_____

_____

_____

_____

• Look at Key Words

Pay attention to all words in *italics*, the slanted, thinner type; in **boldface**, the heavier, darker type; and underscored. These words have been selected because their meanings are important to your understanding the ideas in the chapter. Key words are essential to your comprehending the information in your nursing textbooks.

Read the list of key words in this chapter.
Write any of the key words you need to learn.

_____   _____   _____

_____   _____   _____

_____   _____   _____

_____   _____   _____

- **Examine All Graphic Aids**

Graphic aids are the illustrations, tables, graphs, and charts found in the chapter. Don't skip over graphic aids. Authors often use graphic aids to explain important ideas in the chapter.

Are there any graphic aids in this chapter?

_____

_____

• EXAMPLE •

Below is an example of how you can use the five prereading strategies to preview an excerpt from a nursing textbook (Iyer et al., pp. 151–153; underscores added). Following this excerpt is an example of questions with answers that demonstrate how prereading strategies can help your reading concentration and comprehension.

Identify Factors Influencing Ability to Learn.   The process of planning teaching interventions includes the recognition that there are a number of factors that affect the client's ability to learn, including pre-existing knowledge, level of education, age, motivation, perceived locus of control, state of health, and lifestyle.

Clients' current *level of knowledge*, including their misconceptions and misinformation, frequently affects their ability to learn. Some knowledge is prerequisite for additional learning. For example, clients who need to change a sterile dressing may encounter great difficulty if they do not know the basics of good hand-washing.

Level of education frequently defines clients' knowledge of health and disease. If the information presented is above that level, the client may be unable to learn. The reverse may also be true. If information is presented at a level significantly below the client's level of education, the client might feel insulted and therefore fail to learn the material.

Age also affects ability to learn. The very young child may have difficulty in grasping concepts unless they are presented in very concrete terms. Some elderly clients may have ingrained ideas or "myths" that affect their ability to accept new changes. Additionally, they may have physiological deficits that interfere with their ability to learn (e.g., vision or hearing problems).

Clients must also be *motivated* to learn. Generally, they will readily learn whatever is most important to them. This substantiates the need for an accurate assessment of the client's perceived needs. However, not all clients desire information. Some prefer to delegate the responsibility for promoting, maintaining, or restoring their health to family members or health care personnel. Others in a state of denial may refuse to acknowledge the need to learn about their illness. Therefore, it is very difficult for these clients to learn effectively.

The client's perceptions about *locus of control* will also affect readiness to learn. Locus of control is defined as the belief in one's ability to control reinforcements or results. If an individual perceives that results come from outside forces, such as luck, fate, or powerful others, this person is said to have an *external* control orientation. An individual with an *internal* control orientation perceives that the outcomes of one's own behavior are contingent upon one's own behavior and abilities. A client who has an internal control orientation will be more likely to be motivated to learn than individuals who believe that fate is in charge of their health status.

The client must be *physically and emotionally prepared* for the teaching–learning experience. The nurse should plan to use interventions directed toward relief of pain, fear, anxiety, or fatigue before attempting to involve the client in learning activities. The state of health of the client may affect ability to learn. The client with a critical illness, severe debilitation, or sensory-perception deficits may be unable to process or absorb information. This may also be the case for clients with terminal disease, since they may lack motivation or ability.

The client's <u>lifestyle</u> may affect ability to learn. This is particularly pertinent when considering low socioeconomic groups and people of certain cultures. The client's learning problem may be associated with deficits in the types of experiences that make learning a desirable outcome. The client may not be stimulated in his or her culture to learn content perceived to be unnecessary or unimportant. Certain personality types—e.g., dependent or irresponsible persons—may also have <u>inherent</u> motivational problems.

Develop Individualized Outcomes.   The learning outcomes for each client involve knowledge, attitudes, and skills. For example, the nurse may be required to teach the client who needs an ostomy so that the client will be able to

- Describe how the surgery has altered the <u>gastrointestinal</u> tract (knowledge)
- Explain how the <u>ostomy</u> will affect the client's relationship with spouse (attitude)
- List types of equipment necessary to manage the ostomy (knowledge)
- Cleanse the stomal area and apply a pouch (skill)
- <u>Irrigate</u> the ostomy (skill)
- Express confidence in the ability to manage the ostomy (attitude)

Outcomes must be realistic. The involvement of the client in outcome decisions helps to assure that they will be realistic. Accurate assessment of the client's motivation and abilities is also critical.

1   What are the headings? (Identify Factors Influencing Ability to Learn; Develop Individualized Outcomes)

2   What is the introductory paragraph about? (It highlights the factors that affect a client's ability to learn. These factors are preexisting knowledge, level of education, age, motivation, perceived locus of control, state of health, and lifestyle.)

3   Is there a summary paragraph? (No)

4   List the key words in this selection. Use the glossary if you need help finding the meanings of these words.

interventions	dressing	lifestyle	ostomy
locus	motivated	inherent	irrigate
sterile	delegate	gastrointestinal	

5   What is this reading selection about? (A nurse must recognize the factors that affect a client's ability to learn and develop realistic outcomes.)

• EXERCISE 2–1 •

Directions. Use the five prereading strategies to get actively involved with the following chapter from a nursing textbook (Iyer et al., pp. 168–172; underscores added). Answer the questions at the end of the chapter.

TYPES OF CARE PLANS

There are several different types of care plans in use. Those that are most common include individually constructed, standardized, and computerized care plans.

Individually Constructed

Care plans written from scratch are documented on forms divided into columns with the usual headings of nursing diagnoses, outcomes, and interventions.

Advantages. The individually written plan enables the documentation of the nursing diagnoses, outcomes, and interventions that are most pertinent to a particular client. No <u>extraneous</u> or inapplicable information is included in the care plan.

Disadvantages. Development and documentation of this type of care plan is time consuming. In recognition of these difficulties, the Joint Commission has softened the requirements for individually constructed care plans. As this book is published there are indications that standardized plans of care will become more common. Other new forms of documenting care planning will emerge.

Standardized

Standardized care plans have been introduced into several types of agencies to facilitate the preparation and use of care plans. According to Mayers (1983), "a standard care plan is a specific <u>protocol</u> of care that is appropriate for patients who are experiencing the usual or predictable problems associated with a given diagnosis or disease process." Standardized care plans consist of actual, or potential nursing diagnoses, outcomes, and interventions that are printed in a care plan format. Individualization is possible through the use of blank spaces as illustrated on Table 2–1. Additional standardized care plans are found in the appendix. The nurse may cross off items that do not apply to the client or add additional nursing diagnoses, outcomes, and interventions. The care plans may be developed by the nursing staff of a particular agency or may be derived from the literature. Sources of published standardized care plans include articles or books. Table 2–1 is a standardized plan for the client with pain.

Standardized care plans may be used in one of two ways: (1) they may be placed in a centrally located area and referred to by nurses when developing handwritten individually constructed care plans, or (2) they may be placed directly on the Kardex, dated, and signed.

Advantages. The advantages of standardized care plans include the following.

1. They are usually developed by clinical experts who have carefully researched the literature. They are useful in educating nurses who are not familiar with a certain medical or nursing diagnosis.

2. They reduce the amount of time spent in writing nursing care plans. This increases the efficiency of nursing care planning.

3. They provide information specific to a particular client and require less time to complete. Additionally, because they outline the expected nursing care, they enhance the quality of the delivery and documentation of care.

TABLE 2–1   Acute Pain

Pain related to effects of surgery, effects of ischemia, inflammatory process, effects of trauma, effects of invasive procedures, and prolonged immobility

Outcomes

Reports pain promptly when experiencing it

Verbalizes decreased pain within 30 minutes following initiation of comfort measures

Interventions

1 Help client identify pain relief measures that have been helpful in the past.
2 Explore with client feelings and attitudes related to use of pain medication and fear of addiction.
3 Instruct client/family:
   ☐ to report pain promptly
   ☐ to describe using 0–10 scale
   ☐ regarding prescribed regimen for pain relief
   ☐ to evaluate and report effectiveness of interventions
4 Assess for pain using verbal and nonverbal messages q _____ including location, quality, intensity, duration, precipitating/aggravating/relieving factors, and associated symptoms.
5 Explain source of pain/discomfort if known
6 Collaborate with physician to establish a pain control regimen:
   ☐ Medications
   ☐ Use of hot/cold application
   ☐ Patient controlled analgesia
   ☐ TENS
7 Provide therapeutic comfort measures based on appropriateness and client willingness/desire
   ☐ Position change (specify position of comfort) _____
   _____
   ☐ Back rub/massage
   ☐ Relaxation techniques and guided imagery
   ☐ Diversional activities (specify) _____
   ☐ Alteration in environment (specify) _____
8 Reassure and support client/family during episodes of pain.
9 Provide quiet environment and organize care to promote periods of uninterrupted rest.
10 Medicate prior to activities to promote participation.
11 Assess and document findings and effectiveness of interventions.

Disadvantages. Using standardized care plans can be limiting because it is rare that all of the client's specific problems will be addressed by one standardized care plan. The nurse must individualize the standardized care plan to reflect the client's unique needs.

Computerized

The basic elements of care plan systems, nursing diagnoses, outcomes, and interventions are also present in computerized systems. The nursing care plan may be prepared at a terminal in the client's room or in a central location. Once data are validated and entered, a printed version may be generated daily, on each shift, or on demand (Fig. 2–1). There are a number of mechanisms by which care plans are

```
                          PATIENT CARE PLAN

GENERAL HOSPITAL              5/16/84 11:41 AM                    PAGE 1
─────────────────────────────────────────────────────────────────────
                        │ TRN-09          000187023 2555555  TRN
                        │ TESTPAT JACK                    SEX: M
                        │ ADM: 5/15/84      SRV:URO       SMK: N
                        │ DOB: 10/06/21 62 COND: G     LEVEL: 1
                        │ HT: 5/11 F/I                WT:180/000 P/O
                        │ 10000 INTERNIST OTHER
                        │ ALG: PENICILLIN
                        │ DX: NEPHROLITHIASIS
─────────────────────────────────────────────────────────────────────
KNOWLEDGE DEFICIT RELATED
TO SURGICAL EXPERIENCE

     OUTCOME:           Describes type of surgery
     OUTCOME:           States usual pre-op preparation
     OUTCOME:           Identifies usual postop routine
     OUTCOME:           Verbalizes feelings about impending surgery

     INTERVENTION:      Assess knowledge of surgery and explore past surgical experience(s)
                        at the time of admission

     INTERVENTION:      Review surgical routine (preps, meds, dressing)

     INTERVENTION:      Reinforce pre-operative teaching
                        re: Sequence of events on day of surgery (pre-op stretcher to OR,
                             RR return to room/ICU)
                            Postop equipment (dsg., IV, tubes)
                            Provisions for relief of pain and other symptoms (include need to
                            request and frequency limitations)
                            Turning, coughing and deep breathing
                            Incentive spirometry if ordered
                            Change in bowel/bladder functions
                            Progressive diet changes
                            Progressive self care
```

FIGURE 2–1 Computerized care plan adapted from HBO & Company's STAR Nursing Documentation System. (Courtesy of HBO & Company, Atlanta, GA. All rights reserved.)

generated. Three commonly used systems are (1) standardized plans based on the medical diagnosis, (2) standardized plans based on the nursing diagnosis, and (3) individually constructed plans.

Medical Diagnoses. In these systems, the computer provides the nurse with nursing diagnoses, outcomes, and nursing interventions commonly associated with the medical diagnoses. These are very similar to the printed standardized care plans discussed earlier. The nurse who is formulating the plan selects the appropriate items from the standardized data base. Additional diagnoses, outcomes, and interventions may be entered to reflect other concerns of the client.

Nursing Diagnoses. Other computerized systems are more directly associated with the specific nursing diagnoses identified at the time of the detailed nursing assessment. The computer lists each diagnosis, and the nurse defines outcomes and nursing interventions by selecting from a menu of appropriate choices. The nurse may add other specific outcomes and interventions for an individual client, if appropriate. Some systems are constructed to allow clients to participate actively in the selection of outcomes and appropriate interventions. The nurse assists clients in choosing outcomes or interventions that they feel will best meet clients' needs. Selections are made from a menu that includes appropriate outcomes or nursing orders.

Individually Constructed. In these systems, the nurse develops the care plan in a fashion similar to that used in a manual individualized plan. The nurse is not prompted to focus on specific diagnoses but uses a menu to select those diagnoses, outcomes, and interventions that apply to the individual client. Additional outcomes or interventions not identified in the menu may also be added when necessary.

Most computerized care planning systems facilitate frequent updating of the plan. The nurse identifies problems that have been resolved, and they are eliminated from the plan. Other options may include (1) revision of diagnoses, outcomes, and interventions to reflect the changing status of the client or (2) addition of new diagnoses, outcomes, and interventions. Printed care plans, which are a permanent part of the medical record, document the client's progress as reflected by the changing plan of care.

Computerized care plans increase the potential for accurate and thorough documentation of the delivery of care. The computer identifies specific nursing approaches listed on the plan and prompts the nurse to <u>document</u> the outcome of the intervention. This process also encourages frequent review of the plan as well as modification, when appropriate.

More sophisticated programs compare the client's data with a list of defining characteristics for specific nursing diagnoses. If the client's data match the defining characteristics, the program will display the nursing diagnosis. The nurse then has the option of choosing the displayed diagnosis or rejecting it and selecting another. If the displayed diagnosis is accepted, the system will present expected outcomes and interventions that would be applicable. The nurse chooses the appropriate outcomes and interventions or enters the individualized ones.

Advantages. The advantages of computerized care plans include the following.
   1. Preparation of a computer-generated care plan from a standardized plan takes less time than handwriting an individualized care plan.
   2. The computerized care plan can be designed to determine the staffing needs of the unit.
   3. Care plans that are prepared on a printer are easy to read.
   4. Automated care planning consistently uses a systematic method to develop care plans, thereby decreasing the possibility of error.
   5. Utilizing computer-assisted care planning permits the identification of common nursing diagnoses for research and planning purposes.

Disadvantages. Along with the many advantages, some disadvantages do exist and include the following.
   1. Adequate number of computers must be available to the nursing staff. If sufficient hardware is not available because of cost or space considerations, the care planning process will become more difficult.
   2. Errors that occur in computerized nursing care plans may be harder to detect. Nurses have a tendency to lend more <u>credence</u> to computer printouts than they would to handwritten records.
   3. The computer may develop a care plan that may be logically consistent but is not applicable to a client.

Summary

The development of nursing interventions is the third stage of the planning phase of the nursing process. Nursing interventions define the activities that assist the client in achieving desired outcomes. Nursing interventions are consistent with the plan of care, based on scientific principles, and individualized to the specific client situation. They are also used to provide a safe and therapeutic environment. Additionally, nursing interventions include teaching-learning opportunities for the client and the utilization of appropriate resources.

Nursing interventions are developed through a scientific approach and include date, signature, precise action verbs, specific aspects of interventions, and modifications in standard therapy. The registered nurse is responsible and accountable for the development of nursing interventions.

The fourth stage of the planning phase consists of documentation of the plan on a nursing care plan. Care plans may be individualized, standardized, or computerized. Much time is wasted when care plans are not developed. Nurses who are unfamiliar with the client's care may spend time in reviewing the client's record and asking questions of other nursing personnel or of the client. This hit or miss approach leads to a great deal of wasted effort and inefficient care, which could be avoided by documentation of the plan. Care plans are necessary to provide a framework for the delivery of care and to ensure continuity.

1 The introductory paragraph is about

_____

2 List the boldface headings.

_____

_____

_____

_____

_____

3 List the key words in the selection.

_____

_____

_____

_____

_____

4 Are there any graphic aids in the selection?

_____

5 What is this selection about?

_____

_____

• VOCABULARY CHECK

Directions.   Below are 10 words taken from the key words section of this chapter. Circle the letter of the best definition from the four choices.

1 Impending
   a   dependent on others
   b   about to occur
   c   independent of others
   d   about to finish

2 Sterile
   a   filled with living microorganisms
   b   resembling the sternum
   c   pertaining to steroids
   d   free from living microorganisms

3 Extraneous
   a   unrelated   **c**   necessary
   b   related   **d**   crucial

4 Ostomy
   a   inflammation of the inner ear
   b   closure of an orifice
   c   hardening of the bones
   d   formation of artificial opening

5 Delegate
   a   to remove   **c**   to appoint
   b   to dismiss   **d**   to appreciate

6 Regimen
   a   the natural renewal of a structure
   b   regulated activity designed to achieve certain ends
   c   an instrument used for measuring the refractive power of the eye
   d   the backward or returning flow

7 Locus
   a   an insect   **c**   a split
   b   a point   **d**   a passage

8 Irrigate
   a   to wash a body cavity or wound using water or fluid
   b   to release pressure in a specific area
   c   to react to an external or internal stimulus
   d   to cause a physical or psychological disorder

9 Document
   a   to check on a chart
   b   to prove with verbal evidence
   c   to support with written information
   d   to disprove a medical theory

10 Dressing
   a a medicinal substance taken orally
   b a daily routine of postoperative exercise
   c a feeding tube to collect specimens from the duodenum
   d materials used for protecting a wound

• SUMMARY

Prereading strategies involve previewing the chapter before your actual reading. Read the title, introduction, summary, and headings. Look up the meanings of italicized words and examine all graphic aids.

These five prereading strategies help you to get started, stay involved, and organize, concentrate on, and comprehend the information in the chapter.

• Chapter 3 •

Monitoring Your Comprehension

OBJECTIVE

KEY WORDS

MONITORING

FIVE STRATEGIES TO MONITOR COMPREHENSION
    Monitoring Strategy No. 1: Reread

    Monitoring Strategy No. 2: Summarize

    Monitoring Strategy No. 3: Defining New Words

    Monitoring Strategy No. 4: Visualization

    Monitoring Strategy No. 5: Research

USING MONITORING STRATEGIES FOR LONGER PASSAGES

QUESTION TO MONITOR COMPREHENSION

VOCABULARY CHECK

SUMMARY

• OBJECTIVE

To become aware of when you are reading without comprehension and to learn five monitoring strategies to regain understanding.

• KEY WORDS

Pay attention to the key words, which are listed on the following page. They are underscored the first time they appear in this chapter. Try to determine the meaning of these words from the surrounding words in the passage. If you need further help, use your dictionary or the glossary in the back of this book.

Look up the medical terminology in your medical dictionary or the glossary. As you read the exercises in this chapter, write additional words you need to learn in the space provided.

GENERAL VOCABULARY	MEDICAL TERMINOLOGY
clarify	basophils
incorporated	blood pressure
maladaptive	cognitive
miscommunication	coping
monitoring	corticosteroid
moral	excitatory
multitude	exogenous
schema	glucose
summarize	neuron
visualize	superego
_____	_____
_____	_____
_____	_____

• MONITORING

An important strategy for improving your concentration is monitoring. When you monitor your comprehension, you are continually asking yourself if you understand what you're reading. Depending on the complexity of the material, you may have to do this every sentence, paragraph, section, or page. When you monitor your comprehension, you become immediately aware of when you are not understanding your textbook. When you monitor your comprehension, you become an active reader rather than a passive one. You become involved with and part of the material rather than just looking at words and remaining removed from your reading selection. Good readers constantly ask, "Am I comprehending?" When the answer is no, and they become alert to the fact that they are not understanding, active readers have various monitoring strategies to correct the situation. These strategies are used to regain understanding. An explanation of five useful strategies to monitor comprehension follows.

• FIVE STRATEGIES TO MONITOR COMPREHENSION

• Monitoring Strategy No. 1: Reread

When active readers become aware that they do not understand what they are reading, the strategy they most commonly use is simply to reread the portion they did not understand. Often on a second reading, complex information becomes clear. If need be, don't hesitate to reread aloud. This practice in itself can help clarify the content.

• EXERCISE 3–1 •

Directions. Read the following passage from Ignatavicius and Bayne (p. 829; underscore added). Then reread, noting how much more you understood with the second reading. Try rereading the passage aloud to see if this strategy further helps your comprehension.

> *Neuron*-to-neuron transmission occurs when an impulse goes from the axon of one neuron to the dendrites, the soma, or the axon of another neuron. A synapse may be either *excitatory* or inhibitory, but not both. An excitatory potential occurs when sodium enters the cell, causing depolarization. An action potential is then initiated, and the impulse is carried by the axon to its destination—a synapse with the dendrites of another neuron.

Did your second reading help you understand
the passage better?   Yes _____ No _____
Was rereading aloud helpful?   Yes _____ No _____

Remember to reread passages so that you can better understand complex textbook readings.

• Monitoring Strategy No. 2: Summarize

When reading nursing texts, you will often encounter technical information that may prove challenging. Sentences may be long, and sometimes the material will appear to be poorly organized. When you read complex text information, your best strategy is to summarize the passage. To summarize, you look only for the main idea and important details (see Chapters 8 and 9) and rewrite them in your own words, a shorter version of the original. Depending on the length of the selection, you can do this as brief margin notes right in the textbook or you can summarize in your notebook. In any case, by summarizing and rewriting complex information in your own words, you simplify the material into ideas that you understand—a first step to learning new information.

• EXAMPLE 3–1 •

Directions. Below is an excerpt from the nursing text by Ignatavicius and Bayne (p. 92; underscores added). Following that is a summary of this passage. Notice that only the main points were included in the summary and the writer's own words were used to rewrite the selection.

> Coping is any behavioral or cognitive activity that is used to deal with stress. If an event is perceived as taxing or dangerous, coping should occur. The concept of coping implies that most people do not remain passive and allow events to happen; rather they react. The reactions to a stress-provoking event can be either to use the problem-solving approach to change the event (problem-focused coping) or to change emotional reactions to the event (emotion-focused coping). The coping strat-

egy or strategies used vary from person to person and event to event. It is thought that individuals generally try to use coping strategies that they have found to be successful in the past. If this coping is not successful in the current situation, other strategies may be considered.

Summary

Coping is what we do to deal with a stressful situation. When someone is coping, they are not passive but instead are actively trying to deal with the situation. There are two general types of coping: problem-focused coping and emotion-focused coping. The use of these two strategies differs from person to person and situation to situation; however, we tend to use coping strategies that worked for us in the past.

• EXERCISE 3–2 •

Directions.   In the space provided, summarize the following paragraph from the nursing text by Arnold and Boggs (p. 299; underscore added). Remember to keep it brief. Focus on the main idea and important details. Paraphrase, using your own words.

A professional nurse is called upon daily to communicate with other professionals in some type of written format. Written communication has several advantages over other forms of communication. Written text provides a potentially permanent record of information and may diminish <u>miscommunication</u>. The natural tendency to distort verbal messages or forget components over time is alleviated when there are written records to refer to, particularly when the topic being discussed is complex or when the communication is directed at larger groups of people.

Summary

_____

_____

_____

_____

_____

• Monitoring Strategy No. 3: Defining New Words

At times, reading a specific nursing passage is difficult because you do not know the meanings of general vocabulary words or medical terminology. The best method for correcting this situation is to look up the words in the dictionary or textbook glossary (see Chapter 6). Looking up unknown words in a dictionary or glossary, although time consuming, will lead you to an accurate and precise definition. Understanding vocabulary is an important factor in comprehending your nursing textbook.

• EXERCISE 3–3 •

Directions. In this exercise taken from Ignatavicius and Bayne (p. 529; underscore added), write the meanings of any unknown words in the space provided. Use your dictionary or glossary to attain a precise definition.

<u>Basophils</u> are the rarest of the granulocytes. These cells make up less than 0.5% of the total white blood cell count. Basophils release histamine and heparin in areas of tissue damage and pathogenic invasion. They appear to be most important in the generation of acute inflammatory reactions.

UNKNOWN WORD	MEANING
1 _____	_____
2 _____	_____
3 _____	_____
4 _____	_____
5 _____	_____
6 _____	_____
7 _____	_____
8 _____	_____
9 _____	_____
10 _____	_____

• Monitoring Strategy No. 4: Visualization

Another major reason for poor reading comprehension is lack of concentration. This inability to focus on textbook selections may account for the greatest degree of reading problems in nursing schools. Many factors can cause concentration problems, but primarily they fall into two categories: internal distractions and external distractions. **Internal distractions** are elements within ourselves that won't let us concentrate, such as hunger, personal problems, and headaches. **External distractions** are elements outside ourselves that won't let us concentrate, such as radio sounds, a noisy little brother, or too warm a room.

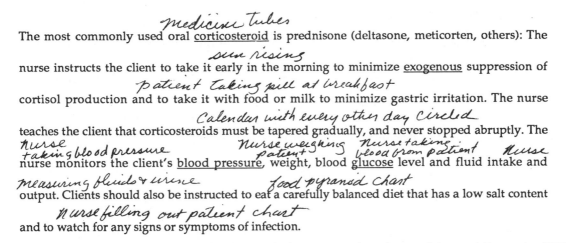

The most commonly used oral <u>corticosteroid</u> is prednisone (deltasone, meticorten, others): The nurse instructs the client to take it early in the morning to minimize <u>exogenous</u> suppression of cortisol production and to take it with food or milk to minimize gastric irritation. The nurse teaches the client that corticosteroids must be tapered gradually, and never stopped abruptly. The nurse monitors the client's <u>blood pressure</u>, weight, blood <u>glucose</u> level and fluid intake and output. Clients should also be instructed to eat a carefully balanced diet that has a low salt content and to watch for any signs or symptoms of infection.

FIGURE 3–1   How one reader visualized a particular passage from Ignatavicius and Bayne (p. 650).

Regardless of the reasons for poor concentration, in nursing school you are expected to understand your textbook. One good strategy for overcoming poor concentration is to <u>visualize</u> what you are reading. When you visualize, you create a mental picture of what you are reading—like a television picture in your mind. As you read each sentence, you adjust the mental image you have, either adding new information or somehow changing the picture to fit each new fact as you read it. In Figure 3–1 pay close attention to the handwritten notes above the printed line. This is one reader's description of what she visualized as she read the passage.

• EXERCISE 3–4 •

Directions.   As you read the following passage from the nursing textbook by Varcarolis (p. 17; underscore added), try to visualize what you are reading and make adjustments to your image according to any new facts provided. As in the previous example, write what you visualize above the line.

The <u>superego</u> consists of two subsystems: the conscience and the ego-ideal. What

parents view as improper and what they punish the child for doing become <u>incor-</u>

<u>porated</u> into the child's conscience. The conscience refers to the capacity for self

evaluation and criticism. When <u>moral</u> codes are violated, the conscience punishes

the person by instilling guilt. A <u>maladaptive</u> example of this behavior is seen in the

extreme condition of depression, in which people berate themselves cruelly for

minor actions and trivial shortcomings.

• Monitoring Strategy No. 5: Research

The best way to learn new information is by having old information or a framework on which to add the new facts. This framework is called a <u>schema</u> and constitutes background information to which you add new knowledge. Many times, the reason you lose comprehension while reading your nursing textbook is that you have insufficient schema or background knowledge on the subject. A solution to this problem may be as simple as reading an encyclopedia entry or consulting another textbook or a nursing journal to get a different perspective on the same subject. Whatever means you choose, once you build up your background knowledge of a difficult subject, your reading comprehension on this subject will improve.

• EXERCISE 3–5 •

Sometimes you need additional information to understand your textbook readings. It's important for you to know which resource material to consult when researching a topic.

Directions. Below is a list of topics you will encounter in nursing school. In the space next to the topic, write whether you would find the best additional information in a general encyclopedia, general nursing textbook, or nursing journal.

1 Latest information on caring for patients with diabetes _____

_____

2 Human sexuality _____

3 General description of the eye _____

4 Writing a care plan _____

5 Newest technique for helping clients with eating disorders _____

_____

6 Cell structure _____

• USING MONITORING STRATEGIES FOR LONGER PASSAGES

When you are actively reading your nursing textbook and you realize that you are not understanding what you have read, you may need to use one, some, or all of the five monitoring strategies discussed in this chapter. Figure 3–2 is an excerpt from the nursing textbook by Arnold and Boggs (p. 215). Above the lines are handwritten notes describing examples of the strategies used. Read carefully, paying close attention to the various ways one reader used these five strategies to monitor comprehension.

Reread

There are times in nursing practice when the principles or activities of the relationship cannot be applied as directly as the nurse would like. The need to communicate in forms other than face *Note: Research communication Channels* to face interpersonal interactions is more likely to occur toward the beginning or end of the *end, close* relationship. There may be times, for instance, when a nurse will have to terminate with a client, *Visualize dead child* because of a sudden transfer, without being able to say good-bye. Or a child dies when a nurse is off duty and the nurse would like to share thoughts with the family. Calling the client or the *to recognize as valid* client's family on the phone or sending a note acknowledges the meaning of the relationship. Letting a client know the relationship has meaning is important even though the interpersonal contact is not of long duration. *summary: when a relationship w/ client ends abruptly, it is okay to recognize relationship with note or phone call.*

FIGURE 3–2 Various ways one reader used the five strategies to monitor comprehension in a passage from Arnold and Boggs (p. 215).

• EXERCISE 3–6 •

Directions. Read the following exercise taken from the nursing textbook by Arnold and Boggs (p. 215). Using the method demonstrated in the previous example, indicate above the printed line the use of the monitoring strategies described in this chapter:

1 Reread

2 Summarize

3 Define new words

4 Visualize

5 Research

Communication strategies take into account the effects of role relationships on the feelings of both participants as they enter into relationships with each other. Knowing "who" your client is and what some of the issues related to role might be gives the nurse greater flexibility in listening as well as responding. For example, relating to clients of high social status is frequently an intimidating experience for students. Establishing a therapeutic relationship with a nurse or physician who is hospitalized with a serious problem can be overwhelming. "What will my client think of me?" is a potent question when the client is perceived as having higher status than the nurse.

Working with clients of lower status affects a relationship if the client's lifestyle differs significantly from what the nurse is accustomed to in other settings. For example, walking onto a public psychiatric long-term unit for the first time is sometimes upsetting to nursing students who might be hearing a poverty-stricken pregnant woman admit she uses laundry starch as a food substitute. Such a practice is a cultural, socioeconomic reality for some people. The variables of socioeconomic status, previous life experience, level of education, and occupation are likely to influence the type of dialogue used in the relationship.

When clients are very angry or very anxious, they usually are less able to engage in productive dialogue. At such times, the nurse might use nonverbal and simple communication techniques to help the client reduce the intensity of feeling before proceeding further.

• QUESTION TO MONITOR COMPREHENSION

As mentioned in the beginning of this chapter, the first responsibility of good readers is to become aware of when they are losing comprehension. They do this simply by continually asking themselves whether they are comprehending. To help you get accustomed to doing this, the following question appears throughout the remaining chapters to remind you to monitor your comprehension:

Comprehending? Yes ___   No ___

When you see this question, please check the response that most accurately reflects how well you understand what you have just read. If the answer is yes, continue reading. If the answer is no, go back and use any of the five strategies to monitor comprehension that you feel will be most helpful. Then continue reading.

• VOCABULARY CHECK

Directions.   Below are 10 words taken from the key words section of this chapter. Circle the letter of the best definition from the four choices.

1 Schema
    a a devious plan
    b part of the care plan
    c a mental code
    d diagnosis of an illness

2 Basophils
    a part of the cell nucleus of a plant or animal
    b structure of plant cell that contains chlorophyll
    c stucture outside the cell nucleus
    d any structures stained readily with basic dyes

3 Miscommunication
    a to talk across a great distance
    b unfinished communication
    c failure to communicate clearly
    d to communicate clearly

4 Coping
    a contending with difficulties in an effort to overcome them
    b feeling closed in, shut in, or removed from a situation
    c not having difficulties or major responsibilities
    d being unable to solve or deal with problems independently

5 Visualize
    a to dream or fantasize
    b to see an object in reality
    c to hear a sound in reality
    d to see or form a mental image

6 Exogenous
    a developed or originating inside the organism
    b developed or originating outside the organism
    c capable of going inside an organism
    d capable of going outside an organism

7 Summarize
    a covering the main points succinctly
    b describing in complete detail
    c reviewing the client's progress
    d describing the client's progress

8 Glucose
   a a factor in protein
   b a complex carbohydrate
   c a simple sugar
   d cellular structure in vegetables

9 Moral
   a relating to principles of right and wrong
   b religious feelings or sentiments
   c disposition to feeling good or bad
   d message at the end of a folk tale

10 Neuron
   a connection between nerve cells
   b chemical transmission of nerves
   c gap between nerve cells
   d the actual nerve cell

• SUMMARY

In this chapter you learned to become aware of when you are losing comprehension while you are reading. You learned five monitoring strategies to help improve your comprehension:

1 Reread

2 Summarize

3 Define new words

4 Visualize

5 Research

You were also introduced to the question that will be used throughout the book to help you monitor your comprehension.

Comprehending? Yes ____ No ____

· U N I T ·

II

VOCABULARY DEVELOPMENT

A well-developed vocabulary, both for medical and for general terminology, is an important asset that will help you through nursing school. A good vocabulary not only will make comprehending your textbook easier but also will enable you to converse better with both patients and colleagues.

This unit will give you strategies for defining unknown words encountered in your textbooks and lectures. Chapter Four, "Affixes," will teach you to analyze word parts for meanings. Chapter Five, "Using Context Clues," will show you how to use surrounding words to figure out the meaning of an unknown word. Chapter 6, "Dictionary, Glossary, and Thesaurus," will instruct you in the use of the dictionary and glossary for obtaining definitions of unknown words and the thesaurus for choosing the more precise word. Finally, Chapter 7, "Word Bank," will suggest a system for memorizing the meanings of unknown words once you have obtained the definitions.

After completing Unit 2, "Vocubulary Development," you will have many techniques that will help you define and remember unknown words. Once these words are no longer unknown, but a part of your normal speaking vocabulary, you will be well on your way to greater nursing school success.

Chapter 4

Affixes

OBJECTIVE

KEY WORDS

INTRODUCTION TO AFFIXES

TYPES OF AFFIXES

AFFIX ANALYSIS IS NOT ALWAYS
APPLICABLE

SUMMARY

• OBJECTIVE

To learn the definition of unknown general vocabulary and medical terminology by analyzing roots, prefixes, and suffixes (affixes).

• KEY WORDS

Pay attention to the key words, which are listed on the following page. They are underscored the first time they appear in this chapter. Try to determine the meaning of these words from the surrounding words in the passage. If you need further help, use your dictionary or the glossary in the back of this book.

Look up the medical terminology in your medical dictionary or the glossary. As you read the exercises in this chapter, write additional words you need to learn in the space provided.

MEDICAL TERMINOLOGY	GENERAL VOCABULARY
agoraphobia	affixes
anti-inflammatory	prefix
appendicitis	pregnant
cardiovascular	pressure
endocrine	purification
hemoglobin	root
hysterectomy	socialism

prematurity   suffix

somatic   transmit

tonsillectomy   unilateral

_____   _____

_____   _____

_____   _____

• INTRODUCTION TO AFFIXES

Part of the experience of being a nursing student is encountering new and unfamiliar words in your nursing textbooks. One of the most efficient ways of unlocking the definitions of these words is by analyzing the meanings of the affixes, or word parts that make up the structure of the word. This technique is useful for both medical and nonmedical vocabulary as long as the words involved possess an affix. Once you have mastered the meanings of a relatively small number of affixes, you will be able to analyze the meanings of thousands of words.

• TYPES OF AFFIXES

Many words in the English language consist of two or more of these word parts: prefix, root, and suffix.

A **prefix** is a word part that comes at the beginning of the word. Its function is to change the meaning of the basic portion of the word. For example, *dis*like (the opposite of like) and *over*protect (to protect too much).

The **root** is the main part of the word and provides the basic meaning of the word. For example, dis*like* (to enjoy) and over*protect* (to guard).

The **suffix** is located at the end of the word and serves two purposes: to change the meaning of the root and to alter the part of speech. For example, dislike*able* (not able to be liked) and overprotect*ive* (tending toward guarding too much). Originally, "dislike" was a verb, but when the "able" suffix was added, it became an adjective. Similarly, "overprotect" is a verb, but adding the suffix "ive" changes it to an adjective.

• EXAMPLE 4–1 •

Look at the following word:

mature

You know that "mature" means "the attainment of maximal development" (Miller and Keane, p. 744).

Now look at the word below:

premature

Add an affix before the main part, or root, of the word. This word part is a prefix and has its own meaning—"before." Combining the meaning of "pre" with that of "mature" you get a new definition—"before maximal development."

Next consider the last example:

<u>prematurity</u>

Now you have added an affix after the root. This word part is the suffix and it refers to "the state of." So adding up all the meanings of the affixes,

pre = before

mature = fully developed

ity = state of

you arrive at the full definition of the words, "the state before maximal development," the meaning of "prematurity." Also note that "premature" is an adjective and "prematurity" is a noun.

• AFFIX ANALYSIS IS NOT ALWAYS APPLICABLE

The technique of analyzing affixes can be used on many of the unknown words you will see in your nursing textbooks. However, you should be cautioned that what may seem to be an affix may in reality be the main part of the word. Consider <u>pregnant</u> and <u>pressure</u>. Both words begin with "pre," but in each case the "pre" is part of the root.

To avoid this type of error, memorize or at least familiarize yourself with the most common prefixes, roots, and suffixes.

Table 4–1 lists the 20 most frequently used prefixes, roots, and suffixes, followed by their definitions and examples of how the affixes are used. The starred (*) entires suggest affixes with a medical use.

• EXERCISE 4–1 •

Directions.   In Table 4–1 under the heading Definition of Example, write the meanings of the example words. Consult a dictionary or glossary if necessary.

• EXERCISE 4–2 •

Directions.   In Table 4–1 under the column labeled Your Example, write another example of a word with the same prefix, root, or suffix as that on the line. If necessary, use your dictionary or glossary.

Comprehending?   Yes ____   No ____

TABLE 4–1 Prefixes, Roots, Suffixes

		Definition	Example	Definition of Example	Your Example
Prefix					
1	anti	against	anti-inflammatory		
2	*dys	bad, difficult	dysfunction		
3	*endo	within	endocrine		
4	ex	out	exhale		
5	fore	before, in front of	foresight		
6	*hem, hemato	relating to the blood	hemoglobin		
7	*hydra, hydro	relating to water	hydrocephalus		
8	*hyper	over, above, beyond	hyperactive		
9	*hypo	under	hypodermic		
10	*idio	relating to the individual organ, distinct	idiomuscular		
11	inter	between	interstate		
12	mal	poor, bad	malpractice		
13	*micro	small	microscope		
14	*neuro	nerve	neurobiology		
15	non	no	nonviable		
16	*ortho	straight, normal	orthodontia		
17	retro	backward	retroactive		
18	semi	half	semicircle		
19	sub	under	subconscious		
20	tele	distant, for	television		
21					
22					
23					
24					
25					
Root					
1	*arteri, arterio	artery	arteriosclerosis		
2	*arthro, arthr	joint	arthritis		
3	*cardi, cardio	heart	cardiovascular		
4	dem, demo	people	democracy		
5	*derm, dermo	skin	dermatologist		
6	fac, fact	make, do	factory		
7	geo	earth	geology		
8	*gyne	woman	gynecology		
9	later	side	unilateral		
10	mit, miss	send	transmit		
11	*nephro, nephr	kidney	nephritis		
12	nil	nothing	nillify		
13	*oste, osteo	bone	osteoporosis		
14	*path	disease	pathology		
15	port	carry	transport		
16	*psych	mind	psychology		
17	*soma	body	somatic		
18	spec, spect	to look at	spectator		

TABLE 4–1   Prefixes, Roots, Suffixes *Continued*

	Definition	Example	Definition of Example	Your Example
Root cont'd				
19 ven, veno	vein	venous		
20 vers	turn	reversible		
21				
22				
23				
24				
25				
Suffix				
1 able, ible	capable of	reachable		
2 ation,	act of	purification		
3 *cide	causing death	pesticide		
4 *cyte	cell	blastocyte		
5 *ectomy	excision	tonsillectomy		
6 er, or, ant	person who	actor		
7 ful	full of	dreadful		
8 graph	picture or record	cardiograph		
9 gram	instrument that records	cardiogram		
10 ism	doctrine	socialism		
11 itis	inflammation of	appendicitis		
12 *meter	measure of	centimeter		
13 ology	study of	biology		
14 *oplasty	plastic surgery	rhinoplasty		
15 *osis	condition of	psychosis		
16 *ostomy	opening	colostomy		
17 *phobia	fear	agoraphobia		
18 rupt	break, burst	interrupt		
19 scope	see	telescope		
20 *tomy	cutting	hysterectomy		
21				
22				
23				
24				
25				

*Affixes with a medical use.

Comprehending?   Yes _____   No _____

• EXERCISE 4–3 •

Directions.   In the blank spaces numbered 21 to 25 in Table 4–1 write in any additional prefixes, roots, or suffixes you may encounter in your readings. Refer back to this table as a quick reference to help you to analyze affixes.

• **EXERCISE 4–4** •

Directions. The following selection is from the Matteson and McConnell nursing textbook (pp. 706-707). Analyze the root and any prefix or suffix of the underscored words and write the definition above the word. The first definition has been added for you. If necessary, check your dictionary or glossary for correct meanings.

after injury

Postinjury Phase. Ideally, accidental injuries should be prevented, but in some instances this simply is not possible. Therefore nurses should attend to optimizing postinjury prevention efforts, to minimize the long-range effects of an injury. Many communities have emergency call systems, such as "Lifeline," that allow older people at risk of falling ready access to postfall assistance. The systems work by activating a central emergency call board (such as in an emergency room) when the client pushes a button. These buttons are generally small and may be worn on light clothing. Other alternatives include daily checking systems, in which neighbors, friends, or family phone the older person each day.

An example of a fall-related injury prevention protocol developed for a nursing home is shown on this page. It includes both preinjury and postinjury interventions to reduce injury.

Evaluation

Criteria for evaluation of nursing care for those with potential for injury are:

1. What is the incidence of injury in the target client population? How does it compare with national averages?
2. What is the incidence of functional impairment attributable to injury in the client population?
3. Are the patients assessed for potential for specific injuries: fall-related injury, other trauma, burns, poisoning?
4. Are steps taken to reduce the at-risk individual's likelihood of sustaining injury?
5. Is the client's lifestyle adversely affected by the injury prevention program?
6. What is the cost of the injury prevention program to the individual, family, and facility or agency?

NONCOMPLIANCE
Definition and Scope of Problem

Noncompliance is a term with many definitions and connotations. Even leading experts on nursing diagnosis offer quite different definitions. Carpenito defines noncompliance as "personal behavior that deviates from health-related advice given by health care professionals." Gordon defines it as "failure to participate in carrying out the plan of care *after indicating initial intention to comply.*" The North American Nursing Diagnosis Association has developed yet another definition: "A person's informed decision not to adhere to a therapeutic recommendation."

Compliance is a concern of nurses because the goal of compliance is improved health status. Despite inconsistencies in definition, there is widespread agreement that achieving compliance is problematic in many different categories of patients. Research on compliance shows that noncompliance is found in patients of all ages, social classes, and ethnic groups; it is found in all types of health care delivery systems and in patients whose symptoms vary from nonexistent to life-threatening.

Noncompliance is most often seen in the community setting, where patients have greater control over their daily routines and are more likely to have competing demands on their time. In institutional settings there are fewer opportunities for noncompliance, because many self-care activities are either closely supervised or done for the patient.

The extent of noncompliance by the elderly is thought to be high by some observers, with medication noncompliance rates averaging about 50 per cent. However, variations in the definition of noncompliance used in studies and measurement difficulties make accurate estimates of the extent of this problem among the elderly difficult to obtain.

Most of the compliance literature focuses on younger adults. Sackett and Snow's review of 31 compliance studies shows that one third of the studies specifically exclude the elderly, and only 2 of 31 are specific to this population. Much of what we know about compliance in the elderly has been extrapolated from studies of age-heterogeneous groups with specific chronic diseases, such as diabetes and hypertension. The literature that considers the elderly as a discrete group calls attention to sensory deficits and memory impairment as two important contributors to noncompliance.

• VOCABULARY CHECK

Directions. Below are 10 words taken from the key word section of this chapter. Circle the letter of the best definition from the four choices.

1 Socialism
   a the state of being with others
   b the system of government in the United States
   c a method by which people are made ready to partake in group activities
   d a system in which there is no private ownership

2 Agoraphobia
   a fear of open and public places
   b fear of spiders
   c fear of close spaces
   d fear of disease and germs

3 Transmit
   a to exchange between individuals
   b to carry from place to place
   c to send from one person to another
   d to change the shape of

4 Cardiovascular
   a pertaining to a device measuring heart function
   b pertaining to the lungs and heart
   c pertaining to the lungs
   d pertaining to the heart and blood vessels

5 Tonsillectomy
   a treatment of tonsils
   b excision of tonsils
   c infection of tonsils
   d pertaining to tonsils

6 Unilateral
  a done by one person or party
  b single handed
  c partial functioning
  d pertaining to an element in the universe

7 Endocrine
  a part of blood constituents
  b pertaining to heart-lung functioning
  c pertaining to internal secretion, hormonal
  d part of the kidneys and their output

8 Prefix
  a an affix found at beginning and end of the word
  b an affix forming the base of the word
  c an affix attached at the end of a word
  d an affix attached to the beginning of a word

9 Somatic
  a pertaining to the body
  b pertaining to the stomach
  c pertaining to the ego structure
  d pertaining to the nervous system

10 Pregnant
  a immediate period right after delivery of unborn young
  b the unborn young
  c containing unborn young within the body
  d the egg containing unborn young

• SUMMARY

In this chapter you have learned a new method for defining unknown general vocabulary and medical terminology: analyzing affixes or word parts. You learned the functions of the following affixes:

- Prefix—a part added to the beginning of the root word that changes its meaning
- Root—the main part of the word
- Suffix—a part added to the end of the root word that changes the meaning of the word and part of speech

You have become familiar with the definitions of these word parts and have had practice learning the meanings of new words by analyzing affixes.

• Chapter 5 •

Using Context Clues

OBJECTIVE

KEY WORDS

DEFINING CONTEXT CLUES

FIVE TYPES OF CONTEXT CLUES

    Direct Definition

    Synonym

    Antonyms

    Appositives

    Examples

CONTEXT CLUES AND THE NURSING STUDENT

VOCABULARY CHECK

SUMMARY

• OBJECTIVES

In this chapter you will learn to use familiar words to figure out the meaning of unknown medical and nonmedical words and to recognize and apply five types of context clues.

• KEY WORDS

Pay attention to the key words, which are listed on the following page. They are underscored the first time they appear in this chapter. Try to determine the meanings of these words in the passage. If you need further help, use your dictionary or the glossary in the back of this book.

Look up the medical terminology in your medical dictionary or the glossary. As you read the exercises in this chapter, write additional words you need to learn in the space provided.

MEDICAL TERMINOLOGY	GENERAL VOCABULARY
antigen	approximate
chronic	dynamic
diabetes	episodes
diagnosed	intractable
dilated	limitation
enzymes	obstacle
exocrine	obstructive
pancreas	precise
plasma	stable
zygote	verify
_____	_____
_____	_____
_____	_____

• DEFINING CONTEXT CLUES

A major obstacle to good reading comprehension is not knowing the meanings of key words. This is especially true for nursing students, who are required to know the meanings of both medical terminology and general vocabulary. One way to arrive at an approximate definition of a word is to use context clues.

• EXERCISE 5–1 •

Directions. Look at the following passage from Brunner and Suddarth (p. 898) and try to fill in the missing words.

Diabetes mellitus is a chronic _____ of major importance in the U.S. today. It is the third leading cause of _____ by disease and currently affects an estimated eleven million _____ . According to the National Diabetes Data Group of the National Institute of Health 5.8 million cases have been diagnosed; the remainder are _____ . About 500,000 new cases of _____ are _____ yearly.

By looking at the entire passage, you should have filled in the words "disease," "death," "people," "undiagnosed," "diabetes," and "diagnosed." What you have done is to use familiar or known words in the sentence to figure out the unknown word. This is what is meant by using the context to arrive at the meaning of an unknown word. The advantage of this process is that you do not have to interrupt the flow of your reading to consult the dictionary for the meaning of a new word.

However, there is a <u>limitation</u> in the use of this strategy when reading nursing texts. When you use context clues, you can arrive at an approximate meaning of a word, in other words, a guess. Although this may be sufficient for general vocabulary, <u>precise</u> definitions are necessary for medical terminology. Therefore use context when possible, but always refer to a medical dictionary or glossary to <u>verify</u> definitions of medical terms. Consider the following example.

• EXAMPLE 5–1 •

The <u>pancreas,</u> located in the upper abdomen, has both <u>exocrine</u> and endocrine gland functions (Ignatavicius and Bayne, p. 947).

Even if you consider the entire sentence, no amount of guessing would allow you to arrive at a definition of exocrine (digestive <u>enzymes</u>) or endocrine (internal secretions) that would be sufficiently precise for your nursing studies. Therefore first use context clues to help you understand both nonnursing and nursing terms, but always double-check the meaning of medical vocabulary by using your medical dictionary or glossary.

• FIVE TYPES OF CONTEXT CLUES

Reading a nursing text can be challenging, especially when you are confronted with unknown words. However, many of these words are defined within the text if you know how to use context clues to look for the definitions. Nursing students should be able to recognize and use five basic types of context clues:

1   Direct definition

2   Synonym

3   Antonym

4   Appositive

5   Example

• Direct Definition

Read the following sentence and see whether you can determine the meaning of the boldface term.

• EXAMPLE 5–2 •

The term **"complement"** refers to circulating <u>plasma</u> proteins made in the liver that can be activated when an antibody couples with its <u>antigen</u> (Brunner and Suddarth, p. 1183).

You can see that the definition for "complement"—circulating plasma proteins made in the liver that can be activated when an antibody couples with its antigen—is found right in the sentence. This sentence where the unknown word is first encountered also supplies the definition. Here are a few more examples of direct definition.

• EXAMPLE 5–3 •

1   *Compliance* is the extent to which a person's behavior coincides with a health practitioner's advice (Kozier et al., p. 43).

2   A *consultation* is a deliberation by two or more people (Kozier et al., p. 114).

3   A *neuritic plaque* is a structure composed of amyloid material surrounded by abnormal neural structures (Kozier et al., p. 114).

• EXERCISE 5–2 •

Directions.   Read each sentence and write a definition in your own words for each boldface word or phrase. Use the direct definition context clue to help you arrive at the meaning.

1   A **fasciculation** is an abnormal contraction (shortening of a bundle of muscle fibers) (Kozier et al., p. 475).

2   A **tremor** is an involuntary trembling of a limb or body part (Kozier et al., p. 475).

3   **Sexual aversion** is the fear of sexual activity leading to avoidance.

4   A **prosthesis** is a replacement for a missing part of the body (e.g., extremity, joint, eye, breast, tooth) (Brunner and Suddarth, p. 237).

5   **Understanding** is a thinking function that combines knowledge with comprehension and application (Lindberg et al., p. 338).

• Synonym

Synonyms are words that have the same or similar meanings. They are often used to avoid the repetition of a word in a passage. Read the following and see whether you can determine the meaning of the boldface term.

• EXAMPLE 5–4 •

Question and **record** verbal orders to avoid miscommunications. In addition to recording the time, the date, the physician's name, and the orders, the nurse documents the circumstances that occasioned the call to the physician, reads the orders back to the physician, and documents that the physician confirmed the orders as the nurse read them back (Kozier et al., p. 94).

It is clear that "record" and "documents" are synonyms; they both mean to write down information or evidence.

• EXAMPLE 5–5 •

Here are a few more examples of synonyms, which are in boldface in each sentence.

1 Whereas, however, the focus of the medical process is on the **disease** process, the nursing process is directed toward a client's response to **illness** (Kozier et al., p. 103).

2 A sense of extreme **hopelessness, despair** or fear may cause disease or even death (Kozier and Erb, p. 82).

3 To **enhance** the ability to collect data and the accuracy of inferences made about the client, the nurse must continually strive to **increase** her or his observational or perceptual field (Kozier et al., p. 107).

• EXERCISE 5–3 •

Directions. Read each sentence, noting the boldface word. Find and circle the synonym for each **boldface** word.

1 A greatly elevated anxiety level can impede learning. Clients or families who are very **worried** may not hear spoken words or may retain only part of the communication (Kozier and Erb, p. 436).

2 On the other hand, clients who appear **uninterested** or unconcerned may need to be told about potential problems to increase their anxiety slightly and thus facilitate their learning (Kozier and Erb, p. 436).

3 Obviously the client who does not understand the nurse's language will find learning seriously impaired. When client values differ from those of the health team, it can also **impede** learning (Kozier and Erb, p. 436).

4 **Rapport** between teacher and learner is essential. A relationship that is both accepting and instructive will best assist learning (Kozier and Erb, p. 437).

5 For example, one episode of angry behavior does not mean that the client is **hostile** (Kozier et al., p. 128).

• **Antonyms**

Read the following sentence and try to determine the meaning of the boldface word.

• EXAMPLE 5–6 •

The diagnosis and orders are **complementary** rather than contradictory (Kozier et al., p. 123).

In this sentence, "complementary" means "mutually supporting," the opposite of "contradictory," which means "to oppose in argument." The clue words "rather than" alert the reader to the use of an antonym as a context clue for determining vocabulary meaning. Antonyms are opposites. By recognizing some connecting words, such as "rather than," "or," "but," "however," and "neither/nor," the reader will become aware of the use of antonyms as context clues.

• EXAMPLE 5–7 •

Following are a few more examples of using antonyms as context clues.

1 Identifying a possible nursing diagnosis alerts other nurses to structure their nursing assessments to gather more data in this area to **confirm** "or" **rule out** their possible diagnosis (Kozier et al., p. 127).

2 For example, heart disease is **common** in middle aged males "but" occurs **infrequently** in younger persons (Kozier and Erb, p. 81).

3 Not uncommonly, people of a **minority** group often lose the cultural characteristics that distinguish them from the **dominant** group (Kozier et al., p. 205).

• EXERCISE 5–4 •

Directions.   Read the following sentences and circle the antonyms of the bold-face words. Look for a possible connecting term that will help you find the antonyms.

1   Activities that were once **enjoyed** with the deceased are now without attraction (Kozier et al., p. 239).

2   The nurse collects data about **dysfunctional** as well as functional behavior (Kozier and Erb, p. 152).

3   Generally, people have a clearer perception of their **problems** or **weaknesses** than of their strengths and assets, which are often taken for granted (Kozier and Erb, p. 165).

4   **Acceptance** and rejection, **sympathy** and pity, **trust** and fear, **curiosity** and revulsion, **valuation** and devaluation face him in countless interpersonal situations (Brunner and Suddarth, p. 174).

5   For example, a high priority of the client might be to become **ambulatory,** however, if the physician's therapeutic regimen calls for extended bed rest, the ambulation must assume a lower priority in the nursing strategy plan (Kozier and Erb, p. 178).

• Appositives

Read the following sentence, paying attention to the boldface term.

• EXAMPLE 5–8 •

Disturbances of **affect** (emotions) become problems in a medical/surgical situation when they are overwhelming or inappropriate (Brunner and Suddarth, p. 188).

You may have noticed that next to the boldface term was a word in parentheses that had the same meaning as "affect"—"emotions." This type of context clue is an appositive, a word or phrase next to, or in apposition to, the unknown word that should help you figure out the meaning of the word. Read the following examples and note that the appositives are usually set off by the word "or," parentheses, commas, or dashes.

• EXAMPLE 5–9 •

1 These criteria are **measurable** or **observable** signs, symptoms and behavioral responses that permit the nurse to evaluate the goals established during the planning phase of the nursing process (Kozier et al., p. 201).

2 Muscle cells are composed of inner **fluid (sarcoplasm)** and an outer membrane (Brunner and Suddarth, p. 336).

3 The pharmaceutical properties of **vegetation—plants, roots, stems, flowers, seeds,** and **herbs**—have been studied, tested, catalogued and used for countless centuries (Potter and Perry, p. 79).

• EXERCISE 5–5 •

Directions. Read the following sentences and circle the appositive for the boldface word or phrase.

1 Areas of **increased color** (hyperpigmentation) and **decreased color** (hypopigmentation) are common (Potter and Perry, p. 248).

2 The **field** or specialty of **cancer** nursing, or oncology nursing, has paralleled the development of medical oncology and the major therapeutic advances that have occurred in the care of the person with cancer (Brunner and Suddarth, p. 262).

3 All humans begin life as a **single cell** (zygote) (Ladewig et al., p. 135).

4 This is particularly important for drugs with a low **therapeutic index** or margin of safety in which minor dosage or absorption changes can result in toxicity or therapeutic failure (Shafler and Marieb, p. 11).

5 Increased levels of other hormones—**epinephrine** and **norepinephrine**—result in increased heart rate, increased blood flow to muscles, increased oxygen intake, and greater mental alertness (Potter and Perry, p. 47).

• Examples

Read the following sentence and notice how the examples in the surrounding words help you to define the unknown word in boldface.

• EXAMPLE 5–10 •

This significance of **spiritual therapy** must not be forgotten. Regardless of the religious affiliation of the patient, the nurse recognizes that faith in a higher power can be as therapeutic as medication (Brunner and Suddarth, p. 309).

The examples given—"religious affiliation", "faith in a higher power," and "therapeutic as medication"—allow you to define the term "spiritual therapy" as help through faith.

Such examples or illustrations allow you to arrive at definitions of unknown words. These details when put together help you to approximate word meanings. In the preceding examples the words "faith in a higher power" and "religious affiliation" refer to the spiritual concepts. "Therapy" and "medicine" allow you to realize that help is implied. Therefore spiritual therapy would be the help offered to a patient through faith.

Notice how the italicized examples help you define the unknown boldface words in the following sentences:

• EXAMPLE 5–11 •

---

1   If the specific gravity of the agent is greater than cerebrospinal fluid (CSF), that is, if the agent is **hyperbaric,** the *drug moves to the dependent position of the subarachnoid space;* if **hypobaric,** *the drug moves away from the dependent position* (Brunner and Suddarth, p. 330).

2   These types of research are commonly called **quality assurance studies.** *Data are collected to determine the impact nurses have on achievement of client care objectives in a particular clinical setting* (Potter and Perry, p. 175).

3   There is a wide variety of **smoking control strategies,** including *prevention, cessation* and *behavior modification* (Brunner and Suddarth, p. 475).

You can apply this strategy in the following exercise.

• EXERCISE 5–6 •

Directions.   Read the following sentences and determine the meaning of the boldface words or phrases from the examples given in the context of each sentence.

1 The air we breathe contains water in the form of vapor. This is referred to as **humidity** (Brunner and Suddarth, p. 502).

2 The blood pressure is measured by the use of the **sphygmomanometer** and the stethoscope. The sphygmomanometer consists of an inflatable cuff and a pressure gauge that communicates with the hollow portion of the cuff (Brunner and Suddarth, p. 520).

3 **Dilated** or **congestive cardiomyopathy** is the most commonly occurring form of the cardiomyopathies. It is distinguished by a dilated and enlarged ventricular cavity along with decreasing muscle wall thickness, left arterial enlargement and stasis of blood in the ventricle (Brunner and Suddarth, p. 560).

4 When the deep veins in legs have incompetent valves following a thrombus, **postphlebitic syndrome** may develop. This disorder is characterized by chronic venous stasis resulting in edema, altered pigmentation, pain, stasis dermatitis and stasis ulceration (Brunner and Suddarth, p. 654).

5 **Minerals** in the diet, such as calcium and iron, are absorbed in the small intestine (Brunner and Suddarth, p. 741).

• EXERCISE 5–7 •

Read the following passages from nursing textbooks. Determine the meaning of each boldface word or phrase from the context. Write the definition of the unknown word.

1 **Intractable pain** is resistant to cure or relief. An example is the pain of arthritis, for which narcotic analgesics are contraindicated because of the long duration of the disease and the risk of addiction. **Behavior modification** is used in some cases of **intractable pain.** Behavior that is not pain-oriented is rewarded, and pain-oriented behavior is ignored. The aim of this technique is to change behavior so that the client can live more comfortably and productively (Kozier et al., p. 603).

behavior modification means_____

intractable pain means_____

2 The instruments and **radioisotopes** (radioactive tracers) used in nuclear medicine are constantly changing but the fundamental principles remain the same. A basic principle is that body constituents are **dynamic** not static. Isotopes enter into the same chemical reactions and metabolic processes as *stable* elements (Kozier et al., p. 492).

radioisotopes means_____

dynamic means_____

3   The **nursing process** has some of the characteristics of an open system. It is open, flexible and dynamic. It is planned and goal directed; it interacts with the environment; and it emphasizes feedback. The nursing process can be viewed as a system with **input,** throughput, **output** and feedback. Input (data) from the client and nurse is transformed by the processes of analyzing, planning and implementing, all of which are throughput. The output (client's response) is then evaluated (Kozier and Erb, p. 143).

nursing process means_____

input means_____

output means_____

4   Using good body mechanics promotes musculoskeletal functioning, reduces the energy required to move and maintain balance and decreases the risks of injury. **Body alignment** is the geometric arrangement of body parts in relation to each other. Good alignment promotes **optimal** balance and maximal body function in whatever position the client assumes. Proper body alignment enhances lung expansion and promotes efficient circulatory, renal and gastrointestinal functions. Conversely, poor body alignment detracts from a pleasing appearance and affects an individual's health **adversely** (Kozier and Erb, p. 558).

body alignment means_____

optimal means_____

adversely means_____

5   **Sleep apnea** is the periodic cessation of breathing during sleep. This disorder needs to be **assessed** by a sleep expert, but it is often suspected when the person has obstructive snoring, excessive daytime sleepiness, and sometimes insomnia. The periods of apnea, which last from 10 seconds to 3 minutes, occur during REM or NREM sleep. **Frequency** of episodes range from 50 to 600 per night. These apneic episodes drain the period of energy and lead to excessive daytime sleepiness (Kozier and Erb, p. 598).

sleep apnea means_____

assessed means_____

frequency means_____

• CONTEXT CLUES AND THE NURSING STUDENT

When reading textbooks, you must determine when context helps you find the meaning of an unknown word and when context clues are not giving you the information you need. In nursing books, much of the medical terminology is defined for you in the text by direct definition. The other context clues—synonyms, antonyms, appositives, and examples—also help you learn the meanings of many general vocabulary words and medical terms. However, while it may be appropriate to approximate meanings for general vocabulary, medical terminology calls for precise meanings. When there are no clues in the context or when the clues do not help you to find exact definitions for medical terms, it is time to turn to the glossary of the textbook or a dictionary. Through practice you will learn to assess when you can use context to define words and when you need to use a glossary, dictionary, or medical dictionary.

• EXERCISE 5–8 •

Directions. Read the following selection from the Iyer et al. nursing textbook (pp. 66-68; boldface added). Fifteen words are in boldface. Fill in the chart at the end of the selection (page 58) to indicate which word meanings you derived from context and which definitions came from a glossary, dictionary, or medical dictionary. The first is done for you.

STEPS IN THE DIAGNOSTIC PROCESS

As mentioned earlier, there are four steps involved in the diagnostic process—data processing, formulation of the diagnostic statement, validation, and documentation.

Data Processing

The information collected by the nurse about an individual client is vital to the development of the nursing diagnosis and subsequent nursing care planning. Before planning can occur, collected data must be processed—classified, interpreted, and validated. Although data processing will be examined as the first step of the diagnostic phase, it is not so specifically isolated. These types of activities occur continuously throughout the nursing process.

Classification

While assessing a client, the nurse accumulates a large volume of data. The nurse may find it extremely difficult to manage this volume in total. The classification process allows the nurse to develop more manageable categories of information. It also stimulates discrimination between data, which helps the nurse to focus on data that are pertinent to the client's needs.

Classification involves sorting information into specific categories. Examples include body systems, functional health patterns, historical data, or significant symptoms. The classification process is facilitated by assessment tools that are organized into specific categories.

Examples

Data ⟶	Classification
Appendectomy three years ago	Past medical history
Sleeps during day	Sleep/rest pattern
Full range of motion	Motor ability
Colostomy	Gastrointestinal system
Mother died of cancer	Family history
Chest pain	Significant symptom
Laxatives every other day	Bowel elimination pattern
Church elder	Spiritual history
Vomiting for three days	History of present illness
Sacral redness	Integumentary system

Placing data into categories also helps the nurse to begin to identify missing data that require further discussion, observation, or physical examination.

Example. Barbara Draper is a 35 year old woman who visits the Women's Health Care Center. During the interview she indicates that her mother died of cancer of the breast (family history) and that she had a breast biopsy two years ago (past medical history).

Classification of this information reveals a missing **component**—current status of breast disease. Therefore, the nurse might (1) question the client regarding the **outcome** of the biopsy and frequency of breast self-examination, (2) pay particular attention to palpation for breast masses during the physical examination, and (3) assess the client's emotional response to this particular health problem.

Interpretation

The second step in data processing is interpretation, which involves identification of significant data, comparison with standards or **norms,** and recognition of patterns or trends. Cues and inferences developed from the scientific nursing knowledge base assist the nurse to interpret the data. A **cue** is a piece of information about an individual client obtained during the assessment process. It is the nurse's **perception** of what exists based on **subjective** and **objective** data obtained from the client and other secondary sources. Cues may include signs which are objective data such as blood pressure and weight or **symptoms** which are subjective data such as pain and sadness.

Examples of Cues

Temperature 102°F
Grimacing
6 ft, 375 lb
White blood count 24,000/mm³ (normal 5000 to 9000/mm³)

"Inferencing" is the assignment of meaning to a cue. An **inference** is a judgment made by the nurse on the basis of education and experience. In the examples identified above, the nurse might make the following inferences based on the cues identified during the assessment of a client.

CUES ⟶	INFERENCE
Temperature 102°F	Elevated temperature
Grimacing	Possible pain, anxiety
6 ft, 375 lb	Obesity
White blood count 24,000/mm	Probable infection

Clusters are groups of cues. The potential for making accurate judgments is increased when the nurse bases an inference on a cluster of cues rather than on a single cue. In the case of the client with a temperature elevation, note that two different inferences could be made based on the particular cluster of cues identified during the assessment of a client.

CLUSTER #1 ⟶	INFERENCE
Temperature 102°F	
White blood count 24,000	
Reddened incision	⟶ Incision is infected
Purulent drainage	

CLUSTER #2 ————————————→ **INFERENCE**

| Temperature 102°F
 Decreased skin turgor
 Dry tongue
 Urine output 200 ml in 8 hr | → Client is dehydrated |

The nurse uses theory, knowledge, experience, and data collected about the client to make correct inferences. Some inferences are very clearly based on **clinical** knowledge. For example, the presence of frequent loose stools, abdominal pain and cramping, and anal irritation suggest a bowel disorder, specifically diarrhea.

Other data may provide fewer **concrete** cues and clusters and require more interpretation. For example, the client with clenched fists and rigid body posture who is crying may be angry, frightened, or experiencing pain. Here, the nurse may (1) make a preliminary interpretation and validate it with the client, or (2) continue to gather additional cues which may help to clarify the inferences based on the identified cues.

The interpretation of data based on cues and clusters is a complex process. Initially, the beginning practitioner may experience difficulty in identifying cues or correctly clustering related cues. However, as nursing knowledge, skill, and expertise increase, the nurse makes accurate clinical judgments more consistently.

WORD	Definition	Context	Glossary	Dictionary	Medical Dictionary
1. classification	sorting information into specific catagories				

Example. Joan Granberry is a nurse on a 24 bed surgical unit. Her clinical knowledge indicates that pain is a common phenomenon in the **postoperative** client. Bob Brown is a 38 year old client who returns to the unit two hours after an **appendectomy**. Mr. Brown denies that he is experiencing pain during his postoperative assessment. However, Joan notes that he is restless, grimaces often, and that his pulse rate and blood pressure are elevated. Based on this cluster of cues, the nurse concludes that the patient may be experiencing pain and continues to gather additional data to support this judgment.

As the nurse becomes more experienced in using the diagnostic process, the ability to anticipate, identify, and interpret specific client responses increases. For example, the experienced postpartum nurse recognizes that most first-time nursing mothers experience anxiety about their ability to breastfeed. On the basis of this knowledge, the nurse assesses for cues that this response might be present and initiates nursing interventions to assist the client to decrease her anxiety.

• VOCABULARY CHECK

Directions. Below are 10 words taken from the key word section of this chapter. Circle the letter of the best definition from the four choices.

1 Diagnosed
  a to have a identified disease
  b to have treated a disease
  c to have cured a disease
  d to have suspected a disease is present

2 Obstacle
  a something that one accomplishes
  b something that one achieves
  c something that impedes progress
  d something that aids progress

3 Diabetes
  a a variety of disorders affecting the liver
  b a variety of disorders characterized by excessive urination
  c a variety of disorders of the nervous system
  d a variety of disorders of the lymphatic system

4 Approximate
  a to accept as satisfactory
  b to reject as unacceptable
  c to be specific
  d to come close

5 Zygote
  a the fertilized ovum
  b the immature sperm
  c the unfertilized ovum
  d the mature sperm

6 Verify
  a to flower or bud
  b serving to eliminate parasites
  c to sign one's name to a document
  d to establish truth or reality of

7 Plasma
  a fluid portion of the blood
  b corpuscles in the blood
  c any factors in the blood
  d immunities in the blood

8 Dynamic

    a marked by danger   **c** pertaining to explosions

    b marked by energy   **d** peaceful; serene

9 Antigen

    a a portion of the cornea

    b a part of the cardiopulmonary system

    c part of one's genetic makeup

    d substance that can induce a specific immune response

10 Intractable

    a not easily relieved or cured   **c** not capable of following

    b not able to detect   **d** not able to comprehend

• SUMMARY

In this chapter you have learned that it is possible to figure out the meanings of unknown words by using the familiar, neighboring words that surround the new term. This is called using context clues. Five examples of context clues were given:

1 Direct definition   **4** Appositive

2 Synonym   **5** Example

3 Antonym

The most common type of context clue used in nursing texts is direct definition. Use direct definition and the other types of context clues whenever possible to help you determine word meanings.

You were also made aware of the possible limitations of context clues. Context clues may not provide a precise enough definition for medical terminology, or the sentence or passage may not contain any context clues.

Therefore, when you need further help in finding word meanings, consult a glossary, dictionary, or medical dictionary.

• Chapter 6 •

Dictionary, Glossary, and Thesaurus

OBJECTIVES

KEY WORDS

USING OTHER SOURCES TO DEFINE WORDS

DICTIONARY

   Purpose of the Dictionary

   Reading a Dictionary Entry

   Locating an Entry

   Guide Words

   Pronunciation Key

   Multiple Definitions

GLOSSARY

THESAURUS

   Reading a Thesaurus Entry

VOCABULARY CHECK

SUMMARY

• OBJECTIVES

To become familiar with the format of the dictionary, glossary, and thesaurus and to learn the way these references can teach the meanings of new words.

• KEY WORDS

Pay attention to the following key words, which are underscored the first time they appear in this chapter. Try to determine the meaning of these words in the passage. If you need further help, use your dictionary or the glossary in the back of this book.

Look up the medical terminology in your medical dictionary or the glossary. As you read the exercises in this chapter, write additional words you need to learn in the space provided.

MEDICAL TERMINOLOGY	GENERAL VOCABULARY
afferent	antonyms
afterbirth	collegiate
bulimia	diacritical marks
cyst	etymology
gynecology	glossary
hematoma	pronunciation
incision	specialized
mysoline	synonyms
myxorrhea	thesaurus
pathogen	unabridged
sclerosis	_____
_____	_____
_____	_____
_____	_____

• USING OTHER SOURCES TO DEFINE WORDS

In the two previous chapters (Chapter 4, "Affixes," and Chapter 5, "Using Context Clues") you learned ways of defining unknown words encountered in your readings without the use of references such as the dictionary. When you use these vocabulary strategies, you do not have to disturb your concentration by stopping to refer to another source. In some instances, however, analyzing affixes and interpreting context clues will not be sufficient. For example, the word may not have an affix, the surrounding words may not suggest the meaning of the unknown word, or the word may be an unknown medical term that requires a precise definition. In these cases you will have to take a momentary break from reading to consult an additional source. Depending on the situation, this may be a dictionary (either collegiate or medical), a glossary, or a thesaurus.

• DICTIONARY

Dictionaries are indispensable to your experience as a nursing student. Most nursing schools require that you buy a medical dictionary, such as the Miller and Keane: *Encyclopedia and Dictionary of Medicine, Nursing, and Allied Health*. This type of dictionary is a <u>specialized</u> dictionary because it focuses on terminology from a particular profession or field—in this case the health profession.

The next type of dictionary that is necessary for your success as a nursing student is a hard-cover <u>collegiate</u> dictionary for general terminology. This dictionary should be used at home and kept in your study area for quick availability.

The last kind of dictionary to buy is a paperback version of a collegiate dictionary. You need a dictionary in this handy form so you can carry it with you to classes and refer to it when necessary. Make sure the paperback dictionary you buy is a complete edition of the hard-cover dictionary, not a shortened version. Otherwise, you may find when you go to look for a word that the entry is not there.

At times you may need to consult an <u>unabridged</u> dictionary in the library. The unabridged dictionary contains most words and is the most complete dictionary.

• Purpose of the Dictionary

Many people think that the dictionary is useful only for learning the meaning of an unknown word. However, the dictionary holds a wealth of other information. Consider some of these further uses:

- *Syllabication*. By reading the main entry you can see how many syllables a word has and where to divide the word at the end of a line.
- *Pronunciation*. By knowing how to use the pronunciation guide, you can find out how to pronounce the word accurately.
- *Parts of speech*. By consulting the appropriate abbreviation within the entry, you can determine the part of speech.
- *Etymology*. By looking at the first line in the entry, you can learn the origin of the word and the year it was first encountered in written form.
- *Spelling*. By checking both the beginning and end of the entry, you can see the correct spelling of the entry and in some instances the variations in spelling when suffixes are added.
- *Synonyms* and *antonyms*. At the end of the entry you may encounter other words that have meanings similar or opposite to the entry word.

• Reading a Dictionary Entry

To use the dictionary skillfully, you must be familiar with the various parts of the entry. Below is an entry taken from *Webster's Ninth New Collegiate Dictionary* (p. 609). The different parts have been numbered:

1.   2.   3. 4.   5.

in·ci·sion \in-'sizh-ən\ *n* (15c) **1** **a** : a marginal notch (as in a leaf) **b** : CUT, GASH; *specif* : a wound made esp. in surgery by incising the body **2** : an act of incising something **3** : the quality or state of being incisive

We will examine each of these parts of the entry more closely:

1   The *main entry or entry word* is usually printed in boldface. The letters of the word can be set undivided, divided by one or more spaces, or, as in this example, divided by hyphens. These divisions tell how many syllables the word has. In the above example, the entry has how many syllables? _____

2   The *pronunciation* is placed next to the main entry and is separated from it by reversed virgules (\   \). Later in the chapter we will explain the use of the pronunciation guide. Write the pronunciation of the entry word. _____

3   The *part of speech* follows the pronunciation and is usually abbreviated in the following manner:

adj   = adjective
adv   = adverb
conj   = conjunction
interj   = interjection
n   = noun
prep   = preposition
pron   = pronoun
vb   = verb
vt   = transitive verb
vi   = intransitive verb

In our example the entry word is what part of speech? _____

4   The *date* tells the earliest recorded use of the word in English. In many entries this is preceded by the *etymology* or origin of the word, that is, the country where the word is believed to have originated and what the word looked like in its original form. Some abbreviations found in the etymology are as follows:

OE   = Old English
ME   = Middle English
L   = Latin
G   = Greek
F   = French

In our example entry the word was first encountered in which century? _____

5   The rest of the entry is the *definitions* of the word. If the word has more than one meaning, the definitions are numbered. Sometimes the definition of the word has two or more shades of meaning or senses. If this is so, the definition is subdivided by letters.

In our example, how many definitions are there? _____

Which definition has different senses? _____

Comprehending?   Yes ___   No ___

• Locating an Entry

The dictionary is designed to help you find an entry as efficiently as possible. Interrupting your reading for several minutes to hunt for a word will discourage you from using the dictionary as a vocabulary builder. Because the dictionary entries are listed in alphabetical order, your first step is to make sure you know the order of the letters in the alphabet so you can quickly locate your word. That means that if the word you are looking for begins with a letter toward the end of the alphabet, you need not begin with "A" and go through the entire alphabet to get an approximate idea of where your word is located. You also must understand how to alphabetize up to the third, fourth, and fifth letters of the word. For various reasons, many students have to review alphabetical order. Once you are proficient in using alphabetical order, you will be able to work with your dictionary more skillfully.

• EXERCISE 6–1 •

Directions.   Below is a list of medical terms. In the space provided, write these words in alphabetical order.

MEDICAL TERMS	ALPHABETICAL ORDER
1 hematoma	1 _____
2 peripheral	2 _____
3 carcinogen	3 _____
4 perioperative	4 _____
5 menopause	5 _____
6 sinusitis	6 _____
7 nematodes	7 _____
8 cardiac	8 _____
9 hemophilia	9 _____
10 peritonitis	10 _____

Comprehending?   Yes ___   No ___

• Guide Words

The dictionary provides a handy tool to make locating an entry easier for you—*guide words*, which are printed at the top of a dictionary page. In the sample page from *Webster's Ninth New Collegiate Dictionary* shown opposite, you can see there are two boldface words, or guide words. (Other dictionaries may have one guide word on the lefthand page and another one on the facing page). The guide words in this example are "caterpillar" and "caucus." This tells you that every word that falls alphabetically between "caterpillar" and "caucus" appears on this page. You will find the page of your entry much faster by focusing on the guide words than by glancing over each page.

• EXERCISE 6–2 •

Directions. Below in the lefthand column are guide words taken from Miller and Keane: *Encyclopedia and Dictionary of Medical, Nursing and Allied Health*. In the righthand column are entries taken from the same dictionary. In the space provided in the center, write the number of the guide words that would be found on the page where the entry appears. The first one is done for you.

GUIDE WORDS		ENTRIES
1	myoplasm / myringotomy	_8_ sclerosis
2	globulinuria / glomerulus	___ cyst
3	buclizine / bundle	___ myotomy
4	dissolution / disulfiram	___ pathogen
5	mysoline / myxovirus	___ glomerulitis
6	afferent / agammaglobulinemia	___ scoliosis
7	cycrimine / cystectasis	___ myxorrhea
8	sclerogenous / sclerous	___ bulimia
9	path(o) / pathway	___ afterbirth
10	scolex / scotochromogen	___ distillation

Comprehending? Yes ___ No ___

• Pronunciation Key

One of the dictionary's functions is to help you pronounce unknown words. You learn pronunciation by consulting the *pronunciation key.* In some dictionaries the pronunciation key can be found at the bottom of each page, in others on the inside front cover, and in still others on a page near the front of the book. Check the dictionary's table of contents if you are having trouble locating the pronunciation key. If you need to buy a new dictionary, you may want to consider one with a pronunciation key at the bottom of each page. This format will help you check pronunciation easily.

Caterpillar *trademark* — used for a tractor made for use on rough or soft ground and moved on two endless metal belts
cat·er·waul \'kat-ər-,wȯl\ *vi* [ME *caterwawen*] (14c) **1 :** to make a harsh cry **2 :** to quarrel noisily — **caterwaul** *n*
cat·fac·ing \'kat-,fā-siŋ\ *n* (1940) **:** a disfigurement or malformation of fruit suggesting a cat's face in appearance
cat·fish \-,fish\ *n* (1612) **:** any of numerous usu. stout-bodied large-headed fishes (order Ostariophysi) with long tactile barbels

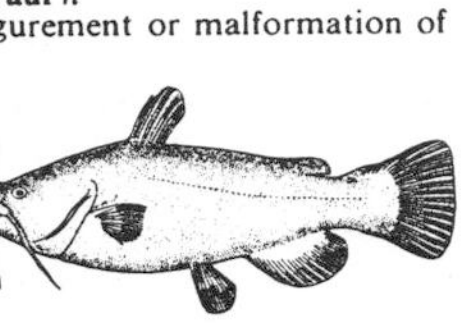
catfish

cat·gut \-,gət\ *n* (1599) **:** a tough cord made usu. from sheep intestines
cath- — see CATA-
Cath·ar \'kath-,är\ *n, pl* **Cath·a·ri** \'kath-ə-,rī, -,rē\ *or* **Cathars** [LL *cathari* (pl.), fr. LGk *katharoi*, fr. Gk, pl. of *katharos* pure] (1637) **:** a member of one of various ascetic and dualistic Christian sects flourishing in the later Middle Ages teaching that matter is evil, and professing faith in an angelic Christ who did not really undergo human birth or death — **Cath·a·rism** \'kath-ə-,riz-əm\ *n* — **Cath·a·rist** \-rəst\ *or* **Cath·a·ris·tic** \,kath-ə-'ris-tik\ *adj*
ca·thar·sis \kə-'thär-səs\ *n, pl* **ca·thar·ses** \-,sēz\ [NL, fr. Gk *katharsis*, fr. *kathairein* to cleanse, purge, fr. *katharos*] (1803) **1 :** PURGATION **2 a :** purification or purgation of the emotions (as pity and fear) primarily through art **b :** a purification or purgation that brings about spiritual renewal or release from tension **3 :** elimination of a complex by bringing it to consciousness and affording it expression
[1]**ca·thar·tic** \kə-'thärt-ik\ *adj* [LL or Gk; LL *catharticus*, fr. Gk *kathartikos*, fr. *kathairein*] (1612) **:** of, relating to, or producing catharsis
[2]**cathartic** *n* (1651) **:** a cathartic medicine **:** PURGATIVE
cat·head \'kat-,hed\ *n* (1626) **:** a projecting piece of timber or iron near the bow of a ship to which the anchor is hoisted and secured
ca·thect \kə-'thekt, ka-\ *vt* [NL *cathexis*] (1925) **:** to invest with mental or emotional energy
ca·thec·tic \kə-'thek-tik, ka-\ *adj* [NL *cathexis*] (1927) **:** of, relating to, or invested with mental or emotional energy
ca·the·dra \kə-'thē-drə\ *n* [L, chair — more at CHAIR] (15c) **:** a bishop's official throne
[1]**ca·the·dral** \kə-'thē-drəl\ *adj* (13c) **1 :** of, relating to, or containing a cathedra **2 :** emanating from a chair of authority **3 :** suggestive of a cathedral
[2]**cathedral** *n* (1587) **1 :** a church that is the official seat of a diocesan bishop **2 :** something that resembles or suggests a cathedral ⟨higher education has been . . . the secular ~ of our time — David Riesman⟩
ca·thep·sin \kə-'thep-sən\ *n* [Gk *kathepsein* to digest (fr. *kata-* cata- + *hepsein* to boil) + E *-in*] (1929) **:** any of several intracellular proteinases of animal tissue that aid in autolysis in some diseased conditions and after death
cath·er·ine wheel \,kath-(ə-)rən-\ *n, often cap C* [St. *Catherine* of Alexandria †*ab*307 Christian martyr] (15c) **1 :** a wheel with spikes projecting from the rim **2 :** PINWHEEL 1 **3 :** CARTWHEEL 2
cath·e·ter \'kath-ət-ər, 'kath-tər\ *n* [LL, fr. Gk *kathetēr*, fr. *kathienai* to send down, fr. *kata-* cata- + *hienai* to send — more at JET] (1601) **:** a tubular medical device for insertion into canals, vessels, passageways, or body cavities usu. to permit injection or withdrawal of fluids or to keep a passage open
cath·e·ter·iza·tion \,kath-ət-ə-rə-'zā-shən, ,kath-tə-rə-\ *n* (1849) **:** the use of or introduction of a catheter (as in or into the bladder, trachea, or heart) — **cath·e·ter·ize** \,kath-ət-ə-,rīz, ,kath-tə-\ *vt*
ca·thex·is \kə-'thek-səs, ka-\ *n, pl* **ca·thex·es** \-,sēz\ [NL (intended as trans. of G *besetzung*), fr. Gk *kathexis* holding, fr. *katechein* to hold fast, occupy, fr. *kata-* + *echein* to have, hold — more at SCHEME] (1922) **:** investment of mental or emotional energy in a person, object, or idea
cath·ode \'kath-,ōd\ *n* [Gk *kathodos* way down, fr. *kata-* + *hodos* way — more at CEDE] (1834) **1 :** the negative terminal of an electrolytic cell — compare ANODE **2 :** the positive terminal of a primary cell or of a storage battery that is delivering current **3 :** the electron-emitting electrode of an electron tube — **ca·thod·ic** \ka-'thäd-ik\ *or* **cath·od·al** \'kath-,ōd-ᵊl\ *adj* — **ca·thod·i·cal·ly** \-i-k(ə-)lē\ *or* **cath·od·al·ly** \-ē\ *adv*
cathode ray *n* (1880) **1 :** one of the high-speed electrons projected in a stream from the heated cathode of a vacuum tube under the propulsion of a strong electric field **2 :** a stream of cathode-ray electrons
cathode–ray tube *n* (1905) **:** a vacuum tube in which cathode rays usu. in the form of a slender beam are projected on a fluorescent screen and produce a luminous spot
cath·o·lic \'kath-(ə-)lik\ *adj* [MF & LL; MF *catholique*, fr. LL *catholicus*, fr. Gk *katholikos* universal, general, fr. *katholou* in general, fr. *kata* by + *holos* whole — more at CATA-, SAFE] (14c) **1 :** COMPREHENSIVE, UNIVERSAL; *esp* **:** broad in sympathies, tastes, or interests **2** *cap* **a :** of, relating to, or forming the church universal **b :** of, relating to, or forming the ancient undivided Christian church or a church claiming historical continuity from it; *specif* **:** ROMAN CATHOLIC — **ca·thol·i·cal·ly** \kə-'thäl-i-k(ə-)lē\ *adv* — **ca·thol·i·cize** \kə-'thäl-ə-,sīz\ *vb*
Cath·o·lic \'kath-(ə-)lik\ *n* (15c) **1 :** a person who belongs to the universal Christian church **2 :** a member of a Catholic church; *specif* **:** ROMAN CATHOLIC
Catholic Apostolic *adj* (1837) **:** of or relating to a Christian sect founded in 19th century England in anticipation of Christ's second coming
ca·thol·i·cate \kə-'thäl-ə-,kāt, -'thäl-i-kət\ *n* (ca. 1847) **:** the jurisdiction of a catholicos
Catholic Epistles *n pl* (1582) **:** the five New Testament letters including James, I and II Peter, I John, and Jude addressed to the early Christian churches at large
Ca·thol·i·cism \kə-'thäl-ə-,siz-əm\ *n* (1613) **1 :** the faith, practice, or system of Catholic Christianity **2 :** ROMAN CATHOLICISM
cath·o·lic·i·ty \,kath-(ə)-'lis-ət-ē\ *n, pl* **-ties** (1704) **1** *cap* **:** the character of being in conformity with a Catholic church **2 a :** liberality of sentiments or views ⟨~ of viewpoint — W. V. O'Connor⟩ **b :** UNIVERSALITY **c :** comprehensive range ⟨the ~ of subjects represented by the press's trade list — *Current Biog.*⟩
ca·thol·i·con \kə-'thäl-ə-,kän\ *n* [F or ML; F, fr. ML, fr. Gk *katholikon*, neut. of *katholikos*] (15c) **:** CURE-ALL, PANACEA
ca·thol·i·cos \kə-'thäl-i-kəs\ *n, pl* **-i·cos·es** \-kə-səz\ *or* **-i·coi** \-'thäl-ə-,kȯi\ *often cap* [LGk *katholikos*, fr. Gk, general] (1625) **:** a primate of certain Eastern churches and esp. of the Armenian or of the Nestorian church
cat·house \'kat-,hau̇s\ *n* (1931) **:** a house of prostitution
cat·ion \'kat-,ī-ən\ *n* [Gk *kation*, neut. of *katiōn*, prp. of *katienai* to go down, fr. *kata-* cata- + *ienai* to go — more at ISSUE] (1834) **:** the ion in an electrolyzed solution that migrates to the cathode; *broadly* **:** a positively charged ion
cat·ion·ic \,kat-(,)ī-'än-ik\ *adj* (ca. 1920) **1 :** of or relating to cations **2 :** characterized by an active and esp. surface-active cation ⟨a ~ dye⟩ — **cat·ion·i·cal·ly** \-i-k(ə-)lē\ *adv*
cat·kin \'kat-kən\ *n* [fr. its resemblance to a cat's tail] (1578) **:** a usu. long ament densely crowded with bracts
cat·like \'kat-,līk\ *adj* (1600) **:** resembling a cat; *esp* **:** STEALTHY ⟨with ~ tread, upon our prey we steal —W. S. Gilbert⟩
cat·mint \-,mint\ *n* (13c) **:** CATNIP
cat·nap \-,nap\ *n* (1823) **:** a very short light nap — **catnap** *vi*
cat·nap·per *or* **cat·nap·er** \'kat-,nap-ər\ *n* [[1]*cat* + *-napper* (as in *kidnapper*)] (1942) **:** one that steals cats usu. to sell them for research
cat·nip \-,nip\ *n* [[1]*cat* + obs. *nep* (catnip), fr. ME, fr. OE *nepte*, fr. L *nepeta*] (1712) **1 :** a strong-scented mint (*Nepeta cataria*) that has whorls of small pale flowers in terminal spikes and contains a substance attractive to cats **2 :** something very attractive
cat–o'–nine–tails \,kat-ə-'nīn-,tālz\ *n, pl* **cat–o'–nine–tails** [fr. the resemblance of its scars to the scratches of a cat] (1665) **:** a whip made of usu. nine knotted lines or cords fastened to a handle
ca·top·tric \kə-'täp-trik\ *adj* [Gk *katoptrikos*, fr. *katoptron* mirror, fr. *katopsesthai* to be going to observe, fr. *kata-* cata- + *opsesthai* to be going to see — more at OPTIC] (1774) **:** of or relating to a mirror or reflected light; *also* **:** produced by reflection — **ca·top·tri·cal·ly** \-trik(ə-)lē\ *adv*
cat rig *n* (1867) **:** a rig consisting of a single mast far forward carrying a single large sail extended by a boom — **cat–rigged** \'kat-'rigd\ *adj*
CAT scan \'kat-, ,sē-,ā-'tē-\ *n* [computerized axial tomography] (1975) **:** an image made by computerized axial tomography
CAT scanner *n* (1975) **:** a medical instrument consisting of integrated X-ray and computing equipment and used for computerized axial tomography
cat's cradle *n* (1768) **1 :** a game in which a string looped in a pattern like a cradle on the fingers of one person's hands is transferred to the hands of another so as to form a different figure **2 :** INTRICACY ⟨the socioreligious *cat's cradle* of small Greek communities — *Times Lit. Supp.*⟩
cat's–eye \'kat-,sī\ *n, pl* **cat's–eyes** (1599) **1 :** any of various gems (as a chrysoberyl or a chalcedony) exhibiting opalescent reflections from within **2 :** a marble with eyelike concentric circles
cat's–paw \'kat-,spȯ\ *n, pl* **cat's–paws** (1769) **1 :** a light air that ruffles the surface of the water in irregular patches during a calm **2** [fr. the fable of the monkey that used a cat's paw to draw chestnuts from the fire] **:** one used by another as a tool **:** DUPE **3 :** a hitch in the bight of a rope so made as to form two eyes into which a tackle may be hooked — see KNOT illustration
cat·sup \'kech-əp, 'kach-; 'kat-səp\ *n* [Malay *kĕchap* spiced fish sauce] (1690) **:** a seasoned tomato puree
cat·tail \'kat-,tāl\ *n* (1548) **:** any of a genus (*Typha* of the family Typhaceae, the cattail family) of tall reedy marsh plants with brown furry fruiting spikes; *esp* **:** a plant (*Typha latifolia*) with long flat leaves used for making mats and chair seats
cat·tery \'kat-ə-rē\ *n, pl* **-ter·ies** (1834) **:** an establishment for the breeding and boarding of cats
cat·tle \'kat-ᵊl\ *n pl* [ME *catel*, fr. ONF, personal property, fr. ML *capitale*, fr. L, neut. of *capitalis* of the head — more at CAPITAL] (13c) **1 :** domesticated quadrupeds held as property or raised for use; *specif* **:** bovine animals on a farm or ranch **2 :** human beings esp. en masse
cattle call *n* (1952) **:** a mass audition (as of actors)
cattle egret *n* (ca. 1899) **:** a small white egret (*Bubulcus ibis*) with a yellow bill and in the breeding season buff on the crown, breast, and back that has been introduced into the eastern U.S. from the Old World
cattle grub *n* (1926) **:** any of several heel flies esp. in the larval stage; *esp* **:** COMMON CATTLE GRUB
cat·tle·man \-mən, -,man\ *n* (1864) **:** a man who tends or raises cattle
cattle tick *n* (1869) **:** a tick (*Boophilus annulatus*) that infests cattle in the southern U.S. and tropical America and transmits the causative agent of Texas fever
cat·tleya \'kat-lē-ə; kat-'lā-ə, -'lē-\ *n* [NL, fr. Wm. *Cattley* †1832 Eng. patron of botany] (1828) **:** any of a genus (*Cattleya*) of tropical American epiphytic orchids with showy hooded flowers
[1]**cat·ty** \'kat-ē\ *n, pl* **catties** [Malay *kati*] (1598) **:** any of various units of weight of China and southeast Asia varying around 1 1/3 pounds; *also* **:** a standard Chinese unit equal to 1.1023 pounds
[2]**catty** *adj* **cat·ti·er; -est** (1903) **1 :** resembling a cat; *esp* **:** slyly spiteful **:** MALICIOUS **2 :** of or relating to a cat — **cat·ti·ly** \'kat-ᵊl-ē\ *adv* — **cat·ti·ness** \'kat-ē-nəs\ *n*
cat·ty–cor·ner *or* **cat·ty–cor·nered** *var of* CATERCORNER
cat·walk \'kat-,wȯk\ *n* (1885) **:** a narrow walkway (as along a bridge)
Cau·ca·sian \kȯ-'kā-zhən, -'kazh-ən\ *adj* (1807) **1 :** of or relating to the Caucasus or its inhabitants **2 a :** of or relating to the white race of mankind as classified according to physical features **b :** of or relating to the white race as defined by law specif. as composed of persons of European, No. African, or southwest Asian ancestry — **Caucasian** *n* — **Cau·ca·soid** \'kȯ-kə-,sȯid\ *adj or n*
Cau·chy sequence \kō-,shē-\ *n* [Augustin-Louis *Cauchy* †1857 Fr. mathematician] (1955) **:** a sequence of elements in a metric space such that for any positive number no matter how small there exists a term in the sequence for which the distance between any two consecutive or nonconsecutive terms beyond this term is less than an arbitrarily small number
[1]**cau·cus** \'kȯ-kəs\ *n* [prob. of Algonquian origin] (1763) **:** a closed meeting of a group of persons belonging to the same political party or faction usu. to select candidates or to decide on policy; *also* **:** a group of people united to promote an agreed-upon cause
[2]**caucus** *vi* (1788) **:** to hold or meet in a caucus

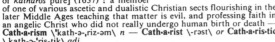

Following is the pronunciation key found at the bottom of each page in *Webster's Ninth New Collegiate Dictionary:*

\ə\ abut	\ᵊ\ kitten, F table	\ər\ further	\a\ ash	\ā\ ace	\ä\ cot, cart	
\aù\ out	\ch\ chin	\e\ bet	\ē\ easy	\g\ go	\i\ hit	\ī\ ice	\j\ job
\ŋ\ sing	\ō\ go	\ò\ law	\òi\ boy	\th\ thin	\t͟h\ the	\ü\ loot	\ù\ foot
\y\ yet	\zh\ vision	\à, k̲, ⁿ, œ, œ̄, ɷ, ɷ̄, ʸ\ *see* Guide to Pronunciation

As you can see, it consists of symbols (diacritical marks) and simple words. Parts of it are printed in boldface. Look more closely at one entry:

$$\backslash \overline{\imath} \backslash \text{ ice}$$

This tells you that when you are reading the pronunciation portion of a dictionary entry and you see the symbol ī, you pronounce that "i" as you would say the beginning "i" in "ice." For a further illustration, consider the following:

$$\text{b}\overline{\imath}\text{l}$$

Again, this diacritical mark is pronounced like the "i" in "ice." Pronounce the ī sound and you come up with the word for liver secretion—bile.

Now look at a more difficult word:

$$\text{g}\overline{\imath}\text{n-ə-käl-ə-Jē}$$

Referring back to the pronunciation key, try to figure out the pronunciation of the underlined letters.

ī = like the "i" in **ice**

ə = like the "a" and the "u" in **abut**

ä = like the "o" in **cot**

ə = like the "a" and the "u" in **abut**

j = like the "j" in **job**

ē = like the "ea" in **easy**

The word is "gynecology"—the branch of medicine that deals with women's health.

• **EXERCISE 6–3** •

Directions. Use the pronunciation key on p. 68 to determine the correct spelling and pronunciation of the following words. Write the word in the space provided.

1 ā-ort-ə _____

2 kə-rē-ə _____

3 dī-(y)ə-ret-ik _____

4 hī-pə-gas-trik _____

5 fȧs-fāt _____

6 spī-nə bĭ-fed-ə _____

7 tĕk-nŏl-ō-jĭst _____

8 kŏn-vō-lū-shŭn _____

9 dĭs-grăf-ĭ-ă _____

10 mer-kū-rī _____

Comprehending? Yes ____ No ____

• **Multiple Definitions**

Many medical and nonmedical terms have more than one meaning. When a word has multiple definitions, the individual meanings in the entry will be numbered. It is important that you choose the correct definition for your purpose when you are using the dictionary to determine the meaning of an unknown word. To do this you must consider how the unknown word is used in the sentence. For example, you may read the word "callus" in the following context or sentence:

She got a *callus* on her heel from walking barefoot.

You check your medical dictionary and you see two definitions—1. localized hyperplasia of the horny layer of the epidermis due to pressure or friction. 2. an unorganized network of woven bone formed about the ends of a broken bone (Miller and Keane, p. 197).

From the sentence, the context clues "heel" and "walking barefoot" let you know that you are not concerned with broken bones, but rather with roughened skin from going shoeless. The first definition is the more appropriate. Again, when searching for the correct definition of an unknown word, make sure the meaning fits the sense of the sentence.

• **EXERCISE 6–4** •

Directions. Following are sentences with an unknown word or phrase in bold-face. Read the sentence and determine the correct use of the word. Then look up the definition in the page from *Webster's Ninth New Collegiate Dictionary* shown on p. 71. In the blank, write the number of the correct definition.

1 The doctor's **succinct** way of talking made him easy to listen to. _____

2 The child dropped the lemon **sucker** the pediatrician gave him. _____

3 Eventually, he will **succumb** to cancer. _____

4 A cactus in the hospital is a **succulent** plant. _____

5 The mother will **suckle** her baby. _____

6 The calf will **suckle** the cow. _____

7 Nurse Smith is first in line of **succession** to be dean. _____

8 The chubby man tried to **suck in** his stomach. _____

9 The **suction** on the vacuum tube was broken. _____

10 Her **sudden death** at 30 was alarming. _____

Comprehending? Yes _____ No _____

When analyzing affixes and context clues is not sufficient, having a good collegiate dictionary and a medical dictionary is crucial to your success in learning unknown words. The efficient use of a dictionary enables you to locate the meanings of unknown words effortlessly.

• **GLOSSARY**

The *glossary* is a collection of key words at the back of some textbooks. As in a dictionary, the entries are listed in alphabetical order, but unlike a dictionary, the glossary usually provides only the definition of the entries. Syllabication, pronunciation, etymology, dates, and synonyms and antonyms are usually omitted. The advantage of looking up words in the glossary instead of a dictionary is that the

suc·cess \sək-'ses\ *n* [L *successus,* fr. *successus,* pp. of *succedere*] (1537) **1** *obs* : OUTCOME, RESULT **2 a** : degree or measure of succeeding **b** : favorable or desired outcome; *also* : the attainment of wealth, favor, or eminence **3** : one that succeeds

suc·cess·ful \-fəl\ *adj* (1588) **1** : resulting or terminating in success **2** : gaining or having gained success — **suc·cess·ful·ly** \-fə-lē\ *adv* — **suc·cess·ful·ness** *n*

suc·ces·sion \sək-'sesh-ən\ *n* [ME, fr. MF or L; MF, fr. L *succession-, successio,* fr. *successus,* pp.] (14c) **1 a** : the order in which or the conditions under which one person after another succeeds to a property, dignity, title, or throne **b** : the right of a person or line to succeed **c** : the line having such a right **2 a** : the act or process of following in order : SEQUENCE **b (1)** : the act or process of one person's taking the place of another in the enjoyment of or liability for his rights or duties or both **(2)** : the act or process of a person's becoming beneficially entitled to a property or property interest of a deceased person **c** : the continuance of corporate personality **d** : unidirectional change in the composition of an ecosystem as the available competing organisms and esp. the plants respond to and modify the environment ⟨the highlights of the ~ were the weed, grass, and forest communities developed in that order⟩ **3 a** : a number of persons or things that follow each other in sequence **b** : a group, type, or series that succeeds or displaces another — **suc·ces·sion·al** \-'sesh-nəl, -ən-ᵊl\ *adj* — **suc·ces·sion·al·ly** \-ē\ *adv*

succession duty *n, chiefly Brit* (1853) : INHERITANCE TAX

suc·ces·sive \sək-'ses-iv\ *adj* (15c) **1** : following in order : following each other without interruption **2** : characterized by or produced in succession — **suc·ces·sive·ly** *adv* — **suc·ces·sive·ness** *n*

suc·ces·sor \sək-'ses-ər\ *n* [ME *successour,* fr. OF, fr. L *successor,* fr. *successus,* pp.] (13c) : one that follows; *esp* : one who succeeds to a throne, title, estate, or office

suc·ci·nate \'sək-sə-,nāt\ *n* (1790) : a salt or ester of succinic acid

suc·cinct \(,)sək-'siŋ(k)t, sə-'siŋ(k)t\ *adj* [ME, fr. L *succinctus,* pp. of *succingere* to gird from below, tuck up, fr. *sub-* + *cingere* to gird — more at CINCTURE] (13c) **1** *archaic* **a** : being girded **b** : close-fitting **2** : marked by compact precise expression without wasted words ***syn*** see CONCISE — **suc·cinct·ly** \-'siŋ(k)-tlē, -'siŋ-klē\ *adv* — **suc·cinct·ness** \-'siŋt-nəs, -'siŋk-nəs\ *n*

suc·cin·ic acid \(,)sək-,sin-ik-\ *n* [F *succinique,* fr. L *succinum* amber + F *-ique* -ic] (ca. 1790) : a crystalline dicarboxylic acid $C_4H_6O_4$ found widely in nature and active in energy-yielding metabolic reactions

succinic dehydrogenase *n* (1942) : an iron-containing flavoprotein enzyme that catalyzes often reversibly the dehydrogenation of succinic acid to fumaric acid in the presence of a hydrogen acceptor and that is widely distributed esp. in animal tissues, bacteria, and yeast — called also *succinate dehydrogenase*

suc·ci·nyl \'sək-sən-ᵊl, -sə-,nil\ *n* [ISV] (ca. 1868) : either of two groups of succinic acid: **a** : a bivalent group $OCCH_2CH_2CO$ **b** : a univalent group $HOOCCH_2CH_2CO$

suc·ci·nyl·cho·line \,sək-sən-ᵊl-'kō-,lēn, -sə-,nil-\ *n* (1952) : a basic compound that acts similarly to curare and is used intravenously chiefly in the form of a hydrated chloride $C_{14}H_{30}Cl_2N_2O_4{\cdot}2H_2O$ as a muscle relaxant in surgery

[1]suc·cor \'sək-ər\ *n* [ME *succur,* fr. earlier *sucurs,* taken as pl., fr. OF *sucors,* fr. ML *succursus,* fr. L *succursus,* pp. of *succurrere* to run up, run to help, fr. *sub-* up + *currere* to run — more at CURRENT] (13c) **1** : RELIEF; *also* : AID, HELP **2** : something that furnishes relief

[2]succor *vt* **suc·cored; suc·cor·ing** \'sək-(ə-)riŋ\ (13c) : to go to the aid of : RELIEVE — **suc·cor·er** \'sək-ər-ər\ *n*

suc·co·ry \'sək-(ə-)rē\ *n* [alter. of ME *cicoree*] (1533) : CHICORY

suc·co·tash \'sək-ə-,tash\ *n* [of Algonquian origin; akin to Narraganset *msəkwataš* succotash] (1751) : lima or shell beans and green corn cooked together

suc·cour \'sək-ər\ *chiefly Brit var of* SUCCOR

suc·cu·ba \'sək-yə-bə\ *n, pl* **-bae** \-,bē, -,bī\ [LL, prostitute] (1559) : SUCCUBUS

suc·cu·bus \-bəs\ *n, pl* **-bi** \-,bī, -,bē\ [ME, fr. ML, alter. of LL *succuba* prostitute, fr. L *succubare* to lie under, fr. *sub-* + *cubare* to lie, recline — more at HIP] (14c) : a demon assuming female form to have sexual intercourse with men in their sleep — compare INCUBUS

suc·cu·lence \'sək-yə-lən(t)s\ *n* (1787) **1** : the state of being succulent **2** : succulent feed ⟨wild game subsisting on ~⟩

[1]suc·cu·lent \-lənt\ *adj* [L *suculentus,* fr. *sucus* juice, sap; akin to L *sugere* to suck — more at SUCK] (1601) **1 a** : full of juice : JUICY **b** : moist and tasty : TOOTHSOME **c** *of a plant* : having fleshy tissues designed to conserve moisture **2** : rich in interest — **suc·cu·lent·ly** *adv*

[2]succulent *n* (1825) : a succulent plant (as a cactus)

suc·cumb \sə-'kəm\ *vi* [F & L; F *succomber,* fr. L *succumbere,* fr. *sub-* + *-cumbere* to lie down — more at HIP] (1604) **1** : to yield to superior strength or force or overpowering appeal or desire **2** : to be brought to an end (as death) by the effect of destructive or disruptive forces ***syn*** see YIELD

[1]such \(')səch, (,)sich\ *adj* [ME, fr. OE *swilc;* akin to OHG *sulīh* such, OE *swā* so — more at SO] (bef. 12c) **1 a** : of a kind or character to be indicated or suggested ⟨a bag ~ as a doctor carries⟩ **b** : having a quality to a degree to be indicated ⟨his excitement was ~ that he shouted⟩ **2** : of the character, quality, or extent previously indicated or implied ⟨in the past few years many ~ women have shifted to full-time jobs⟩ **3** : of so extreme a degree or quality ⟨never heard ~ a hubbub⟩ **4** : of the same class, type, or sort ⟨other ~ clinics throughout the state⟩ **5** : not specified

[2]such *pron* (bef. 12c) **1** : such a person or thing **2** : someone or something stated, implied, or exemplified ⟨~ was the result⟩ **3** : someone or something similar : similar persons or things ⟨tin and glass and ~⟩ ***usage*** For reasons that are hard to understand, commentators on usage disapprove of *such* used as a pronoun. Dictionaries, however, recognize it as standard; all of the citations upon which our definitions of this word are based are clearly standard.
— **as such** : intrinsically considered : in itself ⟨*as such* the gift was worth little⟩

[3]such *adv* (bef. 12c) **1 a** : to such a degree : SO ⟨~ tall buildings⟩ ⟨~ a fine person⟩ **b** : VERY, ESPECIALLY ⟨hasn't been in ~ good spirits lately⟩ **2** : in such a way

[1]such and such *adj* (15c) : not named or specified

[2]such and such *pron* (1560) : something not specified

[1]such·like \'səch-,līk\ *adj* (15c) : of like kind : SIMILAR

[2]suchlike *pron* (15c) : SUCH 3

[1]suck \'sək\ *vb* [ME *souken,* fr. OE *sūcan;* akin to OHG *sūgan* to suck, L *sugere,* Gk *hyein* to rain] *vt* (bef. 12c) **1 a** : to draw (as liquid) into the mouth through a suction force produced by movements of the lips and tongue ⟨~*ed* milk from his mother's breast⟩ **b** : to draw something from or consume by such movements ⟨~ an orange⟩ ⟨~ a lollipop⟩ **c** : to apply the mouth to in order to or as if to suck out a liquid ⟨~*ed* his burned finger⟩ **2 a** : to draw by or as if by suction ⟨when a receding wave ~*s* the sand from under your feet —Kenneth Brower⟩ ⟨inadvertently ~*ed* into the . . . intrigue —Martin Levin⟩ **b** : to take in and consume by or as if by suction ⟨a vacuum cleaner ~*ing* up dirt⟩ ⟨~ up a few beers⟩ ⟨opponents say that malls ~ the life out of downtown areas —Michael Knight⟩ ~ *vi* **1** : to draw something in by or as if by exerting a suction force; *esp* : to draw milk from a breast or udder with the mouth **2** : to make a sound or motion associated with or caused by suction ⟨his pipe ~*ed* wetly⟩ ⟨flanks ~*ed* in and out, the long nose resting on his paws —Virginia Woolf⟩ **3** : to act in an obsequious manner ⟨when they want votes . . . the candidates come ~*ing* around —W. G. Hardy⟩ ⟨~*ed* up to the boss⟩ **4** *slang* : to be extremely objectionable or inadequate ⟨our lifestyle ~*s* —*Playboy*⟩ ⟨people who went said it ~*ed* —H.S. Thompson⟩

[2]suck *n* (13c) **1** : a sucking movement or force **2** : the act of sucking

[1]suck·er \'sək-ər\ *n* (14c) **1 a** : one that sucks esp. a breast or udder : SUCKLING **b** : a device for creating or regulating suction (as a piston or valve in a pump) **c** : a pipe or tube through which something is drawn by suction **d (1)** : an organ in various animals for adhering or holding **(2)** : a mouth (as of a leech) adapted for sucking or adhering **2** : a shoot from the roots or lower part of the stem of a plant **3** : any of numerous freshwater fishes (family Catostomidae) closely related to the carps but distinguished from them esp. by the structure of the mouth which usu. has thick soft lips **4** : LOLLIPOP **5 a** : a person easily cheated or deceived **b** : a person irresistibly attracted by something specified ⟨a ~ for ghost stories⟩ **c** — used as generalized term of reference ⟨see if you can get that ~ working again⟩

[2]sucker *vb* **suck·ered; suck·er·ing** \'sək-(ə-)riŋ\ *vt* (1661) **1** : to remove suckers from ⟨~ tobacco⟩ **2** : HOODWINK ~ *vi* : to send out suckers

suck in *vt* (15c) **1** : to contract, flatten, and tighten (the abdomen) esp. by inhaling deeply **2** : DUPE, HOODWINK

suck·ing *adj* (bef. 12c) : not yet weaned; *broadly* : very young

sucking louse *n* (ca. 1907) : any of an order (Anoplura) of wingless insects comprising the true lice with mouthparts adapted to sucking body fluids

suck·le \'sək-əl\ *vt* **suck·led; suck·ling** \-(ə-)liŋ\ [prob. back-formation fr. *suckling*] (15c) **1 a** : to give milk to from the breast or udder ⟨a mother *suckling* her child⟩ **b** : to nurture as if by giving milk from the breast ⟨was *suckled* on pulp magazines⟩ **2** : to draw milk from the breast or udder of ⟨lambs *suckling* the ewes⟩

suck·ling \'sək-liŋ\ *n* (15c) : a young unweaned animal

su·crase \'sü-,krās, -,krāz\ *n* [ISV, fr. F *sucre* sugar, fr. MF — more at SUGAR] (ca. 1900) : INVERTASE

su·cre \'sü-(,)krā\ *n* [Sp, fr. Antonio José de *Sucre*] (1886) — see MONEY table

su·crose \'sü-,krōs, -,krōz\ *n* [ISV, fr. F *sucre* sugar] (1862) : a sweet crystalline dextrorotatory disaccharide sugar $C_{12}H_{22}O_{11}$ that occurs naturally in most land plants, is obtained from sugarcane or sugar beets, and unlike glucose and galactose does not reduce Fehling's solution to produce a colored precipitate

suc·tion \'sək-shən\ *n* [LL *suction-, suctio,* fr. L *suctus,* pp. of *sugere* to suck — more at SUCK] (1626) **1** : the act or process of sucking **2 a** : the act or process of exerting a force upon a solid, liquid, or gaseous body by reason of reduced air pressure over part of its surface **b** : force so exerted **3** : a device (as a pipe or fitting) used in a machine that operates by suction — **suc·tion·al** \-shən-ᵊl, -shnəl\ *adj*

suction pump *n* (1825) : a common pump in which the liquid to be raised is pushed by atmospheric pressure into the partial vacuum under a retreating valved piston on the upstroke and reflux is prevented by a check valve in the pipe

suction stop *n* (1887) : a voice stop in the formation of which air behind the articulation is rarefied with consequent inrush of air when articulation is broken

suc·to·ri·al \,sək-'tōr-ē-əl, -'tȯr-\ *adj* [NL *suctorius,* fr. L *suctus,* pp.] (1833) : adapted for sucking; *esp* : serving to draw up fluid or to adhere by suction ⟨~ mouths⟩

suc·to·ri·an \-ē-ən\ *n* [NL *Suctoria,* fr. neut. pl. of *suctorius* suctorial] (ca. 1842) : any of a class (Suctoria) of complex protozoans which have cilia only early in development and in which the mature form is fixed to the substrate, lacks locomotor organelles or a mouth, and obtains food through specialized suctorial tentacles

Su·dan grass \sü-'dan-, -'dän-\ *n* [the *Sudan,* region in Africa] (1911) : a vigorous tall-growing annual grass (*Sorghum vulgare sudanensis*) widely grown for hay and fodder

Su·dan·ic \sü-'dan-ik\ *n* [the *Sudan*] (1925) : the languages neither Bantu nor Hamitic spoken in a belt extending from Senegal to southern Sudan — **Sudanic** *adj*

su·da·to·ri·um \,süd-ə-'tōr-ē-əm, -'tȯr-\ *n* [L, fr. *sudatus,* pp. of *sudare* to sweat — more at SWEAT] (1756) : a sweat room in a bath

su·da·to·ry \'süd-ə-,tōr-ē, -,tȯr-\ *n, pl* **-ries** (1615) : SUDATORIUM

sudd \'səd\ *n* [Ar, lit., obstruction] (1874) : floating vegetable matter that forms obstructive masses in the upper White Nile

[1]sud·den \'səd-ᵊn\ *adj* [ME *sodain,* fr. MF, fr. L *subitaneus,* fr. *subitus* sudden, fr. pp. of *subire* to come up, fr. *sub-* up + *ire* to go — more at SUB-, ISSUE] (14c) **1 a** : happening or coming unexpectedly ⟨a ~ shower⟩ **b** : changing angle or character all at once **2** : marked by or manifesting abruptness or haste **3** : made or brought about in a short time : PROMPT ***syn*** see PRECIPITATE — **sud·den·ly** *adv* — **sud·den·ness** \'səd-ᵊn-(n)əs\ *n*

[2]sudden *n, obs* (1558) : an unexpected occurrence : EMERGENCY — **all of a sudden** *or* **on a sudden** : sooner than was expected : at once

sudden death *n* (1548) **1** : unexpected death that is instantaneous or occurs within minutes from any cause other than violence ⟨*sudden death* following coronary occlusion⟩ **2** : extra play to break a tie in a sports contest in which the first to go ahead wins

glossary is handier and easier to use. Having a collection of key words and definitions in the back of your textbook saves invaluable time when you need to learn a new word. The disadvantage of a glossary, however, is that it is usually limited to definitions of the key terms in the textbook. If you need to learn the meaning of a word that the author hasn't selected as a "key" or "major" word, you will not find it in the glossary. Also, if you need to know more than just the definition of an unknown word, for example, the pronunciation, the glossary may not be useful. However, if your book has a glossary, we recommend that you look there first to define unknown words after affix and context analysis fails.

• EXERCISE 6–5 •

Directions. Opposite is a portion of an index/glossary taken from a nursing textbook (Ignatavicius and Bayne, p. 2293). Following are five statements with a term in boldface. Read the statement. Then locate the term in the glossary. In the space provided after the statement, write "T" if the statement is true according to the entry in the glossary and "F" if the statement is false according to the entry in the glossary.

1 **Arthritis** is an inflammation of the muscle of the body. _____

2 **Audiometry** measures hearing sharpness. _____

3 **Asystole** is an irregular heartbeat. _____

4 **Arteriosclerosis** refers to hardening of the arteries _____

5 Hay fever is an **atopic** reaction _____

• THESAURUS

The *thesaurus* is a collection of words and their synonyms (different words that have the same meaning). In most cases the thesaurus is written in dictionary form. Therefore you would look up an entry the same way you would in your collegiate or medical dictionary. However, instead of giving the definition of a word, the thesaurus groups together all words that have similar meanings. The main purpose of the thesaurus is to aid you in your writing. When you are doing a written assignment, you may find yourself using the same words repeatedly or you may need a new word with a slightly different meaning. Consulting the thesaurus will help you solve these writing problems.

Arterial spiders, 1208
Arterial system, 2084. *See also specific structures and disorders.*
  function of, 2084
  structure of, *2083*, 2084
Arteriography. *See also* Angiography.
  Buerger's disease and, 2226
  cardiac, 2107–2108
  ear and, 1084
Arterioles, *2083*, 2084

Arteriosclerosis: hardening of the arteries, 2187–2195

  analysis: nursing diagnosis and, 2194
  aneurysms and, 2219
  assessment and, 2192–2194
    diagnostic tests and, 2194
    history in, 2192–2193
    laboratory findings in, 2193
    physical, 2193
    psychosocial, 2193
    radiographic findings in, 2193–2194
  discharge planning and, 2194–2195
    client/family education and, 2194–2195
    health care resources and, 2195
    home care preparation and, 2194
    psychosocial preparation and, 2195
  etiology of, 2188
  evaluation and, 2195
  incidence of, 2188
  pathophysiology of, 2187, *2188*
  planning and implementation and, 2194
  prevention of, 2188–2189
  risk of, age and cholesterol level and, 2193
Arteriovenous (AV) fistula, 1906
  hemodialysis and, *1905t*, 1906–1907, *1907*

Arteriovenous (AV) shunt: a method of vascular access for clients receiving hemodialysis, 1904, 2084

  care of, 1906
  hemodialysis and, *1904*, 1904–1906, *1905t*

Arthralgia: ache around joints of the body, 704

  serum sickness and, 665

Arthritis: inflammation of one or more joints of the body, 675

  disease-associated, 710–711
  gouty. *See* Gout.
  infectious, 710
  psoriatic, 710
  rheumatoid. *See* Rheumatoid arthritis (RA).
  sexuality and, 180–181
Arthrocentesis, rheumatoid arthritis and, 695, 696t

Arthrodesis: fusion of bone, 688

Arthrography: radiographic visualization of a joint after instillation of a contrast medium, 727–729

Arthroplasty: surgical creation of a new joint, usually by using metal and plastic implants, or prostheses

Arthroscopy: direct visualization into a joint by using an endoscope, 730, *730*

Arytenoid cartilages, 1933
Asbestosis, 2054–2055
Ascending cholangitis, 1456

Ascites: an abnormal accumulation of serous fluid within the peritoneal cavity, 1481

Asepsis, 616
Aseptic necrosis, fractures and, 785

Aspiration: inhalation of solid or liquid into the upper respiratory tract, 474

  gastroesophageal reflux disease and, 1273
  tracheostomy tubes and, 2022
Aspiration biopsy, of breast, 1657

Assessment: the first step of the nursing process in which the nurse systematically collects data about the client for the purpose of identifying potential and actual health problems, 23–25. *See also under specific conditions.*

  data collection and, 23–24
  data sources for, 24–25
  observation and, 24
  subjective and objective data and, 23
Assistive devices, degenerative joint disease and, 689
Assist-control mode (AC), 2027–2028
Associate degree (AD; ADN), 45
Associated cataract, 1038
Association areas, of parietal lobe, 843
Association of Operating Room Nurses (AORN), 20

Asterixis: arm flapping caused by motor disturbance, especially in comatose individuals with liver disease; also known as "liver flap," 1232–1233, 1485

Asthma: a respiratory condition characterized by bronchospasm, bronchoconstriction, wheezing, and recurrent attacks of dyspnea, 663, 1991

  bronchial, 663–664, 1991

Astigmatism: a refractive error of the eye resulting from an alteration in the eye's curvature that causes visual distortion, 997, 1060

Astrocytoma, 948
Astroglia, 830
Asynchronous breathing, 1994

Asystole: absence of heartbeat, 2130–2131

  etiology of, 2131
  incidence of, 2131
  pathophysiology of, *2130*, 2130–2131

Ataxia: muscular incoordination, irregularity of muscle action, 884

Atelectasis: collapsed or airless state of all or part of the lung, 432, 474, 1935, 1977

  absorption, 2004
Atherectomy, abrasive, mechanical rotational, peripheral arterial disease and, 2210

Atherosclerosis: a form of arteriosclerosis in which deposits of yellow plaques containing cholesterol and lipids are formed within the lining of large and medium-sized arteries, 2187, 2225. *See also* Arteriosclerosis.

  coronary artery disease and, 2149
  in young adulthood, 62
ATN. *See* Acute tubular necrosis.
Atopic dermatitis, 1182, 1183

Atopic reaction: an allergy that has an hereditary predisposition, like hay fever, 658–663

Atopic reaction *(Continued)*
  analysis: nursing diagnosis and, 661
  assessment and, 658–661
    diagnostic tests in, 659–661
    history in, 658–659
    physical, 659
    psychosocial, 659
  discharge planning and, 662–663
    client/family education and, 662–663
    health care resources and, 663
    home care preparation and, 662
    psychosocial preparation and, 663
  etiology of, 658
  evaluation and, 663
  incidence of, 658
  pathophysiology of, 658
  planning and implementation and, 661
  prevention of, 658
  skin inflammations and, 1183, 1185
ATP. *See* Adenosine triphosphate (ATP).
Atrial fibrillation, 2123
  etiology of, 2123
  incidence of, 2123
  pathophysiology of, 2123, *2124*
Atrial flutter, 2123
  etiology of, 2123
  incidence of, 2123
  pathophysiology of, 2123, *2124*
Atrial gallop, 2098
Atrial kick, 2075–2076
Atrial systole, 2075–2076
Atrioventricular (AV) blocks, 2125–2127
  etiology of, 2127
    first-degree, *2126*, 2126
  incidence of, 2127
  pathophysiology of, 2125–2127, *2126*, *2127*
    second-degree, *2126*, 2126–2127
    third-degree, *2127*, 2127
Atrioventricular (AV) valves, 2070
Atrium, 2069
Atrophic gastritis, 1304, 1305

Atrophic vaginitis: a condition in which the vaginal mucosa is thin and dry and is easily traumatized; seen frequently in elderly women, 1693–1694, 1701

Atrophy: a wasting of tissue, resulting in decreased size and inability to use, 646

  protein-calorie malnutrition and, 646
Attention, mental status assessment and, 849
Attitudes, sexuality and, 183
Attraction, phagocytosis and, 536
Audiometer, 1085, *1085*

Audiometry: measurement of hearing acuity, 1084–1090, *1085*, 1085t, *1086*

  pure tone, 1085–1089
    air conduction testing and, 1086–1087
    bone conduction testing and, 1087
    guidelines for, 1087
    interpretation and, 1088–1089
  speech, 1086, 1089–1090
    speech discrimination and, 1090
    speech reception threshold and, 1089–1090
Auditory assessment, 1081–1083
  tuning fork tests and, *1082*, 1082–1083
  voice test and, 1081–1082
  watch test and, 1082
Aura, 892
Auricle, 1075

Auscultation: technique used as part of physical assessment in which sounds within the body are heard through a stethoscope, e.g., breath sounds, 24

  endocrine abnormalities and, 1525
  lung cancer and, 2048–2049

- ## Reading a Thesaurus Entry

Below is an example of an entry from *Roget's New Pocket Thesaurus in Dictionary Form* (p. 285):

Nurse, N. attendant, medical, R.N.
(MEDICAL SCIENCE)

Note that the entry word is in boldface type and is followed by the part of speech.

In this example "nurse" is what part of speech? _____

After this, three synonyms are given for "nurse." The entry ends with a term in capital letters and parentheses (MEDICAL SCIENCE). This is an alternative entry to look up if the original entry does not provide you with the synonym you need.

Once you have acquired a thesaurus, you will find it one of the most valuable references for good writing. Keep it in a convenient place in your study area so it will be available when you need it. Remember to use it when you need a better word choice.

• EXERCISE 6–6 •

Directions. Opposite are copies of pp. 234 and 235 from *Roget's New Pocket Thesaurus in Dictionary Form*. Read the following short passage with words in boldface. After referring to the thesaurus pages, choose a better word for each boldface word and print it above the boldface term. Make sure the part of speech for the synonym matches the original word. The first word is done for you.

The nurse drew out her notebook from the desk in the station. She wanted

jot down

to **note** some of the happenings she **noticed** during her shift. In particular

the **nurse** wanted to object to some of the **objectionable** occurrences on the

floor. However, she wanted to be **objective**, so the **objective** of her obser-

vation would not be to **object** to the other nurse, but to get him to change

his **notions** on what it is to **nurse** a patient.

---

pass, defile, cut, gap, neck, gully, passage, gorge.

V. notch, nick, mill, score, cut, dent, indent, jag, scarify, scallop, gash, crimp; crenelate.

Adj. notched, crenate, scalloped, dentate, toothed, palmate, serrate, serrated, serriform, sawlike; machicolated, castellated.

See also HOLLOW, INTERVAL, PASSAGE. *Antonyms*—See SMOOTHNESS.

note, *n.* letter, communication, message (EPISTLE); memorandum (MEMORY); bill, paper money (MONEY); jotting, record (WRITING); commentary, annotation (EXPLANATION).

note, *v.* write, jot down (WRITING); observe, remark, notice (LOOKING); distinguish, discover (VISION).

notebook, *n.* diary, daybook (RECORD).

noted, *adj.* eminent, renowned (FAME).

nothing, *n.* nil, zero, cipher (NONEXISTENCE).

nothingness, *n.* nullity, nihility, void (NONEXISTENCE).

notice, *n.* announcement, proclamation, manifesto (INFORMATION); handbill, poster, circular (PUBLICATION); caution, caveat, admonition (WARNING).

notice, *v.* remark, observe, perceive (VISION, LOOKING).

noticeable, *adj.* conspicuous, marked, pointed (VISIBILITY).

notify, *v.* inform, let know, acquaint (INFORMATION).

notion, *n.* impression, conception, inkling (UNDERSTANDING, IDEA); concept, view (OPINION); fancy, humor, whim (CAPRICE).

notorious, *adj.* infamous, shady, scandalous (DISREPUTE, FAME).

notwithstanding, *adv.* nevertheless, nonetheless, however (OPPOSITION).

nourish, *v.* feed, sustain, foster, nurture (FOOD).

nourishing, *adj.* nutrient, nutritive, nutritious (FOOD).

nourishment, *n.* nutriment, food, stuff sustenance (FOOD).

nouveau riche (F.), *n.* parvenu, arriviste (F.), upstart (SOCIAL CLASS, WEALTH).

novel, *adj.* fresh, off-beat (*colloq.*), original (UNUSUALNESS); original, Promethean (NEWNESS); unusual, atypical (DIFFERENCE).

novel, *n.* fiction, novelette, novella (STORY).

novelist, *n.* fictionist, anecdotist (WRITER).

novelty, *n.* freshness, recency, originality; original, *dernier cri* (F.), wrinkle (NEWNESS); item, conversation piece (MATERIALITY).

novice, *n.* beginner, tyro, neophyte (BEGINNING, LEARNING); novitiate, postulant (RELIGIOUS COMMUNITY).

now, *adv.* at this time, at this moment, at present (PRESENT TIME).

noxious, *adj.* virulent, unhealthy (HARM); unwholesome, pestiferous, pestilent (IMMORALITY).

nozzle, *n.* spout, faucet (EGRESS, OPENING).

nuance, *n.* shade of difference (DIFFERENCE); implication, suggestion (MEANING).

nucleus, *n.* heart, hub, focus (CENTER); meat, pith, principle (PART).

nude, *adj.* stripped, naked, bare (UNDRESS).

nudge, *v.* push, poke, prod (PROPULSION).

nudity, *n.* nakedness, denudation, exposure (UNDRESS).

nuisance, *n.* gadfly, terror, pest (ANNOYANCE).

nullify, *v.* annul, disannul, invalidate (INEFFECTIVENESS).

numb, *adj.* dazed, torpid, stuporous (INSENSIBILITY).

numb, *v.* dull, blunt, obtund (INSENSIBILITY).

number, *n.* amount (QUANTITY); numeral (NUMBER); song (SINGING).

NUMBER—N. number, numeral, figure, symbol, character, numeral, figure, statistic, Arabic number, cipher, digit, integer, whole number, folio, round number; cardinal number, ordinal number, Roman number; decimal, fraction; infinity, googol; numerator, denominator; prime number.

sum, difference, product, quotient; addend, summand, augend; dividend, divisor; factor, multiplier; multiplicand, faciend, multiplier; minuend, subtrahend, remainder; total, summation, aggregate, tally; quantity, amount.

ratio, proportion, quota, percentage; progression, arithmetical progression, geometric progression, power, root, exponent, index, logarithm.

numeration, notation, algorism, cipher, algebra; enumeration, count, tally, census, poll; statistics; numerology.

V. count, enumerate, numerate, reckon, tally; count down, tell, tell out (off, or down).

page, number, foliate, paginate, mark.

Adj. numeral, numerical, numerary, numeric, numerical; numbered, numerate.

proportional, commeasurable, commensurate, proportionate.

See also ADDITION, COMPUTATION, LIST, MULTITUDE, QUANTITY, TWO, THREE, ETC.

numbers, *n.* scores, heaps, lots (MULTITUDE).

numberless, *adj.* countless, innumerable, myriad (MULTITUDE, ENDLESSNESS).

numeral, *n.* symbol, character, figure (NUMBER).

numerical, *adj.* numeral, numerary (NUMBER).

numerous, *adj.* many, multitudinous, abundant (MULTITUDE, FREQUENCE).

nun, *n.* sister, *religieuse* (F.), vestal, vestal virgin (RELIGIOUS COMMUNITY, UNMARRIED STATE).

nunnery, *n.* convent, abbey, cloister (RELIGIOUS COMMUNITY).

nuptial, *adj.* matrimonial, marital, conjugal (MARRIAGE).

nurse, *n.* attendant, medic, R.N. (MEDICAL SCIENCE).

nurse, *v.* attend, tend, care for (CARE); suck, suckle, lactate (BREAST).

nursery, *n.* day nursery, creche (CHILD); garden, greenhouse, hothouse (FARMING); cradle, childhood, infancy (YOUTH).

nurture, *v.* feed, nourish, sustain (FOOD); care for, cherish, foster (CARE).

nuthouse (*slang*), *n.* lunatic asylum, madhouse (INSANITY).

nutritious, *adj.* nourishing, wholesome (FOOD, HEALTH).

nutty (*slang*), *adj.* potty (*colloq.*), touched, crazy (INSANITY).

nuzzle, *v.* nestle, snuggle, cuddle (PRESSURE, REST).

nymph, *n.* dryad, hamadryad, hyad (GOD).

nymphomania, *n.* erotomania, andromania (SEX).

O

oaf, *n.* lummox, lout, gawky (CLUMSINESS); boob, nincompoop, blockhead (FOLLY).

oar, *n.* paddle, scull (SAILOR).

oath, *n.* curse, curseword, swearword (MALEDICTION, DISRESPECT); affidavit, deposition (AFFIRMATION); word of honor, vow (PROMISE).

OBEDIENCE—N. obedience, observance, conformance, conformity, accordance, compliance, docility, servility, subservience, tameness.

[*one who demands obedience*] disciplinarian, martinet, authoritarian, precisian.

[*obedient person*] servant, minion, myrmidon, slave.

discipline, training; military discipline, blind obedience.

V. obey, observe, comply, conform, submit; mind, heed, do one's bidding, follow orders, do what one is told; behave.

discipline, train, tame; enforce, compel, force; put teeth in.

Adj. obedient, compliant, compliable, law-abiding; observant, law-abiding; dutiful, duteous; orderly, quiet, docile, meek, manageable, tractable, biddable, well-behaved; submissive, servile, subservient, tame.

disciplinary, strict, stern, authoritative, authoritarian.

See also DUTY, FORCE, OBSERVANCE, SLAVERY, SUBMISSION, TEACHING. *Antonyms*—See DISOBEDIENCE, NONOBSERVANCE.

obese, *adj.* paunchy, pursy, fat (SIZE).

obey, *v.* observe, comply, submit (OBEDIENCE).

object, *n.* thing, article, commodity (MATERIALITY); matter, phenomenon, substance (REALITY); mission, objective, end (PURPOSE).

object, *v.* demur, protest, remonstrate (OPPOSITION, UNPLEASANTNESS).

objection, *n.* exception, demurral (OPPOSITION); dislike, disesteem (HATRED).

objectionable, *adj.* displeasing, distasteful, unpalatable (UNPLEASANTNESS, HATRED); exceptionable, opprobrious (DISAPPROVAL).

objective, *adj.* impartial, unprejudiced, unbiased (IMPARTIALITY); actual, concrete, material (REALITY).

objective, *n.* mission, object, end (PURPOSE).

object of art, *n.* bibelot (F.), *objet d'art* (F.), curio (ORNAMENT).

object to, *v.* dislike, have no stomach for, be displeased by, protest (HATRED, UNPLEASANTNESS).

obligate, *v.* indebt, bind, astrict (DEBT).

• VOCABULARY CHECK

Directions.   Below are 10 words taken from the key words section of this chapter. Circle the letter of the best definition from the four choices.

1 Unabridged
  a condensed
  b complete
  c inaccurate
  d unfinished

2 Incision
  a sharp tooth
  b foolish ideas
  c a knife
  d a surgical cut

3 Collegiate
  a referring to college
  b referring to a column
  c referring to a professor
  d referring to classrooms

4 Bulimia
  a bile secretions
  b an eating disorder
  c the endocrine system
  d a fear of pregnancy

5 Synonyms
  a words that are opposites
  b words that sound the same but have different meanings
  c words that are contradictory
  d different words that mean the same

6 Myxorrhea
  a flow of mucus
  b flow of blood
  c flow of hormones
  d flow of fluids

7 Antonyms
  a words that are opposites
  b words that sound the same but have different meanings
  c words that are contradictory
  d different words that mean the same

8 Pathogen
   a study of blood diseases
   b factor following path of oxygen in lungs
   c disease-producing agent
   d path of blood circulation

9 Specialized
   a designed for one particular purpose
   b having been put to a specific use
   c related to the unconventional
   d written in a unique way

10 Gynecology
   a branch of medicine that deals with women's health
   b the inner reproductive organ of a flower
   c the study of women's roles in medicine
   d the philosophy that deals with women's rights

• SUMMARY

Using affix analysis and context clues as tactics for learning unknown words can be helpful but may not be appropriate in all instances. It may be necessary to consult a dictionary, glossary, or thesaurus for help with new words. The collegiate dictionary is particularly useful for learning pronunciation, parts of speech, etymology, word meaning, and in some cases synonyms and antonyms. A medical dictionary is best for helping you with specialized vocabulary encountered in nursing school. The glossary of a textbook is convenient for finding the meanings of key words in the textbook. The thesaurus is helpful for choosing a better word for your writing. All these references are invaluable to your task of building a better vocabulary for nursing school success.

• Chapter 7 •

Word Bank

OBJECTIVE
KEY WORDS
ENCOUNTERING UNKNOWN WORDS
INDICATING UNKNOWN WORDS
REMEMBERING NEW WORDS
CREATING YOUR WORD BANK
VOCABULARY CHECK
SUMMARY

• OBJECTIVE

To learn a method for remembering the definitions of new words.

• KEY WORDS

Pay attention to the following key words, which are underscored the first time they appear in this chapter. Try to determine the meaning of these words from the surrounding words in the passage. If you need further help, use your dictionary or the glossary in the back of this book. As you read the exercises in this chapter, write additional words you need to learn in the space provided.

GENERAL VOCABULARY

arbitrary	reinforce
conversely	repertoire
deposit	variety
flexibility	_____
idioms	_____
maximize	_____
portable	_____
	_____

• ENCOUNTERING UNKNOWN WORDS

In nursing school you encounter many unknown words, both medical and general. During lectures and clinical experiences you constantly hear new terms and phrases. As you read your textbooks, for both nursing and liberal arts courses, you come across more unfamiliar words. Even when socializing and conversing with your fellow nursing students, you hear words and expressions you do not understand. When this happens, do not ignore these new terms but instead indicate the words you need to learn.

• INDICATING UNKNOWN WORDS

During lectures, copy any unknown words from the board and mark them with a question mark (?). This signal will indicate that you should look these words up later in a dictionary or glossary. Similarly, when you are reading your textbooks, place a question mark over any unknown vocabulary terms. When you finish reading that section, take a brief break and check the definitions of the unknown words in your dictionary or glossary. Even when you are with your friends in nursing school, you should not be embarrassed to ask them to explain the meanings of any expressions you do not understand. Remember that you all have the same goal—increasing your vocabulary to <u>maximize</u> your nursing school success. Carry a small notebook with you so you can jot down new expressions and <u>idioms</u>.

• REMEMBERING NEW WORDS

Once you have the meaning of a new word, write the definition in your lecture notes, textbook margin, or notebook. This will ensure that you have a record of the word meaning. But this written note won't be sufficient to help you learn and remember the word. To learn a new medical term or general vocabulary word, you must have a strategy to help you memorize its meaning. This method should allow you to visualize the word repeatedly to <u>reinforce</u> the learning until you can remember the word and it becomes a natural part of your speaking and reading <u>repertoire</u>.

• CREATING YOUR WORD BANK

An excellent means of learning new words is to create a word bank. To do this, buy a package of index cards on which one side is ruled and the other side blank.

On the blank side, clearly write the unknown word. You may find it helpful to write the pronunciation underneath the word. Use a pronunciation key that you understand, either one you make up yourself or one copied from the dictionary. Make sure that the pronunciation key you use will help you say the word correctly.

On the ruled side of the index card, write the precise definition of the word. Underneath the definition, use the word in a sentence, either your own or one copied from the textbook. This way, when you refer to the card later, you will be reminded of how the word is actually used. See Figure 7–1.

What you have created is a flashcard with which you can practice new words over and over again. The word is on one side of the flashcard and its definition is

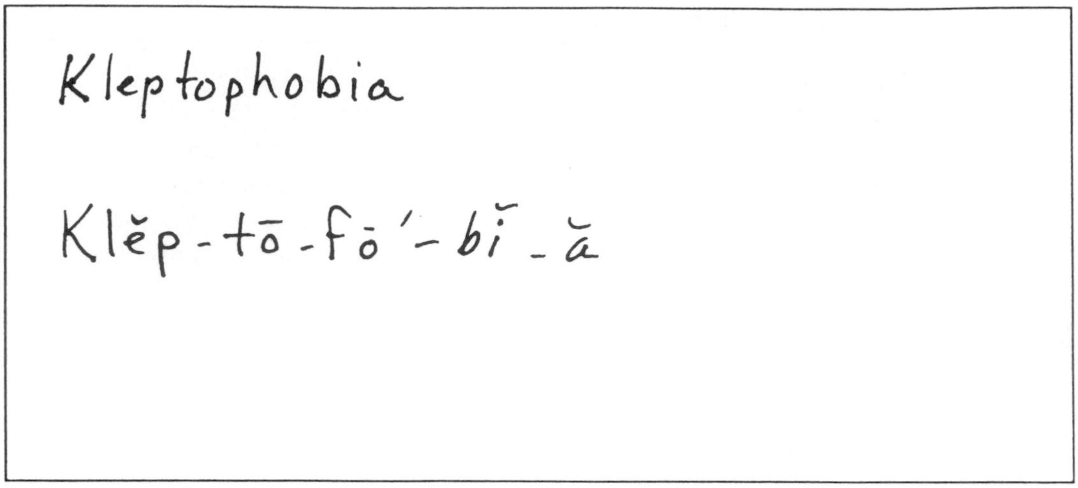

Kleptophobia

Klĕp-tō-fō´-bĭ-ă

SIDE ONE

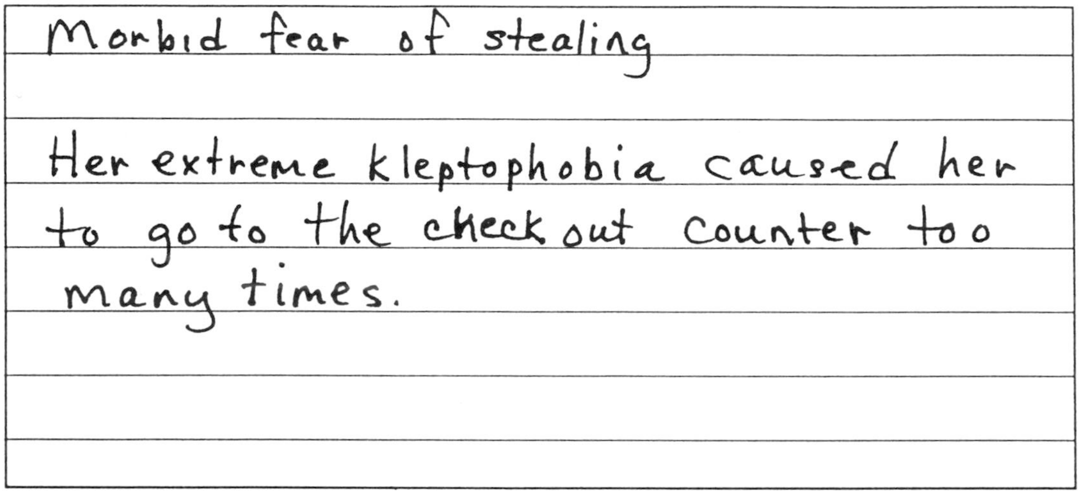

Morbid fear of stealing

Her extreme kleptophobia caused her to go to the check out counter too many times.

SIDE TWO

FIGURE 7-1 Sample item for word bank.

on the other side. The first advantage of the word bank is that it is personalized. These are words that you decide you need to know, not some arbitrary list of words assigned to you by an instructor.

The second advantage of the word bank is that it is portable. Put a rubber band around your cards and you can carry them anywhere. You can use the cards to practice learning new words anytime, on the subway to nursing school, during a lunch break, or while waiting for a doctor's appointment. At home you should "deposit" your words in a file or container to which you can add more new words as you encounter them.

A third advantage of the word bank is its variety. Try to be creative in its use. For instance, show yourself the word side and quiz yourself by supplying the definition. Or conversely, ask yourself the definition and try to recall the correct word. Be imaginative. Create games that will help you memorize the meanings of these words as pleasantly as possible. Learning vocabulary does not have to be a chore.

The last advantage of the word bank is its <u>flexibility</u>. The index card format allows you to group the words according to your needs. For instance, you can place all the new terms learned in a lecture on pediatrics with any other pediatric terms you came across when reading in your textbook on the same subject. You can also separate words you have learned very well from those that still need more work or that you don't know at all.

Considering the simplicity of making a word bank and all of its advantages, this is one of the richest ways of developing vocabulary appropriate for nursing school. Use your word bank daily and you will be wealthier for it.

• EXERCISE 7–1 •

Directions. From this textbook or any of your other books, choose 25 words you don't know. Create the beginning of a word bank, using the example in the illustration. Practice learning these words by following the suggestions from this chapter or invent your own ways of learning the meanings of unknown words.

• VOCABULARY CHECK

Directions. Below are 10 words taken from the key words section of this chapter. Circle the letter of the best definition from the four choices.

1 Arbitrary
   a pertaining to judging or determining
   b pertaining to settling a controversy
   c pertaining to sale of securities
   d pertaining to individual preference or convenience

2 Deposit
   a to place for safekeeping
   b to remove from authority
   c to build railroads
   d to testify under oath

3 Idioms
   a ideas related to a specific field
   b people who are not bright
   c language peculiar to a people or class
   d specific grammars

4 Portable
   a pertaining to a seaport
   b capable of being carried
   c the ability to dock a ship
   d stationary

5 Repertoire

   a a drama series

   b a list or supply of capabilities

   c constant repetition

   d a series of tricks or stunts

6 Conversely

   a ability to talk on a social level

   b ability to change or adapt

   c able to carry from place to place

   d reversed in order, relation, or action

7 Flexibility

   a capability of making a brief movement

   b ability to strike with a light motion

   c ability to lengthen or strengthen

   d capability to adapt to new requirements

8 Maximize

   a to relate a proverb

   b to adjust the upper jaw

   c to make the most of

   d to make the least of

9 Reinforce

   a to make someone bend to one's will

   b to strengthen by additional assistance

   c to create again in a more permanent manner

   d to act in a decisive way

10 Variety

   a having different forms

   b having similar forms

   c having possession of the truth

   d having ability to change

• SUMMARY

In this chapter you were reminded to indicate any new words you come across while listening to class lectures, reading your textbooks, or talking with classmates. Techniques for indicating unknown words include marking these words with a question mark (?) and jotting down words in a small notebook. Once you have indicated the words you need to learn, you can look up these words in the dictionary or glossary to get their precise meanings. So that you will remember these words and make them a natural part of your vocabulary, you were taught how to make a word bank using index cards and how to use these cards to increase your word knowledge.

• U N I T •
III

READING COMPREHENSION

One of your major responsibilities in nursing school is to read and comprehend your textbooks with ease. Unless you have this ability, your reading assignments will take a long time to complete and will seem incomprehensible. Unit III, "Reading Comprehension," introduces the skills that will help you read the information in your textbooks with greater understanding and efficiency.

Chapter 8, "Topics and Main Ideas," teaches you to focus on the subject and main point of a passage. Chapter 9, "Details," helps you to identify the important facts that relate to the main idea. Chapter 10, "Paragraph Organization," illustrates how following patterns of organization will help you to concentrate on, comprehend, and retain textbook organization.

Once you have mastered the strategies for organizing textbook information, you can read and comprehend your nursing textbooks with less effort and greater clarity. Improved reading comprehension thus depends on your ability to organize ideas. Unit III, "Reading Comprehension," provides the comprehension strategies needed for success in nursing school.

• Chapter 8 •

Topics and Main Ideas

OBJECTIVE

KEY WORDS

IMPROVING CONCENTRATION

FINDING THE TOPIC

SELECTING THE CORRECT TOPIC

IDENTIFYING THE TOPIC IN PARAGRAPHS

FINDING THE TOPIC AS AN AID TO CONCENTRATION

DETERMINING THE MAIN IDEA

LOCATING THE MAIN IDEA

    End of the Passage

    Middle of the Passage

    Beginning and End of the Passage

FINDING THE UNSTATED MAIN IDEA

READING WITH A PURPOSE

VOCABULARY CHECK

SUMMARY

• OBJECTIVE

To learn to identify the topics and main ideas in textbook material as an aid to concentration and comprehension.

• KEY WORDS

Pay attention to the following words, which are underscored the first time they appear in this chapter. Try to determine the meaning of these words in the passage. If you need further help, use your dictionary or the glossary. As you read the exercises in this chapter, write additional words you need to learn in the spaces provided.

MEDICAL TERMINOLOGY	GENERAL VOCABULARY
affect	assert
Alzheimer's disease	autonomy
asthma	gestures
diaphoresis	mandates
edema	objective
generativity	ombudsmen
hypotension	retirement
inguinal hernia	shrugging
nitroglycerin	spiritual
pallor	validation
_____	_____
_____	_____
_____	_____
_____	_____

• IMPROVING CONCENTRATION

You may find your mind wandering while you read your textbooks. Staying focused is sometimes difficult. Reading with a purpose gives direction to your reading. Your objective should be to find the topics and main ideas. Check yourself as you read. As you do exercises, pay attention to your reading attention span. Did you concentrate throughout the chapter? Did you have any concentration problems? If so, where? Looking for the topics and main ideas keeps you involved with your reading. Keep track of your reading concentration. Stay on task and use identifying the topics and main ideas as a strategy to improve your reading concentration and comprehension.

• FINDING THE TOPIC

The *topic* of a reading selection is its subject. It is *who* or *what* is being talked about. You should identify the topic as the first step toward comprehending the content of any reading selection. The topic is the general subject, and the details in the reading passage fit under it. Practice finding the topic in lists of words.

• EXAMPLE 8–1 •

sight	senses	hearing	touch	smell

Which of the items on the list is the *topic*? The answer is *senses*. All the other items— hearing, touch, smell, and sight—are specific senses that fit under this general topic.

• EXERCISE 8–1 •

Directions.   Select the topic in each list of words:

1 pointing
  <u>gestures</u>
  nodding
  <u>shrugging</u>
  waving   _____

2 inspection
  auscultation
  palpation
  percussion
  examination   _____

3 systems
  respiratory
  gastrointestinal
  cardiovascular
  neurologic   _____

4 rough
  smooth
  leathery
  thin
  texture   _____

5 depth
  measurements
  color
  description
  odor   _____

Comprehending?   Yes ____   No ____

You have now practiced putting specific details under a general topic. Identifying the topic is a first step to finding the *main idea* in any reading selection. Look for the topic when reading paragraphs or longer selections. Ask *who* or *what* this selection is about.

• SELECTING THE CORRECT TOPIC

The following exercise will help you to choose the correct topic. When determining the topic of a passage, your answer choice should cover the information in the passage. In other words, do not select answer choices that are:

- *Too broad.*   The answer choice covers more than is discussed in the passage.
- *Too narrow.*   The answer choice reflects a detail of the passage and does not cover the entire topic.
- *Not mentioned.* The answer choice is not discussed in the passage.

• EXAMPLE 8–2 •

Directions.   Read the following selections and state whether each answer choice is too broad, too narrow, not mentioned, or the correct topic.

Play-age years are important times for moral and <u>spiritual</u> development. Children develop a sense of right and wrong, good and bad, from the actions, attitudes, and to a lesser extent, words of adults around them. The approval and disapproval of significant others determine a child's moral development (Sorensen and Luckmann, p. 284).

a Play-age years of children   _____

b Children's moral development during play-age
years   _____

c Approval of significant others   _____

d Discipline problems during play-age years   _____

Choice a is too broad. More can be said about play-age years than is discussed in this passage. Choice b is correct; it most precisely defines the ideas in the passage. Choice c is just one detail in the passage, so it is too narrow. Choice d is not mentioned; it is not discussed in this passage.

• IDENTIFYING THE TOPIC IN PARAGRAPHS

• EXERCISE 8–2 •

Directions.   Read the following paragraphs and state whether each answer choice is too broad, too narrow, not mentioned, or the correct topic.

1 Adolescent (or teenage) years are traditionally considered difficult and turbulent. Indeed they are critical times of great change and adaptation. These years are a transition from the known existence of childhood to the unknown life of an adult. Despite the changes and the accompanying stress, adolescent years do not have to be as negative as they are often described (Sorensen and Luckmann, 1986, p. 292).

a Transition from childhood   _____

b Changes and stress during adolescent years   _____

c Stress of early childhood   _____

d Teenage years   _____

2 <u>Generativity</u> is really the consequence of success in the person's psychosocial life tasks. Generativity is the creative production or contribution to life. In the most obvious sense it refers to having and raising children. However, generativity also refers to creativity in occupation, social relationships, and other social contributions. It is during the adult years that most people feel they do their "life's work" and make their contribution to society (Sorensen and Luckmann, 1986, p. 295).

    a Creativity   _____

    b Problems during <u>retirement</u> years   _____

    c Definition of generativity   _____

    d Life's work during adult years   _____

3 Alcohol and other substance abuse (e.g. drugs, glue sniffing) often begins in adolescence. Mood swings typical of these years along with susceptibility to peer pressure can lead teenagers to experiment with consciousness altering substances. Health professionals watch for signs of substance abuse. Treatment is difficult requiring supportive counselling and education (Sorensen and Luckmann, 1986, p. 295).

    a Substance abuse   _____

    b Substance abuse by health professionals   _____

    c Teenage involvement with substance abuse   _____

    d Mood swings in teenagers   _____

4 The decision to become parents is one some couples make together while others find it happening without their choice. Pregnancy may be a time of great joy and happy anticipation, or a time of fear, frustration, and even anger. Often there are times of confused feelings. Even for those who have planned the pregnancy and want the baby there are moments of fear and concern (Sorensen and Luckmann, 1986, p. 296).

    a Emotional reaction to pregnancy   _____

    b Anger during pregnancy   _____

    c Pregnancy   _____

    d Birth control to avoid pregnancy   _____

5 People who have built their self-identity around their profession or occupation will have a difficult time with <u>retirement</u>. (Much as a woman whose self-concept is related to being a mother has difficulty when all her children

become adults.) These people need to find self-respect in who they are rather than in what they do (Sorensen and Luckmann, 1986, p. 301).

a Difficulties with retirement   _____

b Difficulty for mothers   _____

c Difficulty when fired from a job   _____

d Building self-respect   _____

Comprehending? Yes ___ No ___

• EXERCISE 8–3 •

Directions.   Read the following selections and establish the correct topic by asking yourself *who* or *what* the selection is about.

1   While assessing a client, the nurse accumulates a large volume of data. The nurse may find it extremely difficult to manage this volume in total. The classification process allows the nurse to develop more manageable categories of information. It also stimulates discrimination between data which helps the nurse to focus on data that are pertinent to the client's needs (Iyer et al., p. 66).

The topic is _____.

2   The final step in data processing is validation. In this phase, the nurse attempts to verify the accuracy of the data interpretation. This is most often accomplished through direct interaction with the client or significant other(s), consultation with other health care professionals, or comparison of data with an authoritative reference (Iyer et al., p. 70).

The topic is _____.

3   The nurse's ability to formulate nursing diagnosis is dependent upon an accurate and complete data base. Several factors may interfere with the collection of data. These may include communication problems, withholding information, and distractions/interruptions (Iyer et al., p. 74).

The topic is _____.

4   Even when the nurse and client speak the same language, either may use language that confuses the other. The client's age, environment, or cultural background may involve the use of expressions that are foreign to the nurse (Iyer et al., p. 75).

The topic is _____.

5 Under the law each nurse is held accountable for his or her action. A nurse cannot evade this responsibility by explaining that a physician or nursing supervisor ordered the nurse to commit the actions which impaired the client. It is expected that the nurse will use judgement to question orders that are inappropriate or likely to result in harm to the client (Iyer et al., p. 257).

The topic is _____.

Comprehending? Yes ____ No ____

• FINDING THE TOPIC AS AN AID TO CONCENTRATION

Many students find it difficult to concentrate while reading textbooks. They have problems maintaining their focus. Establishing the topic of a reading selection will help you to concentrate on the passage.

• EXERCISE 8–4 •

Directions. Read the following selection (Iyer et al., p. 25) and establish the precise topic to help you concentrate while reading.

Four types of data are collected by the nurse during assessment—subjective, objective, historical, and current. A complete and accurate data base usually includes a combination of these types.

Subjective data might be described as the individual's view of a situation or a series of events. This information cannot be determined by the nurse independent of interaction or communication with the individual. Subjective data are frequently obtained during the nursing history and include the client's perceptions, feelings, and ideas about self and personal health status. Examples include the client's descriptions of pain, weakness, frustration, nausea, or embarrassment. Information supplied by sources other than the client—e.g., family, consultants, and other members of the health team—may also be subjective if based on the individual's opinion rather than substantiated by fact.

In contrast, objective data are both observable and measurable. This information is usually obtained through the senses—sight, smell, hearing, and touch—during the physical examination of the client. Examples of objective data include respiratory rate, blood pressure, edema, and weight.

During the assessment of a client, the nurse must consider both subjective and objective findings. Frequently, these findings substantiate each other, as in the case of John Thomas, the client whose incision opened three days after surgery. The subjective information provided by Mr. Thomas, "feels like my stitches are popping," was validated by the nurse's objective findings—pallor, diaphoresis, hypotension, and protrusion of the bowel through the incision.

In the case of Peggy Malletts, the nurse observes the client crying as she stands in front of the nursery two days after premature delivery of her first child. The nurse suggests that Peggy seems "upset," and the client validates that she is "afraid that her baby might die." Here, the objective data observed by the nurse (crying) were substantiated by subjective data obtained from the client (feelings of fear).

At times, subjective and objective data may be in conflict. Juan, a 16-year-old client, denied that he was in pain after surgical repair of an <u>inguinal hernia</u>. Juan's denial would be considered subjective data, since it reflects his feelings of pain. However, the nurses documented several objective findings that are consistent with the usual response to pain (facial grimaces, elevated pulse rate, clutching incision area). In this case the subjective and objective data are in conflict; therefore the nurse must accumulate additional information to resolve the discrepancy.

Another consideration when describing data concerns the element of time. In this context, data may be either historical or current. Historical data involve information about events that have occurred prior to the present, which might include previous hospitalizations, normal elimination patterns, or chronic diseases. In contrast, current data refers to events that are occurring in the present—blood pressure, vomiting, postoperative pain. Again, a combination of both current and historical data may be used to verify problems or to identify discrepancies.

The topic is _____

_____

Comprehending? Yes ___ No ___

• DETERMINING THE MAIN IDEA

Once you have learned to identify the topic, you can next identify the main idea in a reading selection. The main idea answers the question, "What is being said about the topic or subject?"

Finding the main idea is an important method for understanding what you read. Consider the following example.

• EXAMPLE 8–3 •

Rehabilitation facilities provide a wide spectrum of services. Although many rehabilitation centers are for clients with physical deformities or handicaps, such as spinal cord injuries, some are for clients who abuse drugs or alcohol. Clients in these centers are admitted by referring physicians or are transferred from other inpatient facilities. These centers can be free standing utilities or part of a hospital (Ignatavicius and Bayne, p. 38).

As you just learned, to determine the topic of a passage you ask the question, *"Who* or *what* is this passage mostly about?" In this example you would answer, "Rehabilitation facilities or centers." To find the main idea you must further develop the topic. You do this by asking a second question, "What is the most important point that is being made about the topic?" The answer to this second question is the main idea. Look again at the preceding example. We said the topic of this passage was <u>rehabilitation facilities or centers</u>. What is the most important point being made about rehabilitation centers? The most important point being made about rehabilitation centers is that <u>they provide a wide range of care</u>. Which sentence in the example states this? Look again at the first sentence. "Rehabilitation facilities provide a wide spectrum of services." This is a general sentence that means the same as "provide a wide range of care." So the first sentence in this passage is the main idea sentence.

Read the following examples, keeping in mind the two questions for determining the topic and the main idea:

1   Who or what is this passage mostly about? = topic

2   What is the most important point that is being made about the topic? = main idea

The topic is shown in the margin, and the main idea is boldface in the examples here.

• EXAMPLE 8–4 •

Mental patients' rights

1   **Some states, recognizing mental patients' inability to <u>assert</u> their own rights effectively in the psychiatric setting, have developed <u>ombudsmen</u> programs for mental patients.** State law in California <u>mandates</u> an independent patient advocate, and New York provides for mental health legal services. Both programs assure that patients' constitutional rights are protected and that their expressed interests are represented (Varcarolis, p. 56).

Trust between nurse and client

2   **Clients can also jeopardize the trust a nurse has in them.** Sometimes, clients may "test" a nurse's trustworthiness. They may try to send the nurse on unnecessary errands or talk endlessly about superficial topics. As long as nurses recognize testing behaviors and set clear limits on their role and the client's role, trust will ensue (Arnold and Boggs, p. 181).

Teaching strategies used by the nurse

3   **The teaching strategies utilized by the nurse should be individualized to the client's need and the type of outcome desired.** Knowledge outcomes frequently require the mastery of facts and concepts. These are most effectively taught by using written materials and audio-visual aids reinforced by discussion (Iyer et al., p. 153).

• EXERCISE 8–5 •

Directions. Read each of the short passages below. In the space provided indicate the topic and underline the main idea. Remember to ask the following questions:

1 Who or what is this passage mostly about? = topic

2 What is the most important point that is being made about the topic? = main idea

1 There are several types of angina pectoris. The most common type is chronic stable angina that is usually precipitated by physical exertion or emotional stress, lasts 3-5 minutes, and is relieved by rest and nitroglycerin. Other types include unstable or crescendo angina, varient of Prinzmetal's angina, nocturnal angina, angina decubitus, and intractable or refractory angina. These various types differ in relation to severity of the attack, refractoriness of the pain, and typical precipitants of the attack (Ulrich, p. 298).

Topic: _____.

2 Other reasons for mental illness are considered physical or physiological. For instance, many contemporary health professionals believe that senile plaques in the brain cause Alzheimer's disease, or senile dementia, that excessive alcohol intake results in delirium tremens, and that chemical imbalance may cause depression or manic-depressive reactions (Varcarolis, p. 67).

Topic: _____.

3 Churches and other religious institutions serve the elderly in many ways. In addition to their primary role of providing organized worship, they sponsor many activities that bring elderly together with their peers as well as with younger people. Clergy persons, rabbis, and other spiritual leaders are often excellent counselors, and other members of the congregation or religious group are often willing to help older members in time of trouble (Ignatavicius and Bayne, p. 83).

Topic: _____.

4 In many ways, hospitalization creates an identity crisis for the client. Clients are uprooted from a normal, active life and suddenly find themselves categorized according to diagnosis, level of care, room number, and team assignment. Many of the self-images clients have held about personal autonomy, identity and role have to be reworked (Arnold and Boggs, p. 52).

Topic: _____.

5 Clients with antisocial personality disorders, when hospitalized, evoke strong emotions in nurses. Frustration, anger, disappointment, and despair are usually experienced by health care professionals when caring for these clients. Being aware of these feelings and responses to antisocial clients can assist nurses in understanding and caring for them (Varcarolis, p. 407).

Topic: _____.

Comprehending?   Yes ____   No ____

• LOCATING THE MAIN IDEA

In the preceding examples and exercises, the main idea was located at the beginning of each passage. The main idea sentence was the first sentence in each passage, followed by details or examples. However, this will not always be the case. The main idea sentence can be found in several places in the passage besides the beginning. Look at some of these other places. In the following examples, the topic is written in the space provided and the main idea sentence is in boldface type.

• End of the Passage

Sometimes the main idea sentence is the last sentence of the paragraph. When this is so, the writer begins the paragraph with details and the main idea sentence at the end draws together all the facts.

• EXAMPLE 8–5 •

The inner world of the client is encased by feelings, thoughts, and previous learning. At times, the inner and outer reality may be worlds apart and an individual is said to have a "distorted perception of reality." **When the distortion either continues over a significant period of time or is carried to an extreme, it is considered a mental illness** (Arnold and Boggs, p. 81).

Topic: _____.

• Middle of the Passage

Another place to look for the main idea sentence is in the middle of the passage. Often writers begin a passage with interesting facts or details to capture the reader's interest. Then they insert the main idea sentence and finally end the selection with more details to support the main idea.

• EXAMPLE 8–6 •

When outward signs of stress, such as headaches, high blood pressure, muscle tension, and heart palpitations, occur frequently, are debilitating or may be dangerous, biofeedback can be an effective treatment. **Biofeedback works by training the individual to reverse the subtle changes that lead to a somatic response.** For instance, if a headache is the result of muscle tension in the forehead, the client can be trained to relax that tension before a headache results (Ignatavicius and Bayne, p. 103).

Topic: _____.

• Beginning and End of the Passage

In some cases the main idea is found both at the beginning and at the end of the paragraph. As shown in the first examples introducing the main idea, the paragraph begins with the general main idea sentence, followed by specific details that support the main idea. However, now the paragraph also ends with a main idea sentence that reiterates or restates in different words the idea or ideas expressed in the first main idea sentence.

• EXAMPLE 8–7 •

Trust, however, can be broken. For example, an alcoholic or abusive parent may be gentle one minute and explode with anger the next, leaving children and others unsure of how the parent will behave. The community-health nurse who is always late for client appointments and interviews and the pediatric nurse who indicates falsely that an injection will not hurt, are at risk of jeopardizing their therapeutic relationships. In order for a trusting relationship to continue, trust must be reinforced. **Otherwise, trust may be destroyed during a negative experience** (Arnold and Boggs, p. 181).

Topic: _____.

• FINDING THE UNSTATED MAIN IDEA

Many times you will read a paragraph that has no main idea sentence. Instead, the passage will consist of only a series of details, facts, or examples. In this situation it is your responsibility to create the main idea sentence. You use the same strategy you used to find the main idea—asking the two questions:

1   Who or what is this passage mostly about? = topic

2   What is the most important point being made about the topic? = main idea

---

• EXAMPLE 8-8 •

Clients who talk about only the positive aspects of their situation may not be denying, but rather using *positive reappraisal* as a coping strategy. Clients who blame themselves for their illness or hospitalization may be using the coping strategy of *self-blame.* Clients who use *faith* as a coping strategy may request clergy visits, use religious paraphernalia, and engage in prayer, which are signs that the nurse can observe (Ignatavicius and Bayne, p. 100).

1   **Who or what is this passage mostly about?** Patients using coping strategies = topic

2   **What is the most important point being made about coping strategies?** Clients use a variety of coping strategies to deal with illness and hospitalization = main idea sentence

---

• EXERCISE 8-6 •

Read the following short passages. Determine the topic and write it in the space provided. Underline the main idea. If there is no main idea sentence, create your own in the space provided.

1   All nurses are liable for their own acts of negligence, but those acts can be imputed to the hospital or employer under the doctrine of *respondent superior.* Under this theory, the employer will be held liable for the negligent acts of its employees performed within the scope of their employment. As a practical matter, this theory is most frequently used because the hospital has assets to satisfy a judgment in the plaintiff's favor (Varcarolis, p. 47).

Topic: _____.

Unstated main idea: _____.

2   Silence also can be used to accent an important point in a verbal communication. By pausing briefly after presenting a key idea, before preceding to the next one, the nurse encourages the clients' notice of the most important elements of the communication. Used prudently, a brief silence following an important verbal message dramatizes the significance of the nurses' statement (Arnold and Boggs, p. 241).

Topic: _____.

Unstated main idea: _____.

3 An estimated 8% to 10% of the U.S. population suffers from allergic rhinitis. There is a high familial correlation, with most clients coming from an atopic family, i.e. with a family history of allergies, rhinitis, eczema, <u>asthma</u>, or urticaria. The symptoms almost always appear before the fourth decade of life and gradually diminish with age. Hayfever, or ragweed allergy, and allergy to grass pollen are the most common seasonal allergies. Hayfever is a misnomer because no fever is involved and the allergy is not to hay (Ignatavicius and Bayne, p. 658).

Topic: _____.

Unstated main idea: _____.

4 For example, in social situations, it may be very difficult for juvenile diabetics to regulate fast-food intake when all of their friends are able to eat what they want. When peer pressure is at its peak in adolescence, the teenager with a newly diagnosed nonconvulsive seizure disorder may find it difficult to tell peers he no longer can ride his bicycle or drive a car. Unless appropriate interpersonal support is provided by the family and nurse, such children have to cope with an indistinct assault to the self-concept all by themselves. The social realities the child has to contend with are forces that compel the nurse to consider the child's illness from a broad interpersonal perspective (Arnold and Boggs, p. 421).

Topic: _____.

Unstated main idea: _____.

5 A person who is depressed sees the world through "gray colored" glasses. Posture is poor; the client may look older than his or her stated age, facial expressions reflect sadness and dejection, and the person may be given to frequent bouts of weeping. Feelings of hopelessness and despair are readily reflected in the person's <u>affect</u> (Varcarolis, p. 438).

Topic: _____.

Unstated main idea: _____.

Comprehending? Yes _____ No _____

• READING WITH A PURPOSE

You can now focus on the topic and main idea as aids to concentration when doing textbook assignments. You will be reading with a purpose, which is to create and locate the topic and main idea. Reading with a purpose reduces distractions and helps you to focus on what you are reading.

• EXERCISE 8–7 •

Read the following excerpt from a nursing textbook (Iyer et al, p. 265). Think about the topic and underline the main idea of each paragraph. Then, in the space provided, write the topic and main idea of the entire reading.

1 The nurse is often placed in the role of client advocate in order to protect the rights of clients. While it is important for the nurse to understand the points contained in the Code for Nurses, the nurse needs more substance in order to make ethical decisions. Ethical theories describe approaches for resolving dilemmas commonly faced by nurses. . . . Ethical theories help answer these questions.

2 There are two major ethical theories used to help nurses resolve health care dilemmas: deontology and utilitarianism. The *deontologic* approach states that the rightness or wrongness of actions is determined by how the interventions conform to a rule. For instance, breaking a promise to a client would be considered wrong. Deontologists use rules because they are right, irrespective of the consequences they may produce in a particular situation. This position requires the nurse to be committed to the principle of universalizability. When the nurse makes a moral judgement in one given situation, the nurse will make the same judgement in any similar situation regardless of time, place, and persons involved.

3 One of the flaws with this approach is that most situations have extenuating circumstances. For example, in some instances it would be better to break than to keep a promise. A nurse may be asked to keep a promise not to reveal that the client has brought a quart of whiskey to the hospital. After making the promise, the nurse realizes that it is better to break the promise to protect the client from the consequences of consuming alcohol while being treated in the hospital.

4 The *utilitarian* approach states that actions are right or wrong on the basis of the consequences of the actions. Utilitarians focus on the results of actions rather than on their motivations. According to this approach, the nurse would weigh the consequences of telling the truth. Other factors may take priority, such as the nurse's own survival or the continuation of the system for the benefit of future clients. In this case the nurse may not tell the truth in preference to other interests that promote greater happiness. This view is quite different from the deontological position, which would maintain that the nurse must tell the truth without exception.

Topic: ⎯⎯⎯⎯⎯⎯⎯⎯⎯⎯⎯⎯⎯⎯⎯⎯⎯⎯⎯⎯⎯⎯⎯⎯.

Main idea: ⎯⎯⎯⎯⎯⎯⎯⎯⎯⎯⎯⎯⎯⎯⎯⎯⎯⎯⎯⎯⎯.

Comprehending?   Yes ⎯⎯   No ⎯⎯

• VOCABULARY CHECK

Directions. Below are 10 words taken from the key words section of this chapter. Circle the letter of the best definition from the four choices.

1 Pallor
   a redness of skin
   b faint condition
   c lack of iron
   d paleness of skin

2 Spiritual
   a concerned with secular values
   b concerned with religious values
   c concerned with good health
   d concerned with material values

3 Hypotension
   a raised blood pressure
   b lowered blood pressure
   c elevated stress
   d reduction of stress

4 Retirement
   a withdrawal from one's position or occupation
   b disability insurance for nonworkers
   c the state of disliking work
   d condition of aging

5 Asthma
   a a vaccine to prevent sexually transmitted disease
   b a condition caused by spasmodic contraction of the bronchi
   c a serious but never fatal disease
   d a cure for a chronic illness

6 Assert
   a to reply with vigor
   b to argue in a passive manner
   c to state or declare positively
   d to take back a statement

7 Nitroglycerin
   a a heart attack caused by stress and overexertion
   b an allergic reaction to medicine
   c a medically useful chemical that is also well known as an explosive
   d a potentially addictive sleeping pill prescribed for insomnia

8 Autonomy
  a self-directing freedom
  b to be dependent on others
  c rule by a monarchy
  d rule by a governing board

9 Inguinal hernia
  a hernia occurring in the groin
  b hernia surgery
  c a treatment for hernia
  d hernia occurring in the stomach

10 Gestures
  a the expressing of inner thoughts as a means of communication
  b the use of motions of the limbs or body as a means of expression
  c the use of colorful speech as a means of expression
  d the use of hidden actions as a means of miscommunication

• SUMMARY

You have learned that the first step toward reading comprehension is identifying the precise topic. The topic answers the question, "Who or what is being talked about in the selection?" Your statement of the topic should not be too broad or too narrow. It should cover the subject discussed in the passage. Focusing on the topic will help you to concentrate on your textbook assignments.

You have also learned that the most important point being made about the topic is the main idea. The main idea sentence can be found in any of the following locations in the passage:

- The beginning
- The end
- The middle
- The beginning and end
- Unstated—you create your own main idea

Finding the topic and main idea in your reading will help you to concentrate on and comprehend the most essential information in your nursing textbooks.

• Chapter 9 •

Details

OBJECTIVE

KEY WORDS

GETTING THE FACTS

HOW DETAILS RELATE TO THE MAIN IDEA

MAJOR AND MINOR DETAILS

FIVE TYPES OF DETAILS

    Data

    Cause

    Procedure

    Examples

    Description

VOCABULARY CHECK

SUMMARY

• OBJECTIVE

To learn how details relate to the main idea, how to distinguish between important and unimportant details, and how to recognize five types of details:

- Data
- Cause
- Procedures
- Examples
- Description

• KEY WORDS

Pay attention to the following key words, which are underscored the first time they appear in this chapter. Try to determine the meaning of these words from the surrounding words in the passage. If you need further help, use your dictionary or the glossary in the back of this book.

Look up the medical terminology in your medical dictionary or the glossary. As you read the exercises in this chapter, write additional words you need to learn in the space provided.

MEDICAL TERMINOLOGY	GENERAL VOCABULARY
benign	abuse
DNA	anonymity
endogenous opiate	core
hyponatremia	elaborate
immune system	exacerbation
medulla	feedback
mutations	major
neoplasia	minor
remission	overwhelmed
spinal cord	support
_____	_____
_____	_____
_____	_____

• GETTING THE FACTS

Looking through your nursing textbook, you have undoubtedly noticed how much information is to be found on each page. Perhaps your initial reaction is one of feeling overwhelmed. You may ask yourself: Which of these facts am I supposed to learn? How does one fact relate to another fact or to the main idea of the passage? How will these facts help me to understand the information in this textbook?

Learning what facts, or *details,* are all about will assist you in many ways. First, your reading comprehension will improve once you see how details relate to the bigger picture, or *main idea,* of a selection. Second, your textbook note taking and highlighting will improve once you know which details are important. Third and most important, you will be able to study more efficiently so you will do better on your nursing school exams.

• HOW DETAILS RELATE TO THE MAIN IDEA

The function of all details in any passage is to support the main idea. This means that the details will further describe or elaborate on the important point that the main idea is making. The role of details is to help you grasp or visualize more fully what the main idea is stating.

Consider this statement taken from a nursing textbook:

All types of people may be involved in helping individuals in crisis (Varcarolis, p. 212).

Certainly this is an interesting statement and, in itself, serves as the main idea of the paragraph. But it leaves out a lot of information: Who are these people who help others in crisis? How do these people help others in crisis? By reading the rest of the paragraph from the same nursing textbook, which provides the details, you get answers to these questions:

> For example, people from various professional backgrounds are trained in crisis intervention—police, teachers, welfare workers, clergy, social workers, psychologists, as well as nurses. Crisis intervention is often practiced unwittingly by people without formal training such as bartenders, concerned bystanders, friends and neighbors. People can play a crucial role in the successful resolution of a crisis by responding spontaneously with concern and caring (Varcarolis, p. 212).

By reading the details of this passage you can see how details support and give greater scope to the main idea.

• MAJOR AND MINOR DETAILS

Although the role of details is to support the main idea, giving a greater understanding of the essential point of the passage, not all details do so in the same way. Some important, or major, details relate directly to the main idea, as explained above. However, there are other, less important details that do not relate directly to the main idea but instead support or describe a major detail. These details are minor details. Below is a diagram that illustrates these relationships:

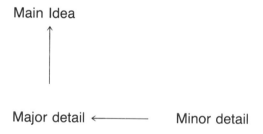

Main Idea

Major detail ⟵———— Minor detail

• EXAMPLE 9–1 •

Read the following paragraph from a nursing text. The main idea is in boldface type.

> **Several theories have been developed to explain the complex phenomenon of pain.** Early theories emphasized the recognition of specific pathways of pain transmission; later ones attempted to uncover the intricate complexity of central processing of pain in specific areas of the brain. More recently, the concept of pain-modulating network has been introduced. This concept describes the various links and connections in the spinal cord and brain, specially the medulla and the midbrain. The identification of special chemical mediators that are involved in the pain response phenomenon, such as the endogenous opiates, has opened new horizons in understanding pain transmission and perception (Ignatavicius and Bayne, p. 108).

Following are two diagrams of how the major and minor details from this passage relate to the main idea. The diagrams help you visualize how the major details support the main idea and how the minor details support the major details. You will see in a concrete way how details are organized.

GENERAL DIAGRAM

Main idea

↑

Major detail

↑

Major detail

↑

Major detail ←   Minor detail

↑

Major detail ←   Minor detail

DETAILS DIAGRAM

Several theories have been developed to explain the complex phenomenon of pain.

↑

Specific pathways of pain transmission

↑

Central processing of pain in specific areas of the brain

↑

Main modulating   ←—————— Describes links and connections in
network   the spinal cord and brain

↑

Identification of   ←—————— Ondogenous opiates
special chemical
mediators

• EXERCISE 9–1 •

Directions. Read the following paragraph from a nursing textbook. Study the general diagram. Then create a details diagram based on the ideas in the selection. Do this in the space provided.

Three types of MS are seen. The *classic* picture of <u>exacerbation</u> followed by <u>remission</u> occurs most often. The course of the disease may be <u>benign</u>, mild, or moderate, depending on the degree of disability. *Progressive MS* is characterized by the absence of periods of remission. Progressive deterioration occurs over several years. The third type, *combined,* begins with the classic presentation of MS and at some point converts to a progressive course (Ignatavicius and Bayne, p. 906).

GENERAL DIAGRAM

Main idea

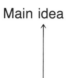

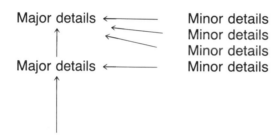

Major details ⟵ Minor details
Minor details
Minor details
Major details ⟵ Minor details

Major details

DETAILS DIAGRAM

Comprehending? Yes ___ No ___

• FIVE TYPES OF DETAILS

Details, both major and minor, support the main idea in different ways. These details relate to and elaborate on the main idea in their own unique fashion. What results are five different styles of paragraphs. The five types of details are:

- Data
- Cause
- Procedure
- Examples
- Description

• Data

Data details are details that prove the main idea. These details consist of facts with numbers, percentages, or statistics.

• EXAMPLE 9–2 •

Read the example below from a nursing text and pay attention to the bold-face data details.

Elder <u>abuse</u>, which by definition, includes neglect, is a crime occurring with increasing regularity. **The number of victims exceeds 500,000 annually and has been as high as 1,200,000.** Abuse can be found in the rural as well as urban areas and is spread throughout the United States (Varcarolis, p. 288).

• Cause

Cause details are details that explain why something is happening or has happened. They give reasons and answer the question, "Why?"

• EXAMPLE 9–3 •

Read the following excerpt, especially noting the boldface cause details.

Advancing age of the individual is probably the single most significant risk factor relating to the development of cancer. Fifty percent of all cancer occurs in individuals older than 65 years. The higher incidence in this age group may reflect **lifelong accumulation of <u>DNA</u> alterations or cell <u>mutations</u>, which result in cell transformation and <u>neoplasia</u>. The body may no longer be able to repair these mutations,** as it did in early years. **The effectiveness of the <u>immune system</u> is also reduced in the elderly population** (Ignatavicius and Bayne, p. 554).

• Procedure

Procedure details are details that explain how something is done. These details give you directions for doing an action.

• EXAMPLE 9–4 •

Pay attention to the boldface procedure details in this next example.

Use of the written process record is an effective but time-consuming process. To obtain maximum benefit from this learning tool, the nurse needs **to record a series of several nurse-client interactions, conducting a self-analysis and obtaining feedbacks with each one.** Over time, both learner and clients will benefit. **Confidentiality must be maintained at all times** to protect the client and the therapeutic nature of the nurse-client relationship. **Anonymity can be ensured by using only client initials rather than proper names and by omitting identifying demographic information on the process record** (Arnold and Boggs, p. 279).

• Examples

Examples details are details that illustrate the main point of the paragraph. These details provide illustrations of the main idea to give you a greater understanding of the essence of the passage. They sometimes appear in list form.

• EXAMPLE 9–5 •

Look at the following paragraph and note that the examples details are in boldface type.

Battered women are present in nearly every health care setting. Examples include **out patient clinics, emergency rooms,** and **obstetric-gynecologic units.** Complaints may be **physical injuries or vague symptoms** such as **sleep disorders, abdominal pain** or **menstrual problems.** Sensitivity on the part of the nurse is required in suspecting the possibility of spouse abuse (Varcarolis, p. 255).

• Description

Description details are details that help you to visualize the main thought of the paragraph. Description details provide a picture that enables you to comprehend the core elements of the paragraph.

• EXAMPLE 9–6 •

Consider the following selection with description details in boldface type.

A malignant tumor is **a large collection of cancer cells, all descendants of a single cell. This ancestor was once a normal cell with a normal function in a particular tissue, which somehow underwent a fundamental change.** As a result of that change, **the ancestor cell began to divide and proliferate in response to directions other than stimuli that result in normal cell reproduction.** Eventually, **the cell parented billions of similarly altered cells composing the tumor mass** (Ignatavicius and Bayne, p. 552).

• EXERCISE 9–2 •

Directions. Underline the main idea in each passage. The type of detail has been identified for you. Use this information to help you locate the major details, those supporting the main idea. Underline the details twice.

1 The term depression is used loosely for a wide range of conditions. It may be used to denote normal, everyday mood variations, mild but pathological depressive disorders, or severe psychotic depression. All have very different etiological natures and varying clinical implications (Varcarolis, pp. 70–71). <u>example</u>

2 Research has identified three body types or configurations and the personality traits most often associated with them. These types are endomorph—heavyset, sociable, friendly, relaxed; mesomorph—sturdy well-developed bone and muscle, vigorous, energetic, assertive; ectomorph—thin, slender, inhibited, private (Ignatavicius and Bayne, p. 159). <u>example</u>

3 There are people who are not able to resolve a particular loss. Between 10% and 20% of newly bereaved persons have serious emotional problems (Ignatavicius and Bayne, p. 202). <u>data</u>

4 The nurse assesses muscle strength by having the client (1) squeeze the nurse's hands, (2) attempt to keep the arms flexed while the nurse pulls downward on the lower arms, and (3) push both feet against a flat surface (a box or a board) while the nurse applies resistance (Ignatavicius and Bayne, p. 283). <u>procedure</u>

5 <u>Hyponatremia</u> has little direct effect on cardiac muscle contractility; however, alterations in cardiac output are associated with hyponatremia. In some instances, cardiac pathologic changes (such as profound conges-

tive heart failure with generalized edema formation) actually cause the hyponatremia (Ignatavicius and Bayne, p. 283). <u>cause</u>

6 Proceeding from a level at age 2 or 3 in which all animals with four legs are horses or some other type of one-dimensional animal, the child is unable to distinguish fantasy from reality, to consider another's viewpoint or to accept the possibility of alternate options in the preschool years (Arnold and Boggs, p. 419). <u>description</u>

7 Don't ask irrelevant questions. Respond to the client in brief concise sentences and don't introduce a lot of explanation. Let the client tell you what he or she is experiencing (Arnold and Boggs, p. 460). <u>procedure</u>

8 Chronic disease is America's primary health problem. Approximately 50% of the population (110 million people) have one or more chronic illnesses, and nearly 32.4 million people have limitations in performing selfcare activities (Ignatavicius and Bayne, pp. 490–491). <u>data</u>

9 Intellect does not decline solely as a result of aging. However, a decrease in intellectual level may be caused by insufficient oxygen supply to the CNS (Ignatavicius and Bayne, p. 847). <u>cause</u>

10 Generally, clients with swallowing problems are able to tolerate or swallow soft or semisoft foods and fluids (mechanically soft or dental diet, junior baby foods) better than thin liquids (water, juice, or broth) or a regular meal (Ignatavicius and Bayne, p. 890). <u>description</u>

Comprehending? Yes ___ No ___

• EXERCISE 9–3 •

Below is a passage from a nursing textbook. In each paragraph, underline the stated main idea. If the main idea is unstated, create your own in the margin. Underline twice the major details that support the main idea.

The adult body contains about 50 mg of iron per 100 mL of blood. Total body iron ranges between 2 and 6 g, depending on the size of the individual and the amount of hemoglobin the client's cells contain. Approximately two-thirds of this iron is contained in hemoglobin; the other third is stored in the bone marrow, the spleen, the liver, and muscle. If an individual has an iron deficiency, the iron stores are depleted first, followed by a reduction in hemoglobin. As a result, RBCs are small in size (microcytic) and diminished in number to the extent that the client has relatively mild manifestations of anemia, including weakness and pallor.

Iron deficiency anemia is the most common type of anemia. It can result from blood loss, increased internal demands (e.g., with pregnancy, adolescence, infection, and high-metabolism states), malabsorption (e.g., in celiac sprue and after partial or total gastrectomy), or dietary inadequacy (e.g., as a result of chronic alcoholism or poverty). In this anemia, the basic problem is a decreased supply of iron for the developing RBC.

Iron deficiency anemia is seen frequently in underdeveloped countries, as well as in technologically advanced societies, such as in the United States. It can occur at any age, but is more frequently noted in women, children, the elderly, and those with restricted diets (e.g., as a result of low income) or unbalanced diets.

The primary treatment of iron deficiency anemia is an increase in the oral intake of iron. Iron is obtained from food. Important sources are red meats, organ meats, kidney beans, whole-wheat products, spinach, egg yolks, carrots, and raisins. An adequate diet supplies the body with about 12 to 15 mg of iron per day, of which only 5% to 10% is absorbed. The amount of iron normally absorbed daily from the diet is sufficient to meet the needs of healthy men and healthy women after the childbearing age, but is not sufficient to supply the greater needs of menstruating women and adolescents during growth spurts. Fortunately, if iron intake is inadequate or if bleeding or pregnancy occurs, the gastrointestinal (GI) tract is capable of increasing the absorption of iron to about 20% to 30% of the total daily intake. When iron deficiency anemia develops in nonmenstruating women or adult men, other possible sources of insidious blood loss should be explored (such as GI lesions) (Ignatavicius and Bayne, p. 2254).

• VOCABULARY CHECK

Directions.   Below are 10 words taken from the key words section of this chapter. Circle the letter of the best definition of the four choices.

1   Benign
  a   not infectious
  b   not malignant
  c   not genetic
  d   not operable

2   Anonymity
  a   the state of being irritating
  b   the state of being irregular
  c   the state of not being named or identified
  d   an explanatory note

3   Hyponatremia
  a   salt deficiency in the blood
  b   oxygen deficiency in the blood
  c   glucose deficiency in the blood
  d   iron deficiency in the blood

4   Exacerbation
  a   to have one's awareness increased
  b   to have one's awareness decreased
  c   to make more pleasant, comfortable
  d   to make more bitter, severe

5 Medulla
   a the outer edge of an organ
   b the central or inner portion of an organ
   c the middle chamber of the heart
   d the outer portion of the skeletal system

6 Feedback
   a the lower portion of the back
   b regurgitated food
   c insulting responses
   d corrective information

7 Neoplasia
   a tumor
   b blood factors
   c the nervous system
   d the endocrine system

8 Overwhelmed
   a ill
   b upset
   c bored
   d tired

9 Remission
   a resubmitting of information
   b diagnosing again; second diagnosis
   c abatement of symptoms of a disease
   d transmission of symptoms of a disease

10 Core
   a outer edges
   b detail
   c central part
   d peripheral element

• SUMMARY

In this chapter you learned how supporting details relate to the main idea. You also saw the difference between major and minor details and how you should focus on the major details for note taking and highlighting in your textbook. You learned a strategy to help you visualize details. Explanations and examples for the following five types of details were given to help you find and understand major details in a passage:

- Data
- Cause
- Procedures
- Examples
- Description

Finally, you were given practice locating these five kinds of details and recognizing how these details support the main idea.

Chapter 10

Paragraph Organization

OBJECTIVE

KEY WORDS

RECOGNIZING PARAGRAPH ORGANIZATION

TYPES OF PATTERN

    Chronological

    Cause and Effect

    Comparison-Contrast

    Simple Listing

VOCABULARY CHECK

SUMMARY

• OBJECTIVE

To use paragraph organization as an aid to concentration, comprehension, and retention.

• KEY WORDS

Pay attention to the following key words, which are underscored the first time they appear in this chapter. Try to determine the meaning of these words from the surrounding words in the passage. If you need further help, use your dictionary or the glossary in the back of this book.

Look up the medical terminology in your medical dictionary or the glossary. As you read the exercises in this chapter, write additional words you need to learn in the space provided.

MEDICAL TERMINOLOGY	GENERAL VOCABULARY
anestheticlike	altered
angina	assumption
auscultation	habitual
epidermis	modification
hemorrhage	optimal
hypertension	potential
melanin	quiescent
metabolic	statute
palpation	supreme
percussion	taxonomy
_____	_____
_____	_____
_____	_____

• RECOGNIZING PARAGRAPH ORGANIZATION

When authors write textbooks, they often organize their ideas in patterns. If you can learn to recognize these patterns, you will concentrate on and comprehend the author's ideas. Recognizing a familiar pattern makes you part of the author's thinking. You are actively participating in the author's arrangement of the ideas in the text. You will also find it easier to retain textbook information if you associate the ideas with a pattern rather than trying to remember random facts.

• TYPES OF PATTERN

There are varying types of organizational pattern. Both single paragraphs and longer selections can be structured in these patterns. Below are listed the patterns most often found in your nursing textbooks. The description and example of each pattern should help you to recognize these patterns as you read your textbooks.

• Chronological (time order)

In a chronological pattern, events are presented in sequence. You can recognize this pattern by such words as first, last, second, later, then, finally, next, ages, and dates.

• EXAMPLE 10–1 •

The second step in the diagnosis review cycle is publication in the *Nursing Diagnosis Journal* which placed the proposed diagnosis in the public domain. Next, it is forwarded for review by a clinical/technical task force with expertise related to the proposed diagnosis. It is then reviewed by the diagnosis review committee, which recommends acceptance, modification or rejection. Next, the proposed diagnosis is reviewed by the NANDA board of directors who forward accepted diagnoses to the general assembly for review and discussion at the biannual National Conference. The final step is a mail ballot to NANDA members (Iyer et al, p. 88).

Underline all the words that indicate a time-order pattern.

• Cause and Effect

Causes are the reasons for events, while effects are results. Clue words to this pattern are since, therefore, thus, as a result, and consequently.

• EXAMPLE 10–2 •

Working to increase self-awareness helps you avoid the often harmful effects of trying to impose your own value system on other people. It also helps you to collect information without making judgements about the information you are given. Thus, you are more likely to receive more accurate, more abundant and more helpful information for professional use (Sorensen and Luckmann, p. 342).

List the word that indicates that the pattern is cause and effect. _____

• Comparison-Contrast

Authors look at similarities and differences. Comparisons describe similarities, while contrasts describe differences. Some paragraphs combine comparison and contrast. Comparisons can be recognized by such words as similarly or likewise. Contrasts can be recognized by such words as but, on the other hand, or however.

• EXAMPLE 10–3 •

Nurses are professionally inadequate if they ignore psychological factors concerning the people they care for. On the other hand, nurses must not use the power of their professional position to pressure people into unwillingly self-disclosing information (Sorensen and Luckmann, p. 338).

Write the phrase that lets you know that the author is contrasting ideas. _____

_____

• Simple Listing

In a simple listing pattern the information in a passage will be in the format of a list. The order is not important. Clue words are and, also, or in addition.

• EXAMPLE 10–4 •

Inspection, <u>palpation</u>, <u>percussion</u> and <u>auscultation</u> are basic maneuvers used during physical assessment. The sense of smell is also used for assessment purposes (Sorensen and Luckmann, p. 360).

Write the clue word that indicates that this pattern is simple listing. _____

• EXERCISE 10–1 •

Directions.   Read each textbook selection and identify the organizational pattern. Write whether each pattern is chronological (time order), cause and effect, comparison-contrast, or simple listing.

1   Adequate rest is necessary for well-being. Physical tiredness and fatigue, exhaustion after minimal muscle activity, difficulty in performing routine tasks, and overall weakness are hallmarks of inadequate rest. In addition, mental activities become difficult because of lapses of attention and decreased ability to concentrate. While not serious in themselves, these manifestations prevent <u>optimal</u> function and high-level wellness (Sorensen and Luckmann, p. 698).

The organizational pattern is _____.

2   Simultaneous monitoring of the EEG, EOG and EMG has shown that sleep is composed of two very distinct types of activity: REM or rapid eye movement and non-REM (NREM) sleep. Far from the traditional view of sleep as a <u>quiescent</u>, <u>anestheticlike</u> state, REM sleep actually involves intense physiologic activation. For this reason, REM sleep is often referred to as "active" or "paradoxic" sleep. Non-REM sleep on the other hand, is associated with progressive relaxation. It is divided into four stages (NREM 1-4). NREM 3 and 4 are often referred to as "slow wave," quiet sleep (Sorensen and Luckmann, p. 699).

The organizational pattern is _____.

3   Nurses, because of their often prolonged and intimate contacts with people, are in a unique position to help those in pain. Providing this help is a challenge, responsibility and privilege. Surely one of the greatest ways of "caring" for people is to prevent or relieve pain, or at least make pain more tolerable. Practicing nurses continue to gain new knowledge and skills for pain prevention and management. Nurses learn about pain not only professionally, but also personally from their experiences with pain (Sorensen and Luckmann, p. 710).

The organization pattern is _____.

4 The intensity of two pains that exist separately, but at the same time, is no greater than that of the more intense of the two. It has long been observed that the existence of one pain may actually raise the threshold for perception of another. Thus, individuals in intense pain may bite their lip or squeeze their fingernails into the palm of their hand. By increasing this "counterpain," they may lessen the intensity of the original pain (Sorensen and Luckmann, p. 714).

The organization pattern is _____.

5 Permanent teeth replace deciduous teeth during these years. The first permanent teeth erupt between ages six and seven. Bones lengthen and harden. Facial bones develop further and sinuses enlarge. The face changes gradually to an adult appearance. Neuromuscular development continues, giving children increasing coordination throughout the school-age years (Sorensen and Luckmann, p. 285).

The organization pattern is _____.

Comprehending? Yes _____ No _____

• EXERCISE 10-2 •

Directions. Read each textbook selection. Identify the organizational pattern. Use this pattern to help you locate the topic, main idea, and major details in each selection.

1 Skin is the largest body organ. It has three continuous layers: epidermis, dermis and subcutaneous tissue. The epidermis (most superficial layer) has several layers called strata. The outermost stratum contains dead cells continuously replaced by cells from deeper layers. Melanin and keratin form in the inner cellular epidermal stratum. Melanin (pigment) provides skin color and protects from ultraviolet sun rays. Keratin contributes to skin acidity.

    The dermis consists of blood vessels, dense connective tissue, nerve fibers, sebaceous (oil) glands and hair follicles. Sebaceous glands are present on all skin surfaces except palms and soles.

    Under the dermis is subcutaneous tissue providing support and blood supply to the dermis. It consists of loose connective tissue, blood and lymph vessels, fat, sweat glands and hair follicles (Sorensen and Luckmann, pp. 661–662).

Organizational pattern: _____.

Topic: _____.

Main idea: _____.

Major details: _____

_____

_____

2 Some people bathe for reasons other than hygiene, e.g. relaxation, therapeutic baths. A warm tub bath can relax and soothe sore tense muscles. For some people bathing is a time for being alone to screen out external stimuli or relieve generalized tension. For others, bathing is a stimulant to "get started in the morning," e.g. a cool shower to "get going." In care facilities, wherever possible, maintain an individual's <u>habitual</u> bathing practices (Sorensen and Luckmann, p. 663).

Organizational pattern: _____.

Topic: _____.

Main idea: _____.

Major details: _____

_____

_____

3 The United States Constitution is the <u>supreme</u> law of the land. The U.S. Constitution gives the courts the power to declare any federal or state <u>statute</u> or other law unconstitutional. Therefore, the U.S. court system can restrict the rights of Congress and the rights of the states to make laws. The theory is that the courts have the right to interpret the law. Therefore, if a conflict is found between a statute and the Constitution, the supreme nature of the Constitution requires that the courts declare the statute invalid. The executive branch which is responsible for enforcing the law is prohibited from doing so if the law is declared unconstitutional (Sorensen and Luckmann, p. 174).

Organizational pattern: _____.

Topic: _____.

Main idea: _____.

Major details: _____

_____

_____

4 Nursing diagnosis is a complex concept to define. Nursing diagnoses are *not* medical diagnoses, although there are similarities between the two. Nursing diagnoses are *similar* to medical diagnoses in that the same basic methods underlie both processes: obtaining the person's history, performing the physical examination, organizing the data base, and analyzing the data obtained. Both nurses and physicians need similar skills to make diagnoses: communication skills, physical assessment skills, observational skills, and intellectual skills. Moreover, the purpose of diagnosis is the same for both professions—to identify the problem and to develop a plan of care to solve the problem or meet the need.

On the other hand, nursing diagnoses *differ* from medical diagnoses in their focus, and consequently in their specific goals and objectives. Physicians are primarily involved in diagnosing disease and its underlying pathologic processes. Physicians examine people to learn the source of their symptoms, and the metabolic, chemical, or pathologic structural changes resulting from the disorder. An example of a medical diagnosis is: "Profound normocytic anemia due to acute hemorrhage."

In contrast to medical diagnosis, Dossey and Guzzetta state that in nursing diagnoses, nurses "describe a combination of signs and symptoms that indicate an *actual* or *potential* problem nurses are licensed to treat and capable of treating." In essence, the nursing diagnosis focuses on the person's *response* (both physical and emotional) to disease and its underlying pathology.

Yura and Walsh describe the nursing diagnosis as the *judgment* or *conclusion* reached by the nurse based on an *accurate data base* that indicates (a) an individual's *potential* for fulfillment of basic human needs and (b) *alterations* that interfere with need fulfillment. Alterations may include an excess (e.g., fluid excess), a deficit (e.g., fluid depletion), a lack or limitation (e.g., insufficient sleep), or an altered pattern in expression (e.g., confusion following surgery).

Many nursing diagnoses are related to, or evolve out of, a person's response to the medical diagnosis. Other nursing diagnoses are independent of the medical diagnoses. For example, a nursing diagnosis related to our medical diagnosis of "profound normocytic anemia due to hemorrhage" might be "actual fluid volume deficit due to hemorrhage." A nursing diagnosis that might be *unrelated* to the medical problems of hemorrhage and anemia would be "sleep pattern disturbance due to excess sensory stimulation in the ICU."

Both medical and nursing diagnoses are necessary and valid. To develop a person's total diagnostic picture, nurses and physicians must work together as well as independently. Also, they must communicate their findings to one another.

Until recently, nurses have not had the benefit of a taxonomy—the systematic organization of knowledge of nursing diagnoses to facilitate communication between themselves. In 1973 the National Group for the Classification of Nursing Diagnosis held its first conference. Its purpose was to identify nursing functions and to establish a classification system suitable for computerization. Since that first meeting, the group (renamed the North American Nursing Diagnosis Association), has met several times and has developed a list of 50 nursing diagnoses. Recognize that this list is growing and being refined as diagnoses are researched and tested. It is not intended to be complete or final. Indeed, much of the growth and development in nursing in the years to come will be directed toward defining and adding to this list of nursing diagnoses (Sorensen and Luckmann, p. 217).

Organizational pattern: _____.

Topic: _____.

Main idea: _____.

Major details: _____

_____

_____

5 Identify the organizational pattern in Figure 10–1.

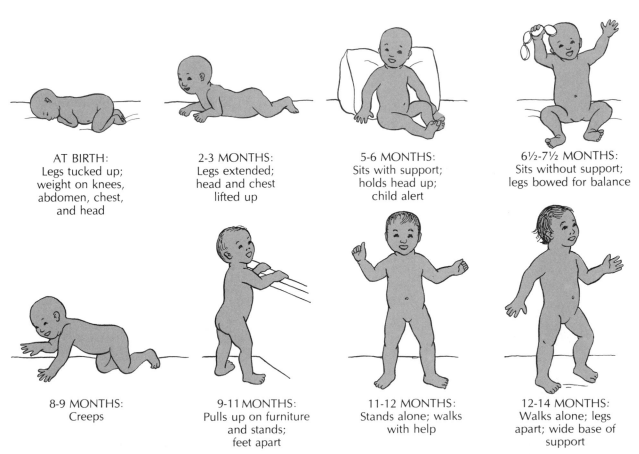

AT BIRTH:
Legs tucked up;
weight on knees,
abdomen, chest,
and head

2-3 MONTHS:
Legs extended;
head and chest
lifted up

5-6 MONTHS:
Sits with support;
holds head up;
child alert

6½-7½ MONTHS:
Sits without support;
legs bowed for balance

8-9 MONTHS:
Creeps

9-11 MONTHS:
Pulls up on furniture
and stands;
feet apart

11-12 MONTHS:
Stands alone; walks
with help

12-14 MONTHS:
Walks alone; legs
apart; wide base of
support

FIGURE 10–1 Development of infant posture and locomotion. (Adapted from Ingalls, A.J., and Salerno, M.C.: Maternal and child health nursing, ed. 5, St. Louis, 1983, The C.V. Mosby Co.)

Organizational pattern: _____.

Topic: _____.

Main idea: _____.

Major details: _____

_____

_____

Comprehending?   Yes ___   No ___

• **EXERCISE 10–3** •

Directions.   Read the following excerpt from a chapter in a nursing textbook (Sorensen and Luckmann, p. 247). As you read, focus on the organizational pattern. Use this pattern to help you concentrate on and comprehend the author's main ideas. Then answer the questions following the selection.

Malcolm Knowles, a leading authority on adult learning theory, has identified four assumptions that characterize adult learning.[20]

The first assumption is that as individuals mature, they become increasingly *self-directed* regarding learning. Knowles identifies those changes in self-concept that take the learner from a state of learning dependency to a state of increasing *self-directedness*. This self-direction is reflected in adults who first identify their learning needs and then take direct action to acquire the needed knowledge. Consider two adults who want (need) to learn how to use a word processor to increase their employment potential. One enrolls in a formal course at a local junior college; the other buys a book on word processing and devises a self-study program that combines reading the book and practicing the skill at the local library, using computerized instruction. Both of these adults identified their need/desire to learn to use the word processor, and chose a method of study that best suited their own learning style. They exhibited self-directed learning behavior.

The second assumption is that the adult learner approaches new learning experiences in light of a *lifetime of accumulated learning*. As adults, "we are what we learn." We define or characterize ourselves in terms of our experiences. This process is quite different for children, who view experiences as something that happens *to* them. The older we become, the more varied (and ingrained) are our learning experiences. Therefore, to facilitate adult learning, we should convey respect for people by making use of their past learning and drawing upon their experiences as a resource to enhance present learning.

Third, the adult learner is often characterized by a *readiness to learn.* For the adult, learning becomes more meaningful as it relates to what the person needs to know in order to perform effectively in a social role: spouse, parent, nurse, mechanic, professor, and so forth. It is often a challenge to structure health education in terms of developmental readiness to learn. People learn more readily when the information is useful and relevant to them socially, professionally, or personally. Mutual exploration and planning enables you and the adult learner to set learning priorities.

Closely related to readiness to learn is the fourth assumption that adult learning is based on solving *real-life problems* and the necessity for getting results immediately. This problem-centered orientation to learning is in contrast to the subject-orientation typical of a child's learning. Children study math, science, and English because they must in order to pass a test or enter high school, college, or graduate school. Subject-oriented learning has a delayed application.

Adults are more inclined to spend time, effort, and money to obtain knowledge that has *immediate* application to their circumstances. Also, when adults cope ineffectively with some of life's problems, they are motivated to seek new information. People who experience angina that interferes with job performance and activities of daily living, for example, may be motivated to learn how to modify their stress level, lose weight, and stop smoking. The executive who has hypertension may be less motivated to learn these things because the disease process does not presently interfere with job performance. Thus, to spend time performing these activities does not seem relevant to this person's present goals. Your task is to convince the person that performing the health behaviors will ultimately lead to a more productive life. On the other hand, the person needs to realize that by ignoring a serious health problem, complications can develop that may impede work performance altogether, e.g., a stroke. Helping people achieve immediate short-term goals that are positively rewarded reinforces learning. In turn, this success motivates people to continue healthy behaviors.

These characteristics of the adult learner should not be viewed as negative qualities. In fact, they are strengths *if* they are integrated sensitively into the learning process. You can provide a supportive learning environment by applying these assumptions when interacting with adult learners.

TO FACILITATE ADULT LEARNING:

- Recognize that adults need to be self-directed
- Integrate past learning experiences into the present learning situation
- Be sensitive to developmental readiness to learn
- Make learning applicable to current life problems

---

1 The organization pattern of this selection is:
   a chronological
   b cause and effect
   c simple listing
   d comparison-contrast

2 This selection is mainly about:
   a learning
   b assumption about learning
   c assumptions about adult learning
   d difficulties adults face when returning to school

3 Adults require:
   a direction from their textbooks
   b self-direction
   c no direction
   d direction from their instructors

4   When adults go back to school, they should:
   a   make use of past learning
   b   start a new career
   c   forget information learned in previous courses
   d   learn from their children

5   Adults learn best when they:
   a   are forced to go back to school
   b   cram for tests
   c   are in poor health
   d   are ready to learn

6   Adults learn best when the learning is:
   a   subject-oriented
   b   problem-centered
   c   delayed
   d   ineffective

7   Adults are motivated to achieve goals which are:
   a   immediate
   b   short-term
   c   positively rewarded
   d   all of the above

8   The older we become, our experiences are more:
   a   varied
   b   limited
   c   restricted
   d   irrelevant

9   People learn best when information:
   a   helps them to escape from life's problems
   b   helps them to forget about priorities
   c   is relevant
   d   is on tape

10   To retain the information in this selection, you should try to remember that the number of points presented by the author is:
   a   one
   b   two
   c   three
   d   four

Comprehending?   Yes ____   No ____

• VOCABULARY CHECK

Directions.   Below are 10 words taken from the key words section of this chapter. Circle the letter of the best definition from the four choices.

1   Metabolic
   a   the process of the digestion of minerals and vitamins
   b   nutrients found in the four food groups
   c   the process of nutrients absorbed into the blood following digestion.
   d   an organ that aids in the digestion of minerals and vitamins

2   Potential
   a   something in the past
   b   something that can develop
   c   something already formed
   d   something that is an obstacle to development

3   Angina
   a   spasmodic choking
   b   sharp pain
   c   heart failure
   d   an inflammation

4   Optimal
   a   obstructive
   b   most satisfactory
   c   dangerous
   d   upset

5   Hemorrhage
   a   a blood vessel near the lungs
   b   the flow of blood to and from the heart
   c   the escape of blood from a ruptured vessel
   d   a blockage that stops the flow of blood

6   Statute
   a   a decision of the jury that changes laws
   b   a signature needed to verify a document
   c   a decorative object, usually made of stone or metal
   d   a law enacted by the legislative branch of a government

7   Hypertension
   a   low blood pressure
   b   high blood pressure
   c   frenetic activity
   d   extreme anxiety

8 Altered
   a to maintain the integrity of a chemical
   b a chemical reaction involving more than one element
   c an abrupt implosion of energy
   d to make different without changing into something else

9 Epidermis
   a the outermost layer of the skin
   b the innermost layer of skin
   c a tough skin or membrane
   d a skin disease of the extremities

10 Assumption
   a a proven theory or concept
   b a mistake in a theory or concept
   c the supposition that something is true
   d misleading information given in court

• SUMMARY

You have learned how to use organizational patterns to improve your concentration and retention. Four patterns which are commonly used in your nursing textbooks are: chronological (time-order), comparison-contrast, cause-effect, and simple listing. Use clue words to help you recognize these patterns. Paying attention to organizational patterns will help you to become actively involved with the author's thinking process and enable you to read your textbooks with purpose.

• U N I T •

IV

STUDY SKILLS

Learning specific study skills will help you do well in nursing school. Once you have mastered them, the time and effort you put into preparing for exams should produce better results. Unit IV, "Study Skills," will help you learn and practice these techniques. Chapter 11, "Reading the Textbook," will teach you how to read and study from your nursing textbook. Chapter 12, "Graphic Aids," will show you how graphs, pictures, tables, and diagrams can be used to visually reinforce the ideas in the written text. Chapter 13, "Active Listening," will demonstrate how active listening will help you to concentrate on and comprehend information presented during lectures. Chapter 14, "Notetaking in the Classroom," will guide you in writing better lecture notes to ensure greater success on exams. Chapter 15, "Test-Taking Strategies," will provide you with techniques for improving your results on exams in your nursing and liberal arts courses.

Applying the study skills discussed in Unit IV will help you attain better grades. Once you see the positive results, you will be motivated to continue using these study skills to further your academic achievement.

• Chapter 11 •

Reading the Textbook

OBJECTIVE

KEY WORDS

SURVEYING THE TEXTBOOK

    Title Page

    Preface

    Table of Contents

    Glossary

    Bibliography

    Appendix

    Index

STRATEGIES FOR READING THE TEXTBOOK

    Before Reading

    While Reading

    After Reading

VOCABULARY CHECK

SUMMARY

• OBJECTIVE

To learn the active reading strategies required for concentrating on, comprehending, and retaining textbook information.

• KEY WORDS

Pay attention to the following key words, which are underscored the first time they appear in this chapter. Try to determine the meaning of these words from the surrounding words in the passage. If you need further help, use your dictionary or the glossary in the back of this book.

Look up the medical terminology in your medical dictionary or the glossary. As you read the exercises in this chapter, write additional words you need to learn in the space provided.

129

MEDICAL TERMINOLOGY	GENERAL VOCABULARY
biologic	alignment
biomechanics	colleagues
disc	friction
fibrocartilage	fulcrum
nonbiologic	gravity
pelvic	kinship
posture	leverage
psychosocial	momentum
sociologic	network
vertebrae	stability
_____	_____
_____	_____
_____	_____

• SURVEYING THE TEXTBOOK

Often the most difficult part of reading the textbook is getting started. Therefore it's a good idea to buy your textbooks as soon as they are assigned. You can then become familiar with your textbook at the beginning of the semester. Don't procrastinate. Open your book and get started! Once you feel comfortable with a text, it will be easier for you to approach each reading assignment. You can learn to use the external structure of your textbook to acquaint yourself with the book and to help you become an active reader. Survey these seven parts of the text to help you read your nursing textbooks:

- Title page
- Preface
- Table of contents
- Glossary
- Bibliography
- Appendix
- Index

• Title Page

The title page is the first printed page of the text and gives the following information:

- Title
- Author
- Edition
- Publisher
- City

• EXERCISE 11–1 •

Directions. Look at the title page opposite. Then answer the following questions.

1 The title of the book is _____

2 The authors are _____

_____

3 The publisher is _____

4 Is the copyright date (date of publication) given on this title page?

Yes _____   No _____

MEDICAL–SURGICAL
NURSING *A Psychophysiologic Approach*

THIRD EDITION

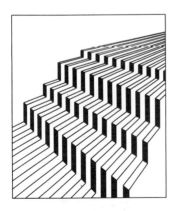

JOAN LUCKMANN, R.N., M.A.
Co-author of Sorensen, K.C., and Luckmann, J.
Basic Nursing: A Psychophysiologic Approach
Philadelphia: W.B. Saunders Company

KAREN CREASON SORENSEN, R.N., M.N.
Co-author of Sorensen, K.C., and Luckmann, J.
Basic Nursing: A Psychophysiologic Approach
Philadelphia: W.B. Saunders Company

1987
W.B. SAUNDERS COMPANY
Philadelphia London Toronto Sydney Tokyo Hong Kong

• Preface

The preface gives the author's objective in writing the text and explains the organization of the text. You can find the preface in the beginning of the book, following the title page.

• EXERCISE 11–2 •

Directions. Read the preface from the Luckmann and Sorensen book opposite and answer the questions that follow.

1 What are the three major sections of the text?

_____

_____

_____

2 List the three unchanging characteristics inherent in nursing today.

_____

_____

_____

• Table of Contents

The table of contents, found in the front of the book after the preface, is the most important part of your survey of your nursing textbook. The table of contents provides you with the author's outline of the entire text. The format of the table of contents usually consists of sections divided into units and units divided into chapters. You will see at a glance how the text is organized.

• EXERCISE 11–3 •

Directions. Survey the table of contents from the Luckmann and Sorensen book, which follows on pages 134-137. Then answer the questions that follow.

1 How many chapters are in Unit II? _____

2 What is the title of Unit IX? _____

3 Which section deals with specific problems in medical-surgical nursing?

_____

4 What page gives you information about nursing people experiencing dependence on alcohol and other drugs? _____

PREFACE

The purpose of human life is to serve and to show compassion and the will to help others.

The Schweitzer Album

Dear Reader:

With great pleasure we offer you the 3rd edition of *Medical-Surgical Nursing: A Psychophysiologic Approach*. Throughout the world, in English and translation, hundreds of thousands of nursing students, faculty, and practitioners have used previous editions of this text. This completely revised, totally updated 3rd edition of the number 1 bestseller in medical-surgical nursing continues to provide valuable information and guidelines.

This edition is divided into three major sections. Section I, *Unifying Concepts of Advanced Nursing Care*, covers the interaction of mind and body, theories of disease, stress management, injury, immunity, infection, fluid and electrolytes, pain, and physiologic shock. Section II, *Specific Problems in Medical-Surgical Nursing*, considers in detail nursing assessment, diagnosis, and intervention for people experiencing medical-surgical conditions. Section III, *A Summation of Holistic Health Assessment*, describes comprehensive nursing assessment. The Appendices contain commonly used laboratory values of clinical significance and information about nursing diagnoses.

The 3rd edition continues to emphasize the essence of nursing—*caring*. It also reflects the many dramatic changes in nursing theory and practice that have occurred in recent years. Therefore, while this edition presents what is new in nursing, it continues to emphasize those unchanging characteristics inherent in nursing, such as empathy, therapeutic communication, and advocacy. In addition to performing technical tasks, nurses must be able to assess an individual's physical, intellectual, emotional, social, and spiritual needs, and to intervene with competence and compassion.

Using this text, you will be able to integrate the five steps of the nursing process into your daily experience of caring for others. The cover of our book symbolically displays these steps in multiple hues. The inside covers present the North American Nursing Diagnosis Association's list of approved nursing diagnoses and a diagrammatic representation of the nursing process. To help you provide comprehensive nursing care, we have carefully integrated the nursing process throughout the content. Each unit begins with a list of relevant nursing diagnoses. Nursing assessment, diagnosis, and intervention is integrated throughout the chapters as they relate to specific medical-surgical disorders.

Each sentence of this book is revised and new material is added throughout. Major new areas of content include stress management, nursing people with infections, nursing people requiring blood transfusions, nursing people experiencing plastic surgery, and nursing people experiencing dermatologic disorders. We have also expanded coverage of women's reproductive health maintenance, human sexuality, and holistic health assessment. We include new and exciting developments in nursing research, and also integrate important findings from allied health fields.

CONTENTS IN BRIEF

SECTION ONE

UNIFYING CONCEPTS OF ADVANCED
NURSING CARE

Unit I
NURSING: A CHALLENGE–1

Chapter 1
NURSING PROCESS: MEETING NEEDS AND
SOLVING PROBLEMS–3

Unit II
HOLISTIC APPROACHES TO HEALTH
CARE–11

Chapter 2
MIND-BODY INTERACTION–14

Chapter 3
HOLISTIC THEORIES OF ILLNESS–20

Chapter 4
STRESSORS AND ILLNESS–31

Chapter 5
STRESS MANAGEMENT: INTERVENTION–45

Unit III
PSYCHOPHYSIOLOGIC RESPONSES TO
DISRUPTED HOMEOSTASIS–61

Chapter 6
NORMAL CELLS AND CELLULAR
IMBALANCES–62

Chapter 7
INJURY: BASIC CONCEPTS AND
INTERVENTION–71

Chapter 8
IMMUNITY: BASIC CONCEPTS AND
INTERVENTION–90

Chapter 9
INFECTION: BASIC CONCEPTS AND
INTERVENTION–118

Chapter 10
FLUID AND ELECTROLYTE IMBALANCES:
BASIC CONCEPTS AND INTERVENTION–134

Chapter 11
PAIN: BASIC CONCEPTS AND
INTERVENTION–174

Chapter 12
PHYSIOLOGIC SHOCK: BASIC CONCEPTS AND
INTERVENTION–214

SECTION TWO

SPECIFIC PROBLEMS IN MEDICAL-SURGICAL
NURSING

Unit IV
NURSING PEOPLE EXPERIENCING
SURGERY–258

Chapter 13
PERIOPERATIVE NURSING: BASIC
CONCEPTS–262

Chapter 14
NURSING PEOPLE BEFORE SURGERY–271

Chapter 15
NURSING PEOPLE DURING SURGERY–280

Chapter 16
NURSING PEOPLE FOLLOWING SURGERY–292

Unit V
NURSING PEOPLE EXPERIENCING
NEOPLASTIC DISORDERS–307

Chapter 17
NEOPLASTIC DISORDERS: BASIC
CONCEPTS–310

Chapter 18
UNDERSTANDING, ASSESSING, AND
PREVENTING NEOPLASTIC DISORDERS–317

Chapter 19
NURSING PEOPLE EXPERIENCING
NEOPLASTIC DISORDERS: INTERVENTION–331

xv

xvi

CONTENTS IN BRIEF

Unit VI
NURSING PEOPLE EXPERIENCING
NEUROLOGIC DISORDERS–356

Chapter 20
NEUROLOGIC STRUCTURE AND
FUNCTION–359

Chapter 21
ASSESSING PEOPLE EXPERIENCING
NEUROLOGIC DISORDERS–367

Chapter 22
MANIFESTATIONS OF ALTERED NEUROLOGIC
STRUCTURE AND FUNCTION–399

Chapter 23
NURSING PEOPLE EXPERIENCING SPECIFIC
NEUROLOGIC DISORDERS–455

Chapter 24
NURSING PEOPLE EXPERIENCING
NEUROSURGERY–527

Unit VII
NURSING PEOPLE EXPERIENCING SENSORY
DISORDERS–543

Chapter 25
NURSING PEOPLE EXPERIENCING EYE
DISORDERS–546

Chapter 26
NURSING PEOPLE EXPERIENCING EAR
DISORDERS–590

Chapter 27
NURSING PEOPLE EXPERIENCING NASAL
AND SINUS DISORDERS–615

Unit VIII
NURSING PEOPLE EXPERIENCING
RESPIRATORY DISORDERS–629

Chapter 28
RESPIRATORY STRUCTURE AND
FUNCTION–633

Chapter 29
ASSESSING PEOPLE EXPERIENCING
RESPIRATORY DISORDERS–644

Chapter 30
RESPIRATORY THERAPEUTIC
INTERVENTION–681

Chapter 31
NURSING PEOPLE EXPERIENCING UPPER
AIRWAY DISORDERS–716

Chapter 32
NURSING PEOPLE EXPERIENCING LOWER
AIRWAY DISORDERS–741

Chapter 33
NURSING PEOPLE EXPERIENCING CHEST
INJURIES–802

Chapter 34
NURSING PEOPLE EXPERIENCING CHEST
SURGERY–818

Unit IX
NURSING PEOPLE EXPERIENCING
CARDIOVASCULAR DISORDERS–849

Chapter 35
CARDIOVASCULAR STRUCTURE AND
FUNCTION–852

Chapter 36
ASSESSING PEOPLE EXPERIENCING
CARDIOVASCULAR DISORDERS–861

Chapter 37
NURSING PEOPLE EXPERIENCING CHRONIC
CONGESTIVE HEART FAILURE–886

Chapter 38
NURSING PEOPLE EXPERIENCING CARDIAC
ARRHYTHMIAS–901

Chapter 39
NURSING PEOPLE EXPERIENCING CORONARY
ARTERY DISEASE–927

Chapter 40
NURSING PEOPLE EXPERIENCING ARTERIAL
HYPERTENSION–948

Chapter 41
NURSING PEOPLE EXPERIENCING
INFLAMMATORY CARDIOVASCULAR
DISEASE–969

Chapter 42
NURSING PEOPLE EXPERIENCING
CARDIOVASCULAR STRUCTURAL
DISORDERS–982

Chapter 43
NURSING PEOPLE EXPERIENCING HEART
SURGERY–998

Unit X
NURSING PEOPLE EXPERIENCING
HEMATOLOGIC DISORDERS–1014

Chapter 44
HEMATOLOGY: BASIC CONCEPTS–1017

Chapter 45
NURSING PEOPLE REQUIRING BLOOD
TRANSFUSIONS–1022

Chapter 46
NURSING PEOPLE EXPERIENCING
ERYTHROCYTE DISORDERS–1036

Chapter 47
NURSING PEOPLE EXPERIENCING OTHER
MAJOR HEMATOLOGIC DISORDERS–1060

Unit XI
**NURSING PEOPLE EXPERIENCING
PERIPHERAL VASCULAR DISORDERS–1083**

Chapter 48
PERIPHERAL VASCULAR STRUCTURE,
FUNCTION, AND ASSESSMENT–1086

Chapter 49
NURSING PEOPLE EXPERIENCING ARTERIAL
DISORDERS–1097

Chapter 50
NURSING PEOPLE EXPERIENCING VENOUS
AND LYMPHATIC DISORDERS–1113

Chapter 51
NURSING PEOPLE EXPERIENCING EXTREMITY
AMPUTATION–1130

Unit XII
**NURSING PEOPLE EXPERIENCING URINARY
DISORDERS–1144**

Chapter 52
URINARY STRUCTURE AND FUNCTION–1147

Chapter 53
ASSESSING PEOPLE EXPERIENCING URINARY
DISORDERS–1157

Chapter 54
NURSING PEOPLE EXPERIENCING URETERAL,
URINARY BLADDER, AND URETHRAL
DISORDERS–1174

Chapter 55
NURSING PEOPLE EXPERIENCING RENAL
DISORDERS–1198

Unit XIII
**NURSING PEOPLE EXPERIENCING
GASTROINTESTINAL DISORDERS–1245**

Chapter 56
GASTROINTESTINAL STRUCTURE AND
FUNCTION–1248

Chapter 57
GASTROINTESTINAL ASSESSMENT AND
INTERVENTION–1258

Chapter 58
NURSING PEOPLE EXPERIENCING ORAL
DISORDERS–1272

Chapter 59
NURSING PEOPLE EXPERIENCING
SWALLOWING AND ESOPHAGEAL
DISORDERS–1280

Chapter 60
NURSING PEOPLE EXPERIENCING GASTRIC
DISORDERS–1289

Chapter 61
NURSING PEOPLE EXPERIENCING INTESTINAL
DISORDERS–1303

Unit XIV
**NURSING PEOPLE EXPERIENCING
DISORDERS OF THE LIVER, BILIARY TRACT,
AND PANCREAS–1333**

Chapter 62
LIVER, BILIARY TRACT, AND PANCREATIC
STRUCTURE AND FUNCTION–1336

Chapter 63
ASSESSING PEOPLE EXPERIENCING LIVER,
BILIARY TRACT, AND PANCREATIC
DISORDERS–1342

Chapter 64
NURSING PEOPLE EXPERIENCING HEPATIC
DISORDERS–1353

Chapter 65
NURSING PEOPLE EXPERIENCING
GALLBLADDER AND BILE DUCT
DISORDERS–1375

Chapter 66
NURSING PEOPLE EXPERIENCING EXOCRINE
PANCREATIC DISORDERS–1384

Unit XV
**NURSING PEOPLE EXPERIENCING
DISTURBANCES OF ENDOCRINE AND
METABOLIC FUNCTION–1396**

Chapter 67
ENDOCRINE STRUCTURE, FUNCTION, AND
ASSESSMENT–1399

Chapter 68
NURSING PEOPLE EXPERIENCING
ENDOCRINE DISORDERS OF THE
PANCREAS–1404

xviii   CONTENTS IN BRIEF

Chapter 69
NURSING PEOPLE EXPERIENCING THYROID
AND PARATHYROID DISORDERS–1438

Chapter 70
NURSING PEOPLE EXPERIENCING ADRENAL,
PITUITARY, AND GONADAL DISORDERS–1456

Unit XVI
NURSING PEOPLE EXPERIENCING
MUSCULOSKELETAL DISORDERS–1479

Chapter 71
MUSCULOSKELETAL STRUCTURE AND
FUNCTION–1483

Chapter 72
NURSING PEOPLE EXPERIENCING
MUSCULOSKELETAL ASSESSMENT AND
INTERVENTION–1490

Chapter 73
NURSING PEOPLE EXPERIENCING
MUSCULOSKELETAL INJURIES AND OVERUSE
PROBLEMS–1516

Chapter 74
NURSING PEOPLE EXPERIENCING OTHER
MUSCULOSKELETAL DISORDERS–1540

Unit XVII
NURSING PEOPLE EXPERIENCING
INTEGUMENTARY DISORDERS–1561

Chapter 75
NURSING PEOPLE EXPERIENCING
DERMATOLOGIC DISORDERS–1563

Chapter 76
NURSING PEOPLE EXPERIENCING BURNS–1614

Chapter 77
NURSING PEOPLE EXPERIENCING PLASTIC
SURGERY–1640

Unit XVIII
NURSING PEOPLE EXPERIENCING
REPRODUCTIVE DISORDERS–1667

Chapter 78
SEXUALITY AND REPRODUCTIVE
HEALTH–1669

Chapter 79
MEN'S REPRODUCTIVE HEALTH
MAINTENANCE–1700

Chapter 80
ASSESSING WOMEN EXPERIENCING
GYNECOLOGIC CONDITIONS–1731

Chapter 81
MANAGING MENSTRUATION–1741

Chapter 82
NURSING CARE OF WOMEN EXPERIENCING
NONMALIGNANT GYNECOLOGIC DISORDERS
AND GYNECOLOGIC SURGERY–1750

Chapter 83
NURSING WOMEN EXPERIENCING
GYNECOLOGIC CANCER–1791

Chapter 84
NURSING PEOPLE EXPERIENCING BREAST
DISORDERS–1808

Unit XIX
NURSING PEOPLE EXPERIENCING
DEPENDENCE ON ALCOHOL AND OTHER
DRUGS–1836

Chapter 85
NURSING PEOPLE EXPERIENCING
DEPENDENCE ON ALCOHOL AND OTHER
DRUGS–1840

Unit XX
NURSING PEOPLE EXPERIENCING MEDICAL-
SURGICAL EMERGENCIES–1867

Chapter 86
NURSING PEOPLE EXPERIENCING MEDICAL-
SURGICAL EMERGENCIES–1870

SECTION THREE

A SUMMATION OF HOLISTIC HEALTH
ASSESSMENT

Unit XXI
HOLISTIC HEALTH ASSESSMENT–1945

Chapter 87
HOLISTIC HEALTH ASSESSMENT–1947

Appendix A: Nursing Diagnoses Approved by
NANDA Through 1984–2023

Appendix B: Additional Nursing Diagnoses
Approved by NANDA in 1986–2049

Appendix C: NANDA Nursing Diagnoses
Taxonomy I–2055

Appendix D: Common Laboratory Values of
Clinical Importance–2059

INDEX–2073

- **Glossary**

A glossary, located in the back of the textbook, gives you an alphabetical listing of the vocabulary that is important for understanding the ideas in the text.

• EXERCISE 11–4 •

Directions. Answer the following question:

How many of your other nursing textbooks contain glossaries?

_____

_____

_____

_____

- **Bibliography**

The bibliography is found in the back of the text or at the end of each chapter. A bibliography lists the sources used by the author when compiling your textbook.

• EXERCISE 11–5 •

Directions. Look at the bibliography page opposite from the Luckmann and Sorensen nursing textbook. Notice that the items are listed alphabetically by the last names of the authors. Then answer the following questions.

1   What is the title of the book written by Boucher, I.A., and Morris, J.S.?

_____

2   Write the name of the journal in which the article by I. Baily is found.

_____

BIBLIOGRAPHY

1. Alexander, B.: Taking the sexual history. *American Family Physician* 23:147, March 1981.
2. American Nurses' Association: *Standards of Psychiatric and Mental Health Nursing Practice.* American Nurses' Association, 1973.
3. Anderson, M.S.: Assessment under pressure: when your patient says, "My head hurts." *Nursing 84* 14:34, September 1984.
4. Anstett, R.E., and Chishold, R.N.: Practical mental status testing by the primary care physician. *Hospital Medicine* 21:214, May 1985.
5. Assessment head to toe. *Transition* 1:53, February 1983.
6. Bailey, I.: Tell me who you are. *Nursing 85* 15:53, October 1985.
7. Barosinek, K., et al.: Assessment under pressure: when your patient says, "My stomach hurts." *Nursing 84* 14:34, November 1984.
8. Barry, P.D.: *Psychosocial Nursing Assessment and Intervention.* Philadelphia: J.B. Lippincott Co., 1984.
9. Bates, B.: *A Guide to Physical Examination,* 3rd ed. Philadelphia: J.B. Lippincott Co., 1983.
10. Beck, M.L.: Guiding your patient a step at a time through a colonoscopy. *Nursing 81* 11:28, June 1981.
11. Beck, M.L.: Preparing your patient psychologically for an esophagogastroduodenoscopy. *Nursing 81* 11:28, January 1981.
12. Beck, M.L.: Three more gastrointestinal tests—and how to help your patient through each. *Nursing 81* 11:22, May 1981.
13. Bell, S.J.: Health risks of obesity. *Physician and Patient* 4:18, September-October 1985.
14. Berger, K.J., and Fields, W.L.: *Pocket Guide to Health Assessment.* Reston, VA: Reston Publishing Co., 1980.
15. Birdsall, C.: How do you interpret pulses? *American Journal of Nursing* 85:785, July 1985.
16. Blumsohn, D.: Clubbing of the fingers with special reference to Schamroth's diagnostic method. *Heart and Lung* 10:1069, November-December 1981.
17. Bostwick, J., III: Breast reconstruction following mastectomy. *Contemporary Surgery* 27:15, July 1985.
18. Boucher, I. A., and Morris, J. S.: *Clinical Skills. A System of Clinical Examination.* Philadelphia: W.B. Saunders Co., 1982.

- **Appendix**

The appendix, also found in the back of the book, lists supplemental material that may be useful when you are reading and studying from your textbook.

• EXERCISE 11–6 •

Directions. Survey the appendix example below and opposite from the Iyer et al. nursing textbook. Then answer the following questions.

1 What is the subject matter of the appendix?

_____

2 How many items are listed under the heading "Respiratory System?"

_____

_____

_____

_____

BODY SYSTEMS ASSESSMENT CRITERIA

General Appearance
- ☐ *Observations*—age, sex, race, height, weight, nutritional status, development

Vital Signs
- ☐ Temperature
- ☐ Pulse (rate)
- ☐ Respirations
- ☐ *Blood pressure*—supine, sitting, right and left arms

Neurological System
- ☐ Level of consciousness
- ☐ *Skull*—size, contour, symmetry, color, pain, tenderness, lesions, edema
- ☐ *Eyes*—acuity, visual loss, glasses, contacts, prosthesis, diplopia, photophobia, color vision, pain, burning, eyelid ptosis, edema, styles, exophathamos, extraocular movement, position and alignment, strabismus, nystagmus, conjunctival color, discharge, vascular changes, corneal reflex, scleral color, vascularity, jaundice, pupil size, shape, equality, reaction to light
- ☐ *Neck*—symmetry, movement, range of motion, masses, scars, pain, stiffness, lymph node size, shape, mobility, tenderness, enlargement
- ☐ *Reflexes*—Deep tendon reflexes (DTRs), Babinski, posturing

Musculoskeletal System
- ☐ *Activity level*—prescribed, actual, range of motion
- ☐ *Extremities*—size, shape, symmetry, temperature, color, pigmentation, scars, hematoma, bruises, rash, ulceration, numbness, paresis, swelling, prosthesis, fracture
- ☐ *Joints*—symmetry, active and passive mobility, deformities, stiffness, fixation, masses, swelling, fluid, bogginess, crepitation, pain, tenderness
- ☐ *Muscles*—symmetry, size, shape, tone, weakness, cramps, spasms, rigidity, tremors
- ☐ *Back*—scars, sacral edema, spinal abnormalities, kyphosis, scoliosis, tenderness, pain

Respiratory System
☐ *Nose*—smell, nasal size, symmetry, flaring, sneezing, deformities, mucosal color, edema, exudate, bleeding, furuncles, pain, tenderness, sinus pain
☐ *Chest*—size, shape, symmetry, deformities, pain, tenderness, expansion, crepitation, tactile fremitus
☐ *Trachea*—deviation, scars
☐ *Breathing patterns*—rate, regularity, depth, ease, use of accessory muscles, cyanosis, clubbing
☐ *Sounds*—normal, adventitious, intensity, pitch, quality, duration, equality, vocal resonance

Cardiovascular System
☐ *Cardiac patterns*—rate, rhythm, intensity, regularity, skipped or extra beats, point of maximum impulse, bruits, thrills, murmurs, rubs
☐ Precordial movements, neck veins, right and left cardiac borders, pacemaker

Gastrointestinal System
☐ *Mouth and throat*—odor, pain, ability to speak, bite, chew, swallow, taste, tongue size, shape, protrusion, symmetry, color, hydration, markings, ulcers, burning, swelling, coating, gum color, edema, bleeding, retraction, pain, number of teeth, absence, caries, caps, dentures, sensitivity to heat, cold, gag reflex, throat soreness, cough, sputum, hemoptysis
☐ *Abdomen*—size, color, contour, symmetry, fat, muscle tone, turgor, hair distribution, scars, umbilicus, striae, rashes, distention, abnormal pulsations, sounds: absent, hypoactive, hyperactive; tenderness, rigidity, free fluid, liver border, air bubble, splenic dullness, air rebound, muscle spasm, masses, guarding, pain
☐ *Rectum*—pigmentation, hemorrhoids, excoriation, rashes, abscess, pilonidal cyst, masses, lesions, tenderness, pain, itching, burning

Renal System
☐ *Urinary patterns*—amount, color, timing, odor, sediment, frequency, urgency, hesitancy, burning, pain, dribbling, incontinence, hematuria, nocturia, oliguria, change in stream, enuresis, flank pain, polyuria, retention, stress incontinence, bladder distention

Reproductive System
☐ *Male*—penis: discharge, ulceration, pain, size, prepuce; *scrotum*: size, color, nodules, swelling, ulceration, tenderness, pain; *testes*: size, shape, swelling, masses, absence
☐ *Female*—labia majora and minora, urethral and vaginal orifices, discharge, swelling, ulcerations, nodules, masses, tenderness, pain, pruritus, Pap smear, menstrual flow, menopause
☐ *Breasts*—contour, symmetry, color, shape, size, inflammation, scars, masses: location, size, shape, mobility, tenderness, pain; dimpling, swelling, nipples: color, discharge, ulceration, bleeding, inversion, pain; axillae: nodes, enlargement, tenderness, rash, inflammation

Integumentary System
☐ *Color*—pink, pale, red, jaundice, mottled, blanched, cyanotic
☐ *Patterns*—pigmentation, vascularity, temperature, texture, turgor, lesions (type, color, size, shape, distribution), bruises, bleeding, scars, edema, dryness, ecchymoses, masses (size, shape, location, mobility, tenderness), odors, petechiae, pruritus, bruises, bleeding, scars, edema

• Index

The index is found in the back of your textbook. The index is an alphabetical listing of important terms in a text with page references. These terms can be the headings of more specific concepts. The index helps you to quickly locate specific information within your text.

• EXERCISE 11–7 •

Directions.   Survey the page from the index opposite from the Luckmann and Sorensen nursing textbook. Then answer the questions that follow.

1   Write the page number on which you would find information about a chronic cough. _____

2   Write the page on which you would find information about cryptitis. _____

Comprehending?   Yes ___   No ___

• EXERCISE 11–8 •

Directions.   You have learned how to survey a textbook. Choose any nursing textbook and answer the following questions.

1   Write the following information from the title page.

Title _____

Author(s) _____

Publisher _____

2   Is there a preface? Yes _____   No _____. If yes, what is the author's objective in writing this text? _____

_____

3   Survey the table of contents.

a   How many sections are in this text? _____

b   How many chapters are in Section 1? _____

4   Look in the back of the text.

Is there a bibliography? Yes _____   No _____

Is there a glossary? Yes _____   No _____

Is there an index? Yes _____   No _____

If yes, write the page number of each. _____

2086

Coronary artery bypass graft (CABG), 998, *1000*
Coronary artery disease (CAD), 927–947
  atherosclerosis and, 927
    pathogenesis of, 929–930, *930*
  complicating abdominal aortic aneurysm surgery, 1099
  incidence of, 927, *928*
  manifestations of, 930–947. See also *Angina pectoris* and *Myocardial infarction.*
  risk factors and, 927–929, 928t
Coronary circulation, 853, *854*
Coronary insufficiency, chest pain and, 862t
Coronary veins, 853
Coroner, jurisdiction of, 1941
Corpus callosum, 362
Corpus luteum, cyst of, 1774
  formation of, 1679
Corset, after spinal surgery, 538
Cortex
  adrenal, 1456, *1457*
    disorders of, 1459–1469
  cerebral, dysfunction of, 505t
    lesions of, pain from, 183
    motor areas of, *496*
  renal, 1147, *1148*
Cortical resection, for seizure, 499
Corticoids, in adaptation, 22
Corticosteroids, 1456
  for myasthenia gravis, 487
  intra-articular injection of, for arthritis, 1548
  intralesional injection of, 1584
  ocular, 561
  systemic, for skin conditions, 1584
  topical 1580t, 1583
Cortisol, plasma levels of, in Cushing's syndrome, 1465
  plasma response of, to ACTH, 1461
  self-administration of, knowledge deficit regarding, 1475
Cortisone, inflammatory response and, 83
Cortisone suppression test, 1465
Costophrenic angle, 665, *666*
Costovertebral angle, percussion over, 1158
Cough, 638, 743–744
  after chest surgery, 830
  anatomy of, *743*
  assessment of, 645, 744
  chronic, 743
    caring for people with, 744
  effective, facilitating, 696, *697*
  physiologic elements of, 638t
  preoperative exercise for, 274
  relieving, intervention for, 744
  splinting for, *697*
Coumadin, self-administration of, *1118*
Coumarin anticoagulants, overdosage with, hypoprothrombinemia and, 1079
Coumarin derivatives, for venous thrombosis, 1116
Coup injury, 506
Cowper's (bulbourethral) glands, 1670
CPAP (continuous positive air pressure), 710–712
CPR. See *Cardiopulmonary resuscitation.*
Cramps, heat, emergency assessment and intervention for, 1908
Crackles, *2004*, 2005t
  with cardiovascular disorders, 872
Cranial nerves, 371t
  damage to, with skull fracture, 507
  disorders of, 522–525

Cranial nerves (*Continued*)
  distribution of, *370*
  examination of, 369, 372–373
  structure and function of, *362, 363*
  tumor involvement of, 460
Cranial neuropathy, diabetic, 1433t, 1435
Craniectomy, 528
Craniocerebral trauma, 504–518. See also *Head injury.*
Craniofacial surgery, 1661
Craniotomy, 528
  suboccipital, *529*
  with osteoplastic bone flap, 528, *528*
Creams, 1568
  administration of, 1583, *1583*
  characteristics of, 1582t
Creatinine, serum levels of, measurement of, 1166
Creatinine clearance, 1165
Credé maneuver, 438, 1183
Cremasteric reflex, 378
CREST syndrome, 1554
Cretinism, 1443
Cribriform plate, fracture of, 1662
Cricoid cartilage, *635, 636*
Cricoid chondritis, 1267
Cricothyroidotomy, 740, 1875, *1875*
Crohn's disease, 1307
  assessment of, 1309
  complications of, 1310
  nursing goals, diagnoses, and intervention for, 1311
  surgical intervention for, 1312
  vs. ulcerative colitis, 1308t
Cromolyn sodium, antiallergic effect of, 684
Crossmatching, 1022
  blood, 1027
    documentation form for, *1027*
    sample collection for, 1026
Crutches, 1500
  fitting, 1500, *1500*
  walking with, 1500, *1501*
Crutchfield tongs, *430*
Cryoextraction, 578, *579*
Cryoprecipitate, 1023
  storage and handling of, 1026, 1030
Cryosurgery, for gynecologic conditions, 1781
  of skin lesion, 1590
Cryothermia, for anesthesia, 290
Crypt abscess, 1309
Cryptitis, 1328
Cryptococcosis, 458, 781
Cryptorchidism, 1708, *1710*
Crypts of Lieberkühn, 1255, 1257
Crystalloid solutions, for hypovolemic shock therapy, 243
Crystalluria, 1165
CT scan, *387*
  for musculoskeletal assessment, 1494
  for neurologic assessment, 386, *388*
  for renal assessment, 1169
  in cancer detection, 324
  of breast masses, 1816
  of chest, 668
  of gastrointestinal tract, 1265
  of liver, biliary tract, and gallbladder, 1350
  of male reproductive system, 1705
Cuff
  endotracheal tube, 702, *702*
    inflation and deflation of, 703
    pressure of, 703
    securing, 702, *702*
  tracheostomy, 746
    inflation and deflation of, 747t
    pressure of, 746

Cuff (*Continued*)
  tracheostomy, problems associated with, 746, *748–749*, 750t
Culdocentesis, 1738
  in ectopic pregnancy, 1771
  in pelvic inflammatory disease, 1765, *1765*
Culdoscopy, 1738, *1739*
Cultural factors, causing illness, 35
  in drug use, 1841
  pain experience and, 185
Culture
  of fungal scrapings, 1576
  of nose, 618, 671
  of sputum, 670
  of throat, 618, 671
  of urine, 1167, 1186
Culture shock, 35
Curative surgery, 264
Curettage, of skin lesion, 1590, *1590*
Curie, 324
Curling's ulcer, intervention to prevent, 1624
Cushing changes, with increased intracranial pressure, 407
Cushing's disease, 1464, 1472
  surgical intervention for, 1466
  therapies prescribed for, 1466t
Cushing's syndrome, 1464–1468
  assessment data for, 1464, *1464*
  surgical intervention for, 1466, *1467*
    nursing diagnoses and intervention for, 1466–1468
  therapies prescribed for, 1465, 1466t
Cushing's ulcers, 511, 1293
Cutaneous (superficial) pain, 180, 180t
Cutaneous T-cell lymphoma, 1609
Cyanosis, 642
  with severe burn, 1622
Cyclocryopexy, 575
Cyclodialysis, 575
Cyclodiathermy, 575
Cycloplegic(s), 560
Cycloplegic refraction, 581
Cyclotherapy, of glaucoma, 575
Cyclotron, in cancer treatment, 339, *340*
Cyst
  epidermoid (sebaceous), 1599
  ovarian, 1774
  pilonidal, 1328
  renal, 1200
Cystectomy, 1190
Cystic disease, congenital, 801
Cystic fibrosis, 767, 1392–1393
Cystinuria, 1210
  medications for, 1214
Cystitis, 1186
  due to radiation therapy, 344t
  emergency assessment and intervention for, 1925
Cystocele, 1779, *1780*
Cystolithotomy, 1188
Cystometrography, 1170, *1170*, 1705
Cystoscopy, 1703
  rigid, 1171, *1171*
Cystourethrography, 1168
  voiding, 1169
Cystourethroscopy, flexible fiberoptic, 1172
Cytology
  cervical, 1735, *1736*
  endometrial, 1737, *1737*
  esophageal, 1264
  exfoliative, 323
    of gastrointestinal tract, 1263
  for cancer, 321
  of sputum, 671
  of urine, 1167

Now that you have had practice surveying a textbook as a whole, you are ready to concentrate on an essential strategy in reading the textbook—previewing the chapter.

• STRATEGIES FOR READING THE TEXTBOOK

Reading a textbook requires concentration strategies that are different from reading books for pleasure. You can learn these specific techniques, which will help you to concentrate on, comprehend, and retain textbook information. Reading concentration requires active reading. You must react to the material to stay focused on the subject.

The following strategies will help you concentrate on textbook information:
- Previewing
- Questioning
- Summarizing

• Before Reading
PREVIEWING

Before reading the assigned textbook material, preview the reading assignment. As you recall from Chapter 2, previewing involves surveying the chapter. Read the *chapter title, introduction,* and *summary.* Notice *typographical clues* such as *boldface type* and *italics,* which are used to emphasize important ideas in the chapter. *Headings* and *key words* will also direct you to the main points discussed in the selection.

QUESTIONING

After previewing the reading assignment, try to anticipate the main ideas that will be discussed in the selection. Formulate questions to help you locate main ideas as you read. When you ask questions, you are reading with a purpose. Searching for the answers to your questions results in active reading. Questioning helps you to concentrate on textbook information.

An effective method for formulating questions is to turn boldface headings into questions. Look at the following example of creating questions from a boldface heading taken from a nursing textbook.

• EXAMPLE 11–1 •

HEADING:

Components of Psychosocial Assessment

SAMPLE QUESTIONS:

1 What are the components of psychosocial assessment?

2 How does psychosocial assessment help the patient?

Looking for the answers to these questions will help you concentrate while you read the text.

- ## While Reading
  ### THE 5 W'S

A strategy for helping you stay actively involved while reading your textbook is to use the 5 W's to lead you to the main idea and major details of a reading selection. The 5 W questions are:

- *Who or What* is the assigned reading about? (The answer to this question leads you to the topic, or subject.)
- *What is the main point* being made about the subject? (The answer to this question leads you to the main idea.)
- *When?*
- *Where?* } Provide the major details
- *Why or How?*

As you read your assignments, thinking about the 5 W questions will help you to concentrate on the author's main ideas and major details. Read the chapter section by section. Ask the 5 W questions. You may want to write the answers to your questions or other comments concerning the text in the margins. Writing notes while you read helps you stay actively involved with the text.

• EXERCISE 11–9 •

Directions. Read the following selection and formulate questions using the 5 W's.

COMPONENTS OF PSYCHOSOCIAL ASSESSMENT

It has been emphasized throughout this chapter that psychologic, sociologic and physical assessment belong together. The three areas overlap and interact so greatly that significant information is lost if they are not considered in relation to each other. As we analyze each component, keep uppermost in your mind that in practice the components are inextricably intertwined (Sorensen and Luckmann, p. 342).

Formulate your questions:

_____

_____

_____

_____

_____

Comprehending?   Yes ____   No ____

SUMMARIZING

Monitor your comprehension by answering your questions. Your answers to the 5 W questions will give you a summary of each topic. Restate the author's information in your own words. This paraphrasing helps you to comprehend the text selection. Be certain that you understand the information before you proceed to the next boldface heading.

- ## After Reading
  UNDERLINING

Highlight the main ideas and details that you want to remember.

WRITING

Prepare a study guide. Write a summary or outline as a review of the chapter as a whole. Work from the general (main ideas) to the specific (details). This written summary or outline will later serve as a study guide.

STUDYING

Use your aids for retention. Review all underlined text material, summaries, and outlines.

Answer the review questions at the end of each chapter. Design a practice test based on your assigned reading. Answer the practice questions and correct your answers. Taking these practice tests is an invaluable method for reinforcing your knowledge of the material. Your improved comprehension and retention of textbook information will result in better test grades.

• EXERCISE 11–10 •

Directions. Use all the reading comprehension strategies you learned in this chapter to concentrate on, comprehend, and retain textbook information. The questions and directions in this exercise will help guide your reading of the following selection from a nursing text (Sorensen and Luckmann, pp. 345–346).

• SOCIOLOGIC ASSESSMENT

Sociologic assessment involves the collection of information about variables that influence an individual's performance of social roles and the person's positions within social systems.[10] As discussed earlier in this chapter, it is impossible to understand a person in a meaningful way without considering the social network within which the individual's life is led.

Social Network

Everyone has a basic human need for *love and belonging.* To fulfill this need, we all establish around ourselves a social network, or a group of people among whom we live our lives. Our social networks have for each of us the potential for fulfilling important functions,[17,25] including:

- *Intimacy,* i.e., a closeness with others in which one can be warm, safe, and expressive. Intimacy is usually found with those others most personally significant or primary to an individual.
- *Social integration,* i.e., cooperative experiences occurring among people sharing similar situations and goals. Often found between friends and colleagues.
- *Nurturing behavior,* i.e., typically the care and responsibility a person has for a child. Also occurs and is important between adults.
- *Reassurance,* i.e., recognition and affirmation of worth and competence.
- *Assistance,* i.e., help and resources from others.

It is true that when people enter the health care system, nurses become temporarily a part of the person's social network. It must be remembered, however, that people still have the right to use their ongoing social networks that are part of their established life styles. In addition, nurses have an obligation to provide care and support for those significant others who are experiencing stress along with a person requiring health care.

Information must be sought, therefore, concerning a person's social network. A nurse needs to know something of the social network structure, along with the person's wishes concerning this structure at the time. Initial information about social network may be gathered by:

- Observing who accompanies a person to and from a health care facility and noting which persons telephone or seek to visit
- Asking the person questions:

Who are the people most significant to you?

What are the names of the people the health care facility should keep in contact with and notify in case of an emergency?

Do you want any restrictions placed on visitors or telephone calls? If so, what people are to be permitted to contact you? (Remember that people may change their minds about any of these matters.)

It is a common tendency to assume that family members are the most primary people for an individual. *This is not always the case.* Social networks and significant others are very personalized, and we can make neither assumptions nor judgments about them.

MacElveen suggests the following areas for social network assessment:

1 Nature of the person's available network
   a Kinship and nonkinship members
   b Members nearby and at a distance
   c Connectedness (loose or close-knit)
2 The person's dominant network style
   a Kinship (i.e., biologic and legal family)
   b Friendship (i.e., nonbiologic and nonlegal relationships)
   c Associate (i.e., organizational relationships)
   d Restricted (i.e., limited relationships in quality and/or number of relationships)
3 The person's relationships that fulfill the following needs:
   a Intimacy
   b Social integration
   c Opportunities for nurturing behavior
   d Reassurance of worth
   e Assistance
4 The network potential to assist with the person's current goals
   a Strengths, resources, and supports
   b The person's history of use of network at previous times of trouble

You will notice that throughout this book we use terms such as *significant others, support systems, concerned others,* and *primary people* instead of "family." This is done to encourage you to seek information about each person's social network rather than make the assumption that everyone functions within a traditional family.

BEFORE READING
Previewing

1 Identify the topic. Use heading and subheadings

_____

_____

2 Read the first and last paragraph.

3 Pay attention to key vocabulary words, which are in italics.

4 After following these preview steps, choose one of the following as the best title for this selection.
   a Social Networks
   b Nurturing Behavior and Sociologic Assessment
   c The Variables That Enable Nurses to Assess a Patient's Social Network
   d The Role of the Nurse as a Primary Figure in a Patient's Social Network

QUESTIONING

5 Based on your preview, formulate questions from the heading of the reading selection.

Examples of questions:
What are the functions of a social network?
How can a nurse assess a social network?

Now formulate your questions:

_____

_____

WHILE READING

6 Ask the 5 W questions. Read the selection with the purpose of answering your questions. Remember to stop at each boldface heading to monitor your comprehension.

Summarizing

Answer your 5 W questions. Remember to monitor your comprehension as you complete each topic. Restate the author's information in your own words. This paraphrasing improves comprehension.

AFTER READING
Underlining

7 Highlight the main ideas and details that you will want to remember. Underline the main ideas and circle the details.

Writing

8 Write a summary or outline of the selection.

Studying

9 Review all underlined material and the written summary or outline. Design a practice test. Correct your answers.

Comprehending? Yes ___ No ___

• EXERCISE 11–11 •

Directions.   Read the following selection from Sorensen and Luckmann, pp. 488–489). Use the strategies for textbook reading discussed in this chapter. These strategies will help you to concentrate on, comprehend, and retain textbook information. Remember to *preview, question, read, underline, summarize, paraphrase, write,* and *study* the information in this excerpt from a nursing textbook.

• INTRODUCTION AND STUDY GUIDE

• Introduction

Physical caregiving skills used by nurses involve appropriate and planned body movements. The nurse and the person being assisted with movement are both governed by principles of physics influencing the effectiveness and ease of body movements.

Body mechanics (biomechanics) is the coordinated, efficient use of the body to move from one position to another. It is important that nurses have a basic understanding of the forces operating during essential movements.

• Study Guide

1   Become familiar with the following terms:

Base of support: Foundation on which an object rests.

Body mechanics: Coordinated and efficient body use to move from one position to another.

Center of gravity: Center of mass, or heaviest part of the body; located in the pelvic area.

Force of movement: Direction toward which energy is exerted.

Friction: Rubbing of one object against another.

Fulcrum: Support on which a lever turns.

Gravity: Weight; attraction of an object to the center of the earth.

Internal girdle: Contraction of muscles that support lower abdomen and back.

Intervertebral disc: Layer of fibrocartilage between vertebrae of the back (backbones); acts as cushion.

Leverage: Use of firm structure (lever) to change direction and motion of object.

Line of gravity: An imaginary line going straight down from the center of gravity.

Load: Weight of an object or person.

Momentum: Force of motion acquired by a moving object.

Stability: Steadiness of position.

Transfer: Move.

2   Spend time in a skills laboratory practicing the various movements described in this chapter. Follow the instructions very carefully and repeat them until you can do them automatically. It is very important that you become highly skilled at using effective body mechanics for your own safety and the safety of people in your care.

3   Take notice of how you feel when you are taking your turn at being the person moved or lifted during your practice sessions. Are you anxious or afraid? Do you feel confident that the person moving or lifting you is strong enough and skilled enough? Do you fear being dropped? Consideration of these questions will help you understand how people you move in nursing situations may feel and enable you to plan sensitive care. Remember that people you care for in nursing situations will be even more anxious than you will be because of their disability, pain, or discomfort.

4   Become familiar with the various equipment described in this chapter (e.g., Surgilift, Hoyer mechanical lifts). Practice until you are thoroughly skilled at their operation before using them with anyone in a nursing situation. Supervised learning is essential for the safe use of this equipment.

5   Take a turn being the person moved by various mechanical lifts. How did it feel? Were you anxious? Did you feel confident in the helper's ability to manage the equipment? Did you have any physical sensations as you were being lifted? Consideration of these questions will help you understand how the people you move may feel and enable you to plan sensitive care. Remember that people requiring the help of mechanical lifts in health care situations will be more anxious than you will be because of their physical helplessness.

6   Become conscious of effective body mechanics and apply them to all your movements. En-

deavor to make effective body mechanics automatic to all your movements wherever you are.

GUIDELINES FOR CORRECT BODY MECHANICS

Correct Body <u>Alignment</u> (<u>Posture</u>)

Body alignment is the proper relationship of body parts to one another. Correct body alignment is important for proper body functioning, reduces strain, and helps maintain balance. When standing in correct alignment (Fig. 11–1) the:
- *Back is straight,* curves of the spine are not exaggerated
- *Head is erect,* not leaning forward, backward, or sideways
- *Chin is tucked in,* not jutting forward
- *Arms are at sides with elbows slightly flexed*
- Lower abdominal area is pulled up and in
- Knees are slightly flexed
- Toes point forward

It is important to practice proper body alignment yourself and demonstrate it to others. Also, it is essential to position those people in your care in proper body alignment. To do so, you must know the correct positioning of body parts.

Guidelines for Effective Body Movements

Effective movement of the body occurs if you follow relatively simple basic guidelines, such as:
- *Plan your movements.* Think about them in advance.
- *Be realistic about the amount of weight you can safely move,* e.g., lift.
- *Assess the amount of assistance the person you are helping can give you during a planned movement.*
- *Maintain a broad "base of support,"* i.e., foundation.
- *Keep your "center of gravity" low,* i.e., heaviest part of your body.
- *Have the "line of gravity" (imaginary line going straight down from the center of gravity) pass through your base of support.*
- *Use smooth and rhythmic movements.*
- *Use leverage to increase the efficiency of the energy you use.*
- *Move in a straight direction.*
- *Use large muscle groups.*
- *Use the "internal girdle of support."*
- *Use pulling or pushing rather than lifting movements when possible.*

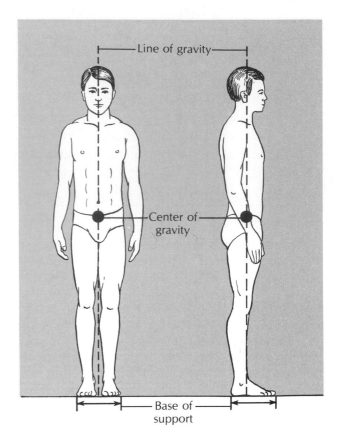

FIGURE 11–1 Correct body alignment. Note: Line of gravity passes through base of support.

- *Keep the load being moved close to your center of gravity.*
- *Use your entire hand, rather than just your fingers.*

The above guidelines are discussed below with examples. It is important that you understand each guideline. Be certain to practice what is discussed. Also, think of additional examples for each guideline.
- *Plan your movements.* Before beginning, assess the situation and determine the best (i.e., safest, most efficient, most comfortable) method of movement. Explain to the person you are assisting: (a) what you are planning to do, and (b) why the move is necessary and what the person can do to help. Listen to the person's suggestions about the move and follow them whenever possible. Provide time to think about the move. Do not hurry unless in an emergency situation. When working with other care providers: (a) identify one of you to be the "leader" (movements are more coordinated when directed by one person); (b) the

leader clarifies what each of you will do during the planned movement, e.g., "Mary, you lift the feet"; (c) let the person being moved participate in the planning; and (d) follow the leader's directions, e.g., "1-2-3-*lift.*" Thus, the move is safe for everyone, it is coordinated, and everyone begins the movement at the same time.

- *Be realistic about the amount of weight you can safely move,* e.g., lift. Be aware of your personal abilities, muscle strengths, and limitations. Assess these factors in relation to the size and weight of each person or object you plan to move. Assess every situation carefully. Determine: (a) the number of people needed to safely and correctly move the person or object, and (b) if mechanical assistance will be helpful, and if so, what type.

- *Assess the amount of assistance the person you are helping can give you during a planned movement.* Assess the movement abilities, strengths, and limitations of the individual you are planning to assist or move.

Participating in movements is usually safer for the individual and the care providers. It also gives the person a sense of personal control.

> Let people move themselves as much as possible. They know what hurts and you do not. They can protect themselves from pain better than you can.

Carefully describe planned moves to the person. Discuss exactly how she/he can participate. Consider the person's suggestions and preferences concerning the move and integrate them into your plans whenever possible.

- *Maintain a broad "base of support."* A person's (or object's) *stability,* i.e., steadiness of position, increases as his/her (its) base of support increases. For example, when you are standing, your base of support is the distance between your feet. Your stability is greater when your feet are spread some distance apart rather than being close together. Thus, when helping a person move up in bed, you can increase your stability by moving your feet apart. This gives you a broad base of support.

Comprehending?   Yes ＿＿   No ＿＿

• VOCABULARY CHECK

Directions.   Below are 10 words taken from the key words section of this chapter. Circle the letter of the best definition from the four choices.

1 Biomechanics
   a the study of biology as applied to the laws of nature
   b the application of mechanical laws to living structures
   c mechanical plants or animals; robotics
   d the study of machines and mechanical laws governing them

2 Gravity
   a weight
   b weightlessness
   c imaginary force
   d a sinking object

3 Discs
   a the backbone
   b a rupture
   c circular flat plates
   d the spine

4 Stability
  a changing conditions
  b the strength to endure
  c the inability to endure
  d a plan of action

5 Posture
  a a mental attitude
  b an attitude of the body
  c problems with the back
  d deviation of the spine

6 Colleagues
  a close relatives
  b casual friends
  c professional associates
  d enduring enemies

7 Psychosocial
  a pertaining to the inability to socialize
  b pertaining to psychic and social elements
  c pertaining to pathological social behavior
  d pertaining to attempts of the mentally ill to seek peers

8 Friction
  a a head-on collision of two vehicles
  b an argument that is easily resolved
  c the rubbing of one body against another
  d a pressure point painful to the touch

9 Vertebrae
  a segments of the spine
  b injuries to the spine
  c segments of the body
  d broken bones

10 Fulcrum
  a support to the spine
  b support to a lever
  c emotional support
  d a psychological crutch

• SUMMARY

Reading a textbook is different from reading books for pleasure. Learn to survey your textbooks. Survey the title page, preface, table of contents, glossary, appendix, and index. Becoming familiar with your text as a whole helps you to get ready to learn the information in each chapter. You can learn the specific strategies that will help you to concentrate on, comprehend, and retain textbook information. These strategies are:

- Previewing
- Questioning
- Summarizing

After reading, underline the main ideas and details you want to remember. Write a summary or outline to use as a study guide. Study all underlined text material, summaries, outlines, and end-of-chapter review questions. Design and take your own practice test.

These active reading strategies will ensure your success in reading nursing textbooks.

• Chapter 12 •

Graphic Aids

OBJECTIVE

KEY WORDS

WHY READ GRAPHIC AIDS?

HOW GRAPHIC AIDS RELATE TO THE WRITTEN TEXT

TYPES OF GRAPHIC AIDS

    Graphs

    Pictures

    Tables

    Diagrams

HOW TO READ GRAPHIC AIDS

TESTING FOR UNDERSTANDING

VOCABULARY CHECK

SUMMARY

• OBJECTIVE

To develop techniques for reading and studying graphs, pictures, tables, and diagrams.

• KEY WORDS

Pay attention to the following key words, which are underscored the first time they appear in this chapter. Try to determine the meaning of these words in the passage. If you need further help, use your dictionary or the glossary in the back of this book.

Look up the medical terminology in your medical dictionary or the glossary. As you read the exercises in this chapter, write additional words you need to learn in the space provided.

MEDICAL TERMINOLOGY	GENERAL VOCABULARY
cal/day	captions
development	concise
gout	enhances
immobility	expedient
nutrition	footnotes
postoperative	graphic
pulse	legends
receptive	potential
thrombus	statistics
vital signs	systematic
_____	_____
_____	_____
_____	_____

• WHY READ GRAPHIC AIDS?

Many students skip over visual materials such as graphs, pictures, tables, and diagrams. It is tempting to look for ways to shorten textbook assignments, but ignoring the visual materials in your nursing textbooks will undermine your efforts to succeed in your studies.

Nursing textbooks are filled with visual materials. These graphs, pictures, tables, and diagrams contain visual information that is pertinent to your understanding the main ideas in a chapter. Furthermore, when you interpret this visual information and paraphrase the ideas in language you understand, you will remember this material. Therefore visual aids serve to improve your:

• Concentration, by visually attracting your attention
• Comprehension, by your interpreting the visual information into verbal language
• Retention, by reinforcing your memory when you learn information visually and verbally

Graphic materials are designed to be clear and accurate so they will help you learn unfamiliar concepts.

Be aware of the help you receive from graphic aids and focus on these materials to help you learn the information in your nursing textbooks.

• HOW GRAPHIC AIDS RELATE TO THE WRITTEN TEXT

Graphic aids make it easier to understand and read the written text. Below are pages copied from a nursing book (Arnold and Boggs, pp. 385–386). Carefully read the text describing the four steps in the advocacy process. Then study Table 12–1. Note especially how the table summarizes, in an easy to read format, the main points of the written text.

TABLE 12–1 Informational Steps in Client Advocacy

Knowledge of the personally held values of nurse and client.

Awareness of treatment, professional, and personal goals.

Information about professional-nursing, environmental and interpersonal protocols, and the bureaucratic structure of the organizational work system.

Knowledge of potential power or recognition needs that could compromise the integrity of the client advocacy process.

• **EXAMPLE 12–1** •

STEPS IN THE ADVOCACY PROCESS

The client advocate pleads or urges the cause of the client based on the four-step informational process presented in Table 12–1.

The first step is for the nurse to learn what is necessary to become an advocate in a specific nursing situation, for the nurse's power base in advocacy is relevant knowledge and information. Basically, the nurse needs to be aware of personal and professional ethics, values, and prejudices. One needs to have a good knowledge and understanding of personal views on "how human beings relate to each other in a framework or philosophy of fairness." For example, if the nurse thinks of elderly clients as helpless and equates aging with being taken care of, then the nurse will be likely to "take charge" of all client health activities, even those the client is still quite capable of performing with little or no assistance. In this situation, personal values have gotten in the way of individualized nursing values associated with client advocacy.

Nurses should have a firm understanding of their personal as well as professional goals in a nursing situation. Frequently, both of these goals are unstated and remain a part of the blind self until called into conscious awareness by circumstance. For example, the nurse may have an unstated personal goal of wanting to be liked by every client or an unspoken professional goal of never making a mistake in the delivery of clinical nursing care. Each implied goal will have as much effect on the nurse's interpersonal behaviors with clients and co-workers as an articulated professional goal of wanting to learn the latest tracheal suction technique.

To be successful as client advocates, nurses also need to know the environmental, interpersonal, and bureaucratic system within which they work, for example, how all the units—nursing and hospital administration, the medical staff, and other health-system disciplines—relate to one another as well as how the system relates to the community at large. It is important to understand how the communication flow filters through the different systems. Usually a combination of formal and informal communication with other staff is necessary for complete understanding.

The new nurse can gain some of this knowledge by observing how communication is passed from person to person and by asking many questions. Knowing how the various units are influenced by outside pressures such as politics, financial constraints, consumer groups, and regulatory agencies is as important as knowing who is in charge and who is influential in facilitating change. All of these understandings add to the nurse's power base in effecting change on the client's behalf. With this knowledge base, the nurse is in a position to accurately inform and assist the client in making the most of health-care choices with the least amount of effort expended.

Finally, the nurse needs to recognize personal power needs within the self that stem from personal insecurities and to analyze how those needs affect professional relationships with clients. To a greater or lesser extent, everyone has power needs and insecurities. The important thing is to recognize their presence. Real interpersonal power comes from having an adequate knowledge base coupled with the courage to take interpersonal risks when the situation requires it.

Comprehending?   Yes ___   No ___

Thus, one major way graphic aids relate to the written text is by summarizing concisely the major points of the selection. Graphic aids make the textbook more comprehensible.

Graphic aids actually save you time in reading. Instead of writing a lengthy description of a concept, the author may choose to use a graphic aid.

Following are pages taken from a nursing book (Arnold and Boggs, pp. 408–409). Pay attention to how the writer introduces an important idea with a graphic aid rather than writing about it at length.

• EXAMPLE 12–2 •

UNDERSTANDING THE ORGANIZATIONAL SYSTEM

Whenever one works in an organization, either as a student or professional, one automatically becomes a part of an organizational system with established political norms of acceptable behavior. Each organizational system defines its own chain of command and rules about social processes in professional communication. Even though your idea may be excellent, failure to understand the chain of command or an unwillingness to form the positive alliances needed to accomplish your objective dilutes the impact on the receiver. For example, if your instructor has been defined as your first line of contact, then it is not in your best interest to seek out staff personnel or other students without also checking with the instructor. Although side-stepping the identified chain of command and going to a higher or more tangential resource in the hierarchy may appear less threatening initially, the benefits of such action may not resolve the difficulty, and the trust needed for serious discussion becomes limited. Some of the reasons for avoiding positive alliances are part of an internal circular process of faulty thinking. Because communication is viewed as part of a system's process, the sender and receiver act on the

TABLE 12–2 Examples of Circular Processes That Block the Development of Cooperative and Receptive Influence Skills

---

Low Self-Disclosure

therefore	→	I don't share my real thoughts, feelings, or needs, and I hide my weaknesses.	→ therefore
↑			↓
I think others would despise me if they knew my weaknesses and I have a low opinion of my inner wishes, dreams and needs.			Others see me as cold, rational, self-sufficient, and as needing little they might be able to give.
↑		Others don't give me sympathy, support, or help or indicate to me that they might be receptive to my needs, weaknesses, and feelings.	↓
therefore ←			← therefore

Unwillingness to Delegate Tasks

therefore	→	I don't believe that others have the energy, drive, commitment, and ability I have	→ therefore
↑			↓
The others withhold energy, commitment, and the full use of their skills in the work.			I communicate mistrust of others' energy, commitment, and ability.
↑		The others feel undervalued, mistrusted, and unappreciated.	↓
therefore ←			← therefore

Overuse of Pressure

therefore	→	I push very hard to get others to accept my ideas, opinions and proposals.	→ therefore
↑			↓
I feel that if I am to make any impact on such resistant people, I must push very hard.			Others feel threatened, believing that if they give an inch, I will dominate and exploit them.
↑		The others resist my ideas and opinions, or they withdraw into passive, unresponsive silence.	↓
therefore ←			← therefore

Overstating Demands

therefore	→	I demand more from others than they feel is reasonable. I always ask for more than I expect to receive.	→ therefore
↑			↓
I feel the others are ungiving, and I must always press for more than I expect to receive.			Others see me as demanding, exploitative, and an unreasonably hard bargainer.
↑		Others resist or withdraw and try to give as little as possible.	↓
therefore ←			← therefore

© 1981. From *The Positive Power and Influence Program,* First Edition, Copyright by Situation Management Systems, Inc., Hanover, Massachusetts, USA. Used by permission.

information received, which may or may not represent the reality of the situation. Examples of the circular processes that block the development of cooperative and receptive influencing skills in organizational settings are presented in Table 12–2.

Often a person is not directly aware of these personal communication blocks in professional relationships. Asking for feedback, self-reflection, and an honest appraisal of personal communication strategies in professional situations help the nurse actualize potential communicative power.

As you can see, it is much more expedient (faster and easier) to look at Table 12–3, "Examples of Circular Processes That Block the Development of Cooperative and Receptive Influence Skills," than to read the many pages it would take to describe the same information. Graphic aids make the textbook easier to read. Rather than ignoring graphic aids when you read your chapters, you should get in the habit of consulting them to make your reading clearer and ultimately faster.

• TYPES OF GRAPHIC AIDS

When looking through your nursing textbooks, you have probably noticed the many varieties of graphic aids. Indeed, it would be hard to find a page without at least one. However, a careful examination would show that they are primarily of four types: graphs, pictures, tables, and diagrams.

• Graphs

Graphs readily show a comparison between two or more facts or items. Look at Figure 12–1 and notice how males and females, whites and others, are being compared in terms of life expectancy in the twentieth century.

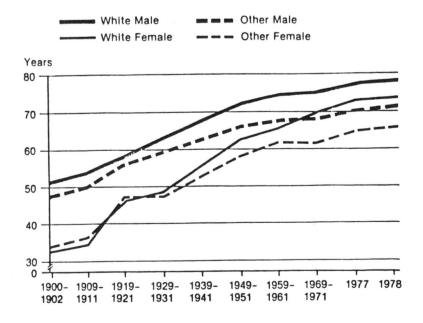

FIGURE 12–1 Changing life expectancy during the twentieth century. (From Allan, C., and Brotman, H. [compilers]: Chartbook on aging in America. Prepared for 1981 White House Conference on Aging, U.S. Government Publication, p. 9.)

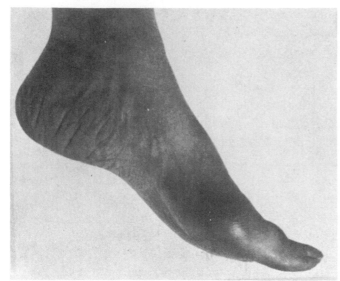

FIGURE 12–2 Acute gouty arthritis involving the first metatarsophalangeal joint (great toe) (podagra). (From Wyngaarden, J.B., and Smith, L.H. [eds.]: Cecil textbook of medicine, ed. 17, Philadelphia, 1985, W.B. Saunders, p. 1137.)

• Pictures

The purpose of pictures is to help you visualize what is being described in the written text. They are included not only to illustrate a major point, but also to add interest to what you are reading. Consider the following example (Matteson and McConnell, p. 187). Note how the picture of acute gouty arthritis enhances the written words (Fig. 12–2).

• EXAMPLE 12–4 •

• GOUTY ARTHRITIS

Gout is characterized by episodes of acute arthritis, followed by chronic damage to joints and other structures. The disease tends to run in families and is seen primarily in middle-aged men. It is rarely seen before the age of 30, and studies have shown that the highest incidence occurs in the thirties, forties, and fifties.

Hyperuricemia, an excess of uric acid in the blood and tissues, is the major cause of gout. Increased serum uric acid levels are related either to increased formation of uric acid or decreased excretion of uric acid. Other related factors include sex, age, genetic factors, obesity, higher social class and intelligence, indulgence in alcohol, and high plasma lipid levels. When hyperuricemia is due principally to an inherited metabolic abnormality, the condition is called _primary gout;_ when it is due to acquired disease or some environmental factor, it is known as _secondary gout._ Primary gout

is seen primarily in men; however, men and women are equally affected by secondary gout.

An acute attack of gouty arthritis is an inflammatory reaction resulting from the presence of sodium urate crystals within a joint. It most often occurs in the great toe, which is affected in 50 per cent of the cases. Acute gout also may appear in other joints, mainly in the periphery, such as the feet and ankles, hands, knees, and elbows. Precipitating factors are loss of body weight, high-fat diet, ingestion of certain drugs (penicillin, thiamine chloride, vitamin B_{12}, insulin, folic acid, sulfa, ergotamine tartrate, and mercurial and thiazide diuretics), joint trauma, emotional turmoil, surgery, or overindulgence in food or alcohol.

Each acute episode lasts for a short period of time and is followed by intervals during which there is freedom from symptoms. Some people have only one or two attacks during their lifetime, while others may have repeated occurrences of increasing duration, severity, and frequency with multiple joint involvement. The affected joint becomes reddened, tender, swollen, and hot (Fig. 12–2). Individuals may have a sensation of discomfort that, over a period of hours, develops into excruciating pain. Larger joints, such as the knee, may have accumulations of inflammatory effusion. Chalky deposits of urate (tophi) form around joints and areas associated with cartilage, such as the ear: in the elderly, tophi are prone to infection.

Diagnosis is made by means of clinical presentation, serum uric acid levels, identification of uric acid crystals in aspirated synovial fluid, examination of tophi, and radiographs. Serum uric acid levels are elevated to 8 to 10 mg per 100 ml in gouty arthritis as opposed to normal levels of 7 mg per 100 ml. Treatment for an initial acute attack is with colchicine, which is 95 per cent effective in providing symptomatic relief. This drug also can provide diagnostic confirmation of the disease. Prophylactic management usually consists of colchicine 0.5 mg. and Benemid (probenemid) 0.5 mg every day, weight loss, restriction of foods high in purines (liver, kidney, sweetbreads), and a high fluid intake; however, treatment of asymptomatic hyperuricemia with uric acid-lowering agents is rarely necessary. The drugs must be used judiciously in the elderly because they tend to experience toxicity and adverse reactions.

• Tables

The function of tables is to present data (statistics, facts, or numbers) in a systematic way for efficient reading and studying. In Table 12–3, see how the table is organized into columns and headings. Make sure you read all title and column headings. Try to see the relationships among the data given.

• Diagrams

Diagrams summarize information that, if written in words, would be lengthy and complicated. From Figure 12–3, try to imagine what it would be like to have to read the same information presented in text form.

Regardless of the different types of graphic aids you may encounter in your nursing textbook, they all serve a similar purpose—to present, in an interesting, concise, and visual way, information that would otherwise be given in long and complicated written text.

Comprehending? Yes ____ No ____

• HOW TO READ GRAPHIC AIDS

1 Look over the graphic aid to get a general impression of the visual material.

2 Read the title carefully to determine the subject of the graphic aid.

3 Pay close attention to:
   Headings—titles found above a graphic aid
   Legends—symbols that explain a graphic aid
   Captions—an explanation accompanying a graphic aid
   Footnotes—an explanatory note found below a graphic aid
   Keys—information used to interpret a graphic aid

4 Determine the purpose of the graphic aid. For example, ask yourself, "What is being compared?"

TABLE 12–3 Recommended Daily Dietary Allowances for Adults* as Revised in 1980 (Designed for the Maintenance of Good Nutrition of Practically All Healthy People in the United States)

NUTRIENT	MEN			WOMEN		
	23-50 YR, 2700 KCAL (RANGE 2200-3000)	51-75 YR, 2400 KCAL (RANGE 2000-2800)	76+ YR, 2050 KCAL (RANGE 1650-2450)	23-50 YR, 2000 KCAL (RANGE 1600-2400)	51-75 YR, 1800 KCAL (RANGE 1400-2200)	76+ YR, 1600 KCAL (RANGE 1200-2000)
Protein, g	56	56	56	56	44	44
Vitamin A, g RE†	5000	1000	1000	4000	800	800
Vitamin D, g		5	5		5	5
Vitamin E, mg a-TE‡	15	10	10	12	8	8
Vitamin C, mg	45	60	60	45	60	60
Thiamine, mg	1.4	1.2	1.2	1	1	1
Riboflavin, mg	1.6	1.4	1.4	1.2	1.2	1.2
Niacin, mg NE§	18	16	16	13	13	13
Vitamin B_6, mg	2	2.2	2.2	2	2	2
Folacin, g	400	400	400	400	400	400
Vitamin B_{12}, mg	3	3	3	3	3	3
Calcium, mg	800	800	800	800	800	800
Phosphorus, mg	800	800	800	800	800	800
Magnesium, mg	350	350	350	300	300	300
Iron, mg	10	10	10	18	10	10
Zinc, mg	15	15	15	15	15	15
Iodine, g	130	150	150	100	150	150

From Recommended Daily Dietary Allowances, 9th rev ed (1980). The National Academy of Sciences, Washington, D.C.
*For men, the average height was 70 inches and the average weight 154 pounds (70 kg). For women, the average height was 64 inches and the average weight 120 pounds (55 kg).
†Retinol equivalents.
‡Alphatocopherol equivalents.
§Niacin equivalent = 1 mg niacin or 60 mg dietary tryptophan.

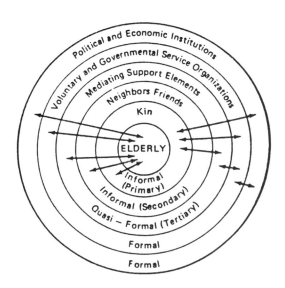

FIGURE 12–3 Schematic model of the social support system of the elderly. (From Cantor, M.: Neighbors and friends: an overlooked resource in the informal support system. Paper presented at the symposium: Natural Support Systems for the Elderly: Current Research Implications for Policy, 30th Annual Meeting of the Gerontological Society, San Francisco, 1977. Reprinted in Cantor, M., and Little, V.: Aging and social care. In Binstock, R. and Shanas, H. [eds.]: Handbook of aging and the social sciences, ed. 2, New York, 1985, Van Nostrand Reinhold, p. 748.)

5 Examine the units of measurement.

6 Ask:

   a What information is given in this graphic aid?

   b How does this information relate to the ideas discussed in the chapter?

   c How does this graphic aid add to or clarify the ideas discussed in the chapter?

7 Try to make a general statement that relates the graphic aid to the ideas covered in the text.

Figure 12–4 is an example that shows you how to read and interpret a graphic aid.

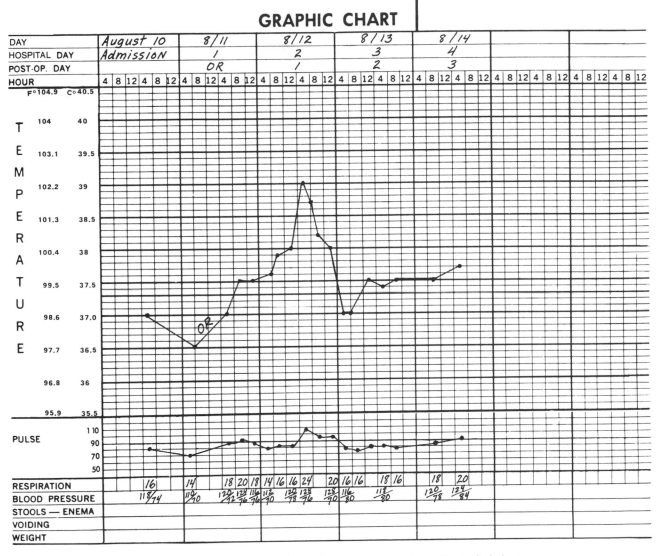

FIGURE 12–4 Sample of a vital signs graphic sheet. Note vital signs when this person has a fever on first postoperative day. Also note increased frequency of measurement as nurse suspects a developing trend. (From Sorensen, K.C., and Luckmann, J.: Basic nursing: a psychophysiological approach, ed. 2, Philadelphia, 1986, W.B. Saunders, p. 547.)

• EXAMPLE 12–7 •

1   What is the subject of the graph? _____
    (a vital signs graphic sheet)

2   What is being compared? _____
    (vital signs and time)

3   How is the temperature listed? _____
    (°F and °C)

4   List the <u>vital signs</u> that are being examined. _____
    (body temperature, <u>pulse</u>, blood pressure, respiration)

5   What is the person's body temperature (°F) on the second <u>postoperative</u>
    day? _____
    (102.2°)

6   Why is this graph included in a chapter titled, "Assessing Pulse, Respi-
    ration and Blood Pressure"? _____
    (to give a visual representation of the concepts in the chapter)

• EXERCISE 12–1 •

Directions.   Read and study the following graphic aid (Fig. 12–5). Answer the
questions and write your answers in the space provided.

1   What is the subject of this picture? _____

2   How many people are in the picture? _____

3   Who are the people? _____

4   What does the equipment suggest? _____

5   What impact does this picture have? _____

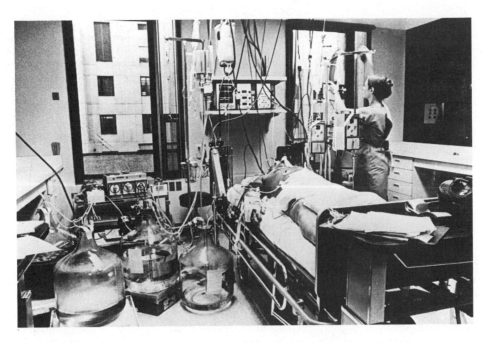

FIGURE 12–5 Intensive care units are very prone to producing sensory overload in people receiving care because of the extra equipment sounds, and people (see text for discussion).

• EXERCISE 12–2 •

Directions. Read and study the following graphic aid (Table 12–4). Answer the questions and write your answers in the space provided.

1 What is the title of this table? _____

2 What ages are discussed in the table? _____

3 At what age is good nutrition 1400 cal/day? _____

4 At what age should a child learn how to cross streets safely? _____

5 What factors of a child's development are examined in this table? _____

TABLE 12–4 Summary of Normal Play-Age Growth and Development

AGE (YEARS)	PHYSICAL COMPETENCY	INTELLECTUAL COMPETENCY	EMOTIONAL-SOCIAL COMPETENCY

General 3-5	Gains 4½ kg (10 lb)
	Grows 15 cm (6 in)
	20 teeth present
	Nutritional require-ments:
	  Energy: 1250-1600 cal/day
	  Fluid: 100 ml/kg/day
	  Protein: 30 gm/day
	  Iron: 10 mg/day
		Becomes aware of self and others
		Vocabulary increases from 900-1200 words
		Piaget's preoperational/intuitive period
			Freud's phallic stage
			  Oedipus complex—boy
			  Electra complex—girl
			Erikson's Initiative vs. Guilt

3	Runs, stops suddenly Walks backwards Jumps: broad jump Pedals tricycle Undresses self Unbuttons front buttons Feeds self well	Knows own sex Desires to please Sense of humor Language-900 words Follows simple direction Uses plurals Names figure in picture Uses adjectives/adverbs	Shifts between reality and imagination Bedtime rituals Negativism decreases Animism and realism: anything that moves is alive
4	Runs well, skips Hops on one foot Heel-toe walks Up and down steps without holding Jumps well Dresses and undresses Buttons well, needs help with zippers, bows Brushes teeth Bathes self Draws with some form and meaning	More aware of others Uses alibis to excuse behavior Bossy Language-1500 words Talks in sentences Knows nursery rhymes Counts to 5 Highly imaginative Name calling	Focuses on present Egocentrism/unable to see the viewpoint of others, unable to understand another's inability to see his/her viewpoint Does not comprehend anticipatory explanation Sexual curiosity Oedipus complex Electra complex
5	Runs skillfully Jumps 3-4 steps Jumps rope, hops, skips Begins dance Roller skates Dresses without assist Ties shoelaces Hits nail on head with hammer Draws man-6 parts Prints first name	Aware of cultural differences Knows name and address More independent More sensible/less imaginative Copies triangle, draws rectangle Knows four or more colors Language-2100 words, meaningful sentences Understands kinship Counts to 10	Continues in egocentrism Fantasy and daydreams Resolution of Oedipus/Electra complex, girls identify with mother, boys with father Body image and body boundary especially important in illness Shows tension in nail-biting, nose-picking, whining, snuffling

Adapted from Tackett, J.J.M., and Hunsberger, M.: *Family-Centered Care of Children and Adolescents: Nursing Concepts in Child Health.* Philadelphia: W.B. Saunders Co., 1981, pp. 912-913.

In Sorensen, K.C., and Luckmann, J.: Basic nursing: a psychophysiological approach, ed. 2, Philadelphia, 1986, W.B. Saunders, p. 283.

NUTRITION	PLAY	SAFETY
Carbohydrate intake approximately 40-50% of calories	Reading books is important at all ages	Never leave alone in bath or swimming pool
Good food sources of essential vitamins and minerals	Balance highly physical activities with quiet times	Keep poisons in locked cupboard; learn what household things are poisonous
Regular tooth brushing	Quiet rest period takes the place of nap time	Use car seats and seatbelts
Parents are seen as examples; if Daddy won't eat it, child won't	Provide sturdy play materials	Never leave child alone in car
		Remove doors from abandoned freezers and refrigerators
1250 cal/day	Participates in simple games	Teach safety habits early
Due to increased sex identity and imitation, copies parents at table and will eat what they eat	Cooperates, takes turns	Let water out of bathtub; don't stand in tub
	Plays with group	Caution against climbing in unsafe areas, onto or under cars, unsafe buildings, drainage pipes
	Uses scissors, paper	
	Likes crayons, coloring books	
Different colors and shapes of foods can increase interest	Enjoys being read to and "reading"	
	Plays "dress-up" and "house"	Insist on seatbelts worn at all times in cars
	Likes fire engines	
Good nutrition	Longer attention span with group activities	Teach to stay out of streets, alleys
1400 cal/day		
Nutritious between-meal snacks essential	"Dress-up" with more dramatic play	Continually teach safety; child understands
Emphasis on quality not quantity of food eaten	Draws, pounds, paints	Teach how to handle scissors
Mealtime should be enjoyable, not for criticism	Likes to make paper chains, sewing cards	Teach what are poisons and why to avoid
As dexterity improves, neatness increases	Scrapbooks	Never allow child to stand in moving car
	Likes being read to, records and rhythmic play	
	"Helps" adults	
Good nutrition	Plays with trucks, cars	Teach child how to cross streets safely
1600 cal/day	Plays with guns, soldiers	Teach child to not speak to strangers or to get into cars of strangers
Encourage regular tooth brushing	Like simple games with letters or numbers	
Encourage quiet time before meals	Much gross motor activity: water, mud, snow, leaves, rocks	Insist on seatbelts
Can learn to cut own food	Matching picture games	Teach child to swim
Frequent illnesses from increased exposure increases nutritional needs		

TABLE 12–5 Problem List

NO.	PROBLEM	DATE ENTERED	DATE RESOLVED
1	Cholecystitis	1963	1963
2	Pneumonia	1972	1972
3	Fractured left hip	2/2/90	
4	Pain	2/2/90	
5	Impaired physical mobility	2/2/90	
6	Potential for trauma	2/2/90	

From Iyer P.W., et al.: Nursing process and nursing diagnosis, ed. 2, Philadelphia, 1991, W.B. Saunders, p. 200.

• EXERCISE 12–3 •

Directions. Read and study the graphic aid above (Table 12–5). Answer the questions and write your answers in the space provided.

1 What is the title of this table? _____

2 How many items are listed in the table? _____

3 The dates begin in what year? _____

4 How many entries were listed for the date 2/2/90? _____

5 How many problems were resolved? _____

• EXERCISE 12–4 •

Directions. Read and study the following graphic aid (Fig. 12–6). Answer the questions and write your answers in the space provided.

1 What is the subject of the diagram? _____

2 List three physical complications of *immobility.* _____

_____

3 List three psychological complications of immobility. _____

_____

_____

4 Thrombus is pointing to what part of the body? _____

5 What general feeling about this patient do you get from this diagram?

_____

6 List the facts that lead you to this general feeling:

_____

_____

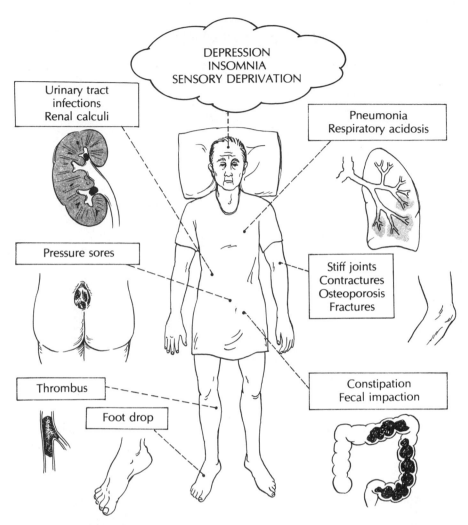

FIGURE 12–6 Some major complications of immobility. (From Sorensen, K.C., and Luckmann, J.: Basic nursing: a psychophysiological approach, ed. 2, Philadelphia, 1986, W.B. Saunders, p. 591.)

• **EXERCISE 12–5** •

Directions. Read and study the following graphic aid (Fig. 12–7). Answer the questions and write your answers in the space provided.

1 What is the title of this graphic aid? _____

2 List the five factors in blocks:

_____

_____

_____

_____

_____

THE NURSING PROCESS

PURPOSES: Maintain health, prevent illness, promote recovery, restore wellness and maximal function, and support in peaceful death

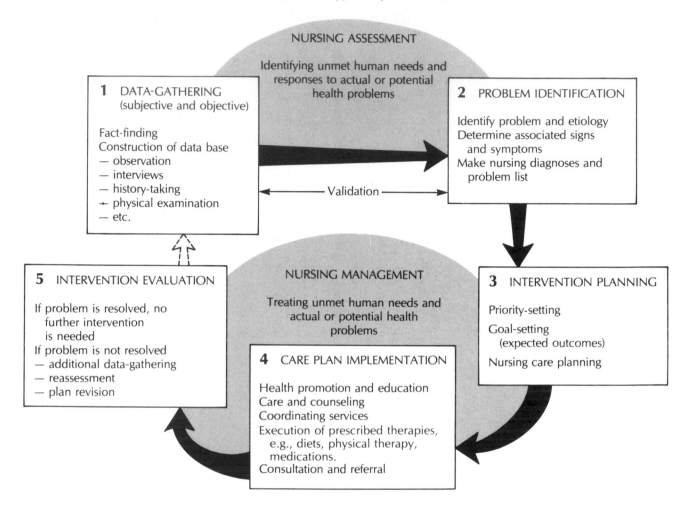

FIGURE 12–7 Diagram of the nursing process. (From Sorensen, K.C., and Luckmann, J.: Basic nursing: a psychophysiological approach, ed. 2, Philadelphia, 1986, W.B. Saunders, inside cover.)

3 What heading is defined as "identifying unmet human needs and responses to actual or <u>potential</u> health problems"?

_____

4 Which block number deals with fact finding? _____

5 Why is this graphic aid on the inside cover of the text?

_____

Comprehending? Yes ____ No ____

• EXERCISE 12–6 •

Directions. Using your own nursing textbook and a separate sheet of paper, copy the format of one graphic aid. Read and study the written text that accompanies this graphic aid. Then fill in as much of the graph, picture, table, or diagram as you remember. When you are finished, check your version with the original. Correct and make changes, if necessary.

• VOCABULARY CHECK

Directions. Below are 10 words taken from the key words section of this chapter. Circle the letter of the best definition from the four choices.

1 Pulse
   a the arteries in which blood flows from the lungs
   b a method of treating heart problems without invading the body
   c damage to the heart because of arterial blockage
   d the beat of the heart as felt through the wall of the arteries

2 Footnotes
   a alphabetized listing of subjects at the back of the text
   b introductory comment or preface
   c the appendix located at the end of the text
   d explanatory notes found at the bottom of the page

3 Postoperative
   a before surgery
   b after surgery
   c during surgery
   d an operation

4 Caption
   a an illustration in a text
   b a design in a journal
   c an addition to a text
   d an explanation accompanying a picture

5 Immobility
   a movement
   b incapacity to be moved
   c a sudden movement
   d ability to move with ease

6 Legend
   a an explanatory list of symbols on a graphic aid
   b the title or heading of a graphic aid
   c a map or chart that acts as a graphic aid
   d the outline or structure of graphic aids

7 Vital signs
   a signs of distress
   b signs of life
   c high temperature
   d respiratory illness

8 Graphic
   a pertaining to a lead substance
   b pertaining to a grape
   c pertaining to a visual representation
   d pertaining to a trauma

9 Gout
   a a clotting disease that affects only males
   b urinary infections brought on by pregnancy
   c a form of arthritis in which uric acid appears in excessive quantities in the blood
   d protein found in the blood

10 Concise
   a brevity of expression
   b expandable
   c elaborately detailed
   d speechless

• SUMMARY

Graphic materials are an important part of your textbook and should not be skipped over. They give you information in a visual form that attracts your attention and holds your concentration. Understanding the visual material and paraphrasing the information into language you comprehend help you to remember the ideas. Graphic aids are easy to read because they are designed to be clear and accurate. When you read graphic aids, focus on the title, all other headings, and descriptions and determine the purpose of the visual aid. Make a general statement that relates the information of the graphic aid to the ideas covered in the chapter. Graphic aids improve your reading concentration, comprehension, and retention. Paying close attention to graphic aids will help you to read your nursing textbooks.

Chapter 13

Active Listening

OBJECTIVE

KEY WORDS

QUESTIONS TO THINK ABOUT BEFORE READING

NEED FOR ACTIVE LISTENING

LISTENING PROBLEMS

STRATEGIES FOR ACTIVE LISTENING

HINTS ON IMPROVING YOUR LISTENING AND NOTE TAKING

BENEFITS OF ACTIVE LISTENING

VOCABULARY CHECK

SUMMARY

• OBJECTIVE

To learn how to become an active listener so that you will concentrate on and comprehend your instructors' lectures.

• KEY WORDS

Pay attention to the following key words, which are underscored the first time they appear in this chapter. Try to determine the meaning of these words from the surrounding words in the passage. If you need further help, use your dictionary or the glossary in the back of this book.

As you read the exercises in this chapter, write additional words you need to learn in the space provided.

GENERAL VOCABULARY

block	impression	preceding	_____
controversial	initial	subjective	_____
deciphered	passive	synonymous	_____
imperative			_____

• QUESTIONS TO THINK ABOUT BEFORE READING

1   Do you daydream during class lectures?   Yes _____   No _____

2   Do you sometimes pretend to pay attention   Yes _____   No _____
    during class?

3   Do you attempt to write every word instead   Yes _____   No _____
    of listening for your instructor's main points?

4   Do you turn off subjects or speakers without   Yes _____   No _____
    giving them a chance?

5   Are you easily distracted?   Yes _____   No _____

• NEED FOR ACTIVE LISTENING

If you've answered yes to the preceding questions, you need to improve your skills in active listening. Many people think that listening is synonymous with hearing, but there is an important difference. Listening involves comprehension. An active listener concentrates on and reacts to a speaker's message. Hearing, on the other hand is passive. The sounds are heard, but they are not deciphered into information that is understood.

When you are listening to an instructor's information during your nursing class lectures, you need to be an active listener. You must pay attention during class lectures because you will be responsible for knowing these facts when you take your exams.

• LISTENING PROBLEMS

Unfortunately, many students have listening problems that interfere with their ability to get the most out of their classroom lectures. Do you have any of the following listening problems?

___ • *Daydreaming.* Your mind wanders during the lecture. You then try to jump back in. You've probably missed several important facts. Daydreaming is the most common listening problem. You daydream because your mind works faster than the speaker can talk. In this chapter you will learn strategies to use this extra mental time to focus on a person's ideas, rather than letting your mind wander.

___ • *Pretending attention.* You are pretending to pay attention in class, but you are really mentally asleep behind open eyes. This is even worse than daydreaming because you are missing all the information and you are not fooling your instructor. Your instructor knows from your blank expression that you are not concentrating. An active listener reacts to a speaker's ideas. The facial muscles move.

___ • *Rote note taking.* You can think faster than a speaker can talk, but you can't write as fast as the speaker can talk. If you try to write every word, without thinking about what is being said, you will end up with unfinished sentences. This is a listening problem because you are not focusing on the most important information. Concentrate on writing the most important main ideas and details.

___ • *Closing off the subject or speaker*. We are all <u>subjective</u>. However, if you make up your mind before your class begins that you find the information too <u>controversial</u> or difficult or the subject or speaker boring, you may tune out. If you refuse to listen during class, you are preventing yourself from learning. Your task, as a nursing student, is to concentrate on and comprehend your instructor's information. Learn to put your <u>initial impression</u> aside. Be open to receiving your instructor's message and you will be successful when you take your exams.

___ • *Giving in to distractions*. All students have a tendency to let external noises and events distract them during class lectures. However, it is up to you, the listener, to <u>block</u> out these distractions and concentrate on your instructor's main ideas. Using external distractions as an excuse for losing attention will only result in a loss of information.

• EXERCISE 13–1 •

Directions.   Reread the list of five listening problems. Place a check next to any listening problem that affects you.

• STRATEGIES FOR ACTIVE LISTENING

Now that you are aware of your listening problems, you can try to correct them. Apply the following strategies for active listening:
- Listen for the main idea. Ask yourself, "What is the most important point of the lecture?"
- Listen for major details. Ask yourself, "Which facts support the main idea?"
- Paraphrase the information. Put the information in your own words. Summarize by asking yourself the 5 W questions:
Who or What?
What Happened?
When?
Where?
Why or How?

• EXERCISE 13–2 •

Directions.   Apply the strategies for active listening to your next classroom lecture. Fill in the following information.

1 List any listening problems that you had during the lecture:

_____

_____

_____

_____

2 Write how you tried to correct any of your listening problems.

_____

_____

_____

_____

• HINTS ON IMPROVING YOUR LISTENING

You can be actively involved in improving your listening skills. Focus attention on the speaker by looking directly at your instructor. Ask questions and listen for the answers. Sit in front of the room if you have trouble seeing, hearing, or concentrating. Be aware of your body language. Sit up straight. Slouching in your chair makes it easier for you to fall mentally asleep. Evaluate the instructor's information. Do you agree? Disagree? *React!* Focus on the subject.

• RELATIONSHIP BETWEEN ACTIVE LISTENING AND NOTE TAKING

Study skills research indicates that successful students take good notes. It is imperative to be an active listener to take effective notes. Applying active listening strategies will help you to take good notes.

- Listen for your instructor's main ideas.
- Pay attention to key words that signal important ideas.
- Mentally summarize the information, then write an outline or summary that includes all main ideas and major details.
- Pay extra attention to the beginning and end of your classroom lectures; that's when important points are introduced and summarized.

• BENEFITS OF ACTIVE LISTENING

Use your active listening strategies to help you concentrate on and comprehend the main points discussed in your nursing class lectures. Active listening will help you to improve your grades in nursing school. You will:

- Get more out of class lectures.
- Take better notes.
- Be an active participant in your nursing studies.
- Be actively involved in your success in nursing school.

• VOCABULARY CHECK

Directions. Below are 10 words taken from the key words section of this chapter. Circle the letter of the best definition from the four choices.

1 Preceding
  a coming after
  b coming before
  c following
  d returning

2 Synonymous
  a when words have opposite meanings
  b when words have similar spelling
  c when words have the same or similar meanings
  d when words sound the same but have different meanings

3 Passive
  a active   **c** inactive
  b involved   **d** bored

4 Deciphered
  a interpreted a foreign language
  b figured out the meaning of something obscure
  c repeated information without comprehension
  d decoded a new language

5 Subjective
  a pertaining to a neutral position
  b influenced by one's perception
  c being against something or someone
  d pertaining to unfair treatment

6 Controversial
  a pertaining to an agreement
  b pertaining to harmony
  c arousing strife
  d arousing violence

7 Initial
  a the ending
  b the middle
  c an imitation
  d the beginning

8 Impression
  a a feeling of approval
  b a mirage
  c a stamp of approval
  d an image stamped on the mind

9 Block
  a to progress
  b to hinder progress
  c to tackle a difficult project
  d to improve a situation

10 Imperative
  a something to be avoided
  b unimportant
  c not to be avoided
  d not to be changed

• SUMMARY

Active listening differs from hearing because listening involves comprehension. To improve your listening skills, you have to recognize your listening problems and then correct these problems by applying the strategies of active listening.

You can improve your listening habits and use active listening strategies to take better notes and succeed in nursing school.

• Chapter 14 •

Note Taking in the Classroom

OBJECTIVE

KEY WORDS

CHECKLIST

IMPORTANCE OF GOOD LECTURE NOTES

BE PREPARED

ATTENDANCE

ORGANIZED NOTEBOOK

ORGANIZED NOTE PAPER

HOW MUCH INFORMATION TO WRITE

LESS DETAILED NOTE TAKING

MORE DETAILED NOTE TAKING

   Streamlined Handwriting

   Abbreviations

   Shorthand System

   Symbols

INDICATING MAJOR AND MINOR POINTS

CUES FOR DETERMINING WHAT IS IMPORTANT

   Ideas Written on the Board

   Verbal Tips

   Reading from a Text

   Enumerations and Terminology

   Subtle Tips

END OF LECTURE

REVIEWING YOUR NOTES

TAPING THE LECTURE

STUDYING YOUR NOTES

    Headings

    Questions

OTHER WAYS OF STUDYING FROM YOUR NOTES

VOCABULARY CHECK

SUMMARY

• OBJECTIVE

To learn procedures for the organizing, taking, and studying of notes from nursing school lectures.

• KEY WORDS

Pay attention to the following key words, which are underscored the first time they appear in this chapter. Try to determine the meanings of these words from the surrounding words in the passage. If you need further help, use your dictionary or the glossary in the back of this book.

Look up the medical terminology in your medical dictionary or the glossary. As you read the exercises in this chapter, write additional words you need to learn in the space provided.

MEDICAL TERMINOLOGY	GENERAL VOCABULARY
ambulatory care	abbreviations
anatomy	chronological order
care plan	concepts
charting	conversely
clotting	dilemma
coagulability	former
physiology	regardless
psychotherapy	sabotage
pulmonary	streamlined
self-concept	supplemented
_____	_____
_____	_____
_____	_____

• CHECKLIST

Directions. Evaluate your present note-taking system. Check yes or no.

1 Do I already know something about   Yes _____   No _____
   what the lecture is on?

2   Do I attend all lectures?   Yes _____   No _____

3   Do I use an adequate notebook?   Yes _____   No _____

4   Do I have a system for organizing my   Yes _____   No _____
    sheets of paper?

5   Do I know how much information to   Yes _____   No _____
    write?

6   In a lecture, can I tell the important   Yes _____   No _____
    facts from the unimportant ones?

7   Can I take speedy notes?   Yes _____   No _____

8   Are my notes complete?   Yes _____   No _____

9   Do I take notes to the end of the ses-   Yes _____   No _____
    sion?

10 Do I have methods for studying my   Yes _____   No _____
    notes?

If you answered no to most of these questions, you need help in taking classroom notes. This chapter will teach you techniques for organizing, taking, and studying your lecture notes.

• IMPORTANCE OF GOOD LECTURE NOTES

A good portion of your time in nursing school will be spent listening to lectures on various nursing topics. While these lectures will be supplemented by reading assignments in your textbooks, it is important to take accurate and complete classroom notes for the following reasons:

- Your instructor may want you to learn additional concepts not covered in your nursing book.
- Your instructor may restate facts you have already encountered in your reading, thereby reinforcing learning.
- Your instructor may indicate what information will appear on tests.

Thus taking good lecture notes has many advantages.

• BE PREPARED

Before attending any lecture, read all the textbook assignments that pertain to the lecture topic. By reading beforehand, you will have a foundation of knowledge on which to add the new information you will be getting in lectures. In other words, you will have background knowledge or a framework to which you can relate new facts and ideas. After the lecture, you should reread these same textbook assignments. Not only will you gain a stronger understanding of what you have previously read, but also you may interpret the concepts differently after hearing the lecture. Reading your assignments before and after the lecture will greatly improve your success on exams.

• ATTENDANCE

To take the best possible notes and to get the greatest benefit from lectures, attend all your classes. At times all students are tempted to skip a class; staying home or studying in the library is so much easier. But once you have missed a lecture, you must rely on some secondhand method for obtaining the information you have missed. You may also have lost the chance to gain invaluable information. So make it a point to attend all lectures, regardless of the weather, headaches, or the argument you had with your friend. Eventually you will be glad you were there to record the information yourself.

Plan your schedule so you can arrive on time. Many instructors introduce the main points in the beginning of their lectures. This introduction, of course, is something you would not want to miss.

• ORGANIZED NOTEBOOK

A reliable pen and a well-organized notebook are essential for taking good classroom notes. You should invest in the following:
- A different 8½ × 11 inch spiral-bound notebook for each class, *or*
- An 8½ × 11 inch spiral-bound notebook divided into different sections, *or*
- An 8½ × 11 inch looseleaf notebook with dividers that separate one subject from another

You do not want to mix your anatomy and physiology notes with your nursing notes. So make sure you have organized your notebook so that one subject is distinct from another.

• ORGANIZED NOTE PAPER

In the minutes while you are waiting for your instructor to begin, you should be organizing the sheets of paper on which you will be taking your notes. At the top of the first sheet, on the righthand side, write the date of the lecture. All lecture notes must begin with the date so you can keep them in sequential order. If you are using an individual spiral-bound notebook or one divided into sections, the earlier lectures will be in the front of the notebook and the later lecture notes will be in the back. If you prefer a loose-leaf notebook, you should place the beginning lecture notes in the back with the more current ones in front. Keeping your lecture notes dated and in chronological order is important when it comes time to study for exams.

In addition to dating your sheet of paper while you are waiting for the lecture to begin, you should draw a second lefthand margin line, about 1½ to 2 inches to the right of the first, on all the sheets of paper to be used (Fig. 14–1).

During the lecture you will write only on the portion of the paper marked *B* in Figure 14–1. The area you have created by drawing a second margin line—*A*—should remain blank. The purpose of area *A*, as shown in the figure, is to provide a space for later adding information you have missed, such as summaries, headings, and comments. With this method of organizing your paper, you not only have room to jot down additional information after the lecture, but also have space to write in

A   B

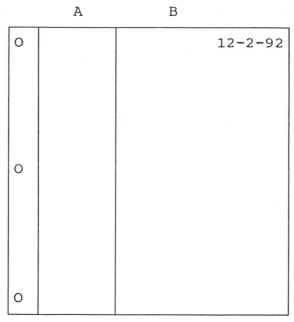

FIGURE 14–1 Hand-drawn second lefthand margin.

when you study or review your notes for a test. Your paper is now ready for the actual lecture notes.

• HOW MUCH INFORMATION TO WRITE

When attending a lecture class, you are faced with a <u>dilemma</u>—how much information should you be writing? Should you try to write down "everything," or will focusing on the main ideas and major details be sufficient? Time, experience, and a little knowledge will help you to judge the situation.

When you get the results of your first exam, you will be able to assess whether your note taking was adequate. If possible, compare the items on your exam to the topics you covered in your notes. If you see that your notes contain the majority of items asked about on your exam, you know your notes are sufficient. If you see many omissions, however, you know you need to write more to be prepared for the next exam. <u>Conversely</u>, if your notes contain many items that were not mentioned on your test, you may want to write more succinctly next time.

Once you are experienced and familiar with your instructor's lecture style, you may have a greater sense of how much to write down in your notes. In fact, your instructor may let you know during the course of her talk just what she feels you should be writing down. So stay alert and listen for an instructor's cues that let you know when and what to write.

Knowing something in advance about the course you are taking will also dictate how detailed your notes should be. If, for example, you are in a nursing lecture and you have heard that the exams are multiple choice focusing on the application of terms and concepts to clinical situations, you will need to write down all definitions and examples given during the lecture. If you have heard that the psychology instructor gives essay tests on major concepts only, it may be necessary only to write down the main points and actively listen to the rest of the lecture.

Reliable ways of finding out about your course are:

- Asking the instructor or your advisor
- Checking with former students who did well in the class
- Reading the course description in the nursing school catalogue

Once you know something about your course requirements, you will be in a better position to judge how much information you should be writing.

• LESS DETAILED NOTE TAKING

When the situation in your lecture class requires that you familiarize yourself with just the broader concepts of the course, the best approach to note taking is to summarize the material. To summarize, you must first listen to what your instructor is saying. Write, *in your own words,* the main points of what was just said. Summarizing consists in a large part of listening and reflecting and, in smaller part, of writing. When you listen, pay attention to the most important concepts and examples the instructor is presenting. You do not have to concern yourself with minor details or incidental facts and examples (see Chapters 8 and 9). When you reflect, you want to quickly translate the instructor's most important points into your own words. You do this by first listening and then silently in your mind phrasing in your own words what you just heard. You capture this paraphrasing by writing it in your notebook.

• EXERCISE 14–1 •

Directions. Below is an excerpt from a nursing textbook (Matteson and McConnell, p. 144). Read it silently, reflect on the content, and in the space provided summarize the main points of the selection.

FREE RADICAL THEORY

Free radicals [consist of] the separated electrons [that] have a large amount of free energy and oxidatively attack adjacent molecules. The O_2 molecule most commonly generates free radicals, and the most vulnerable sites are the mitochondrial and microsomal membranes rich in unsaturated lipids. Lipid molecules are especially vulnerable to attack by free radicals, resulting in structural changes and malfunctions. Chemical and structural changes are progressive with a potential for a chain reaction in which free radicals generate other free radicals. Free radicals do not contain useful biological information and replace genetic order with randomness; thus faulty molecules and cellular debris accumulate in the nucleus and cytoplasm over a lifetime.

Lipofuscin is a pigmented material rich in lipids and proteins that accumulates in many organs with aging. The pigments originate from a peroxidation of components of polyunsaturated acids located in mitochondrial membranes. Lipofuscin appears to have some relationship to free radicals and the process of aging because the substance is associated with oxidation of unsaturated lipids. The accumulation of lipofuscin interferes with the diffusion and transport of essential metabolites and information-bearing molecules in the cells and may play an important part in the aging process.

_____

_____

_____

_____

Comprehending?   Yes ____   No ____

• MORE DETAILED NOTE TAKING

When you are in a course that requires you to know a lot of factual information, your notes will necessarily be more detailed. When taking detailed notes, you listen and write to a large extent and reflect to a lesser extent. You write as quickly as possible to catch as many of the instructor's ideas as possible. This does not mean that you try to copy verbatim what the instructor is saying. That would be impossible, since we can talk much faster than we can write. It does mean, however, that you try to write as much as you can of what is being said in the most concise way. Following are four suggestions for taking notes efficiently.

• Streamlined Handwriting

Eliminating all extraneous, or extra, strokes in your handwriting will make note taking a quicker process. Use script, or cursive, rather than printing, or manuscript. Since you pick up the pen less often when writing script than when printing, your writing speed is naturally increased. Eliminate all fancy loops in your handwriting. A streamlined writing style is more conducive to speed than an ornate one. See the example below.

(too fancy)   *Nursing is a great profession*

(streamlined)   *Nursing is a great profession*

• EXERCISE 14–2 •

Directions.   In the space provided, copy the following short selection. Make sure your handwriting is streamlined—no extra strokes or loops.

Once the plan is formulated, the nurse should share care plans with the rest of the staff. Though the nurse may have consulted the staff about different aspects of the plan, it is useful to summarize initial plans with other staff members. Failure to involve staff in the initial planning stages can <u>sabotage</u> the most careful and creative plan (Arnold and Boggs, p. 140).

_____

_____

_____

_____

_____

Comprehending? Yes _____ No _____.

• Abbreviations

When it is necessary to take many pages of notes as quickly as possible, you should not write out every word in its entirety. Instead, you will want to abbreviate as many of these words as possible. This does not mean that you have to know and use the standard medical <u>abbreviations</u>. Instead you can make up your own system of abbreviations; just be sure that days or weeks later you will know what the abbreviations stand for. Below are suggestions for abbreviating some common nursing terms.

• EXAMPLE 14–1 •

TERM	ABBREVIATION
Nurse	Nrs
Nursing	nrsing
Care plan	C.P.
Ambulatory care	Amb. c.
Cardiac	Card.
Pulmonary	Pulm
Diagnosis	Diag.
Inflammation	Inflam.

• EXERCISE 14–3 •

Directions.   Choose 10 nursing or medical terms from your nursing textbook, and in the space provided create your own abbreviations.

TERM	ABBREVIATION
1 _____	_____

2 _____   _____

3 _____   _____

4 _____   _____

5 _____   _____

6 _____   _____

7 _____   _____

8 _____   _____

9 _____   _____

10 _____   _____

Comprehending?   Yes ____   No ____

• Shorthand System

Another suggestion to help you take more rapid notes is to create your own shorthand system. To do this most simply, eliminate some vowels from key words. See the example below.

• EXAMPLE 14–2 •

Longhand: You must learn to write careful and complete care plans.

Shorthand: You mst lrn to writ carfl and complt cps.

Remember that you must be able to understand your shorthand style days or weeks later.

• EXERCISE 14–4 •

Directions. Below is a short excerpt from a nursing textbook. Practice using the shorthand system above by rewriting the passage in the space provided, leaving out some vowels from key words.

The body also prepares for the possibility of injury by increasing the blood's coagulability and decreasing the clotting time. The faster the blood clots, the less blood is lost. Catecholamines initiate this response to threat (Ignatavicius and Bayne, p. 88).

_____

_____

_____

_____

Comprehending?   Yes ____   No ____

• Symbols

The last suggestion for writing more rapidly is to use symbols instead of words. Some symbols that you might already be familiar with are:

&	for "and"
w/	for "with"
w/out	for "without"
#	for "number"
=	for "equals"
≠	for "not equal to"

• EXERCISE 14–5 •

Directions.   In the space provided, write the symbols for these familiar terms.

1 per cent   _____
2 question   _____
3 feet   _____
4 inches   _____
5 greater than   _____
6 less than   _____

7 at   _____

8 five   _____

9 by   _____

10 money   _____

Comprehending?   Yes ____   No ____

Using a streamlined handwriting, abbreviations, a shorthand system, and symbols will help you to take more pages of detailed notes quickly. You can decide through practice which of these hints for increasing note-taking speed will benefit you.

• INDICATING MAJOR AND MINOR POINTS

While you are taking your lecture notes, you need to make a distinction between the major and minor points being presented. One way to do this is by using an indentation method. Starting at your hand-drawn left margin, write down the main ideas. If the next idea presented is a major detail supporting this main idea, indent a bit to the right as you write it down. If you need to write a minor detail, indent this even more to the right (Fig. 14–2).

```
O |   Main idea
  |
  |           major detail
  |
  |                   minor detail
  |
  |           major detail
  |
O |           major detail
  |
  |   Main idea
  |
  |           major detail
  |
  |                   minor detail
  |
  |                   minor detail
O |
```

FIGURE 14–2

• EXERCISE 14–6 •

Directions.   Read the selection below from a nursing textbook (Matteson and McConnell, p. 155). Following the indentation system described above, take notes in the space provided, indicating the main ideas and major and minor details.

• SKIN GLANDS

The two major types of skin glands are *sebaceous glands* and *sweat glands.* Sebaceous glands originate in the dermis and secrete *sebum,* an oily, colorless, odorless fluid, through hair follicles. Sweat glands originate in the subcutaneous tissue and are of two major types: *eccrine* and *apocrine.* Eccrine sweat glands are unbranched, coiled, tubular glands that are widely distributed and open directly onto the skin surface. They promote body cooling by allowing the sweat secretions to evaporate from the skin surface. The apocrine sweat glands are large, branched, specialized glands located chiefly in the axillary and genital regions that empty into hair follicles. They are responsible for body odor through bacterial decomposition of the sweat secretions.

Sebaceous glands show little atrophy or histological change with age; however, their function tends to diminish as seen by a decrease in sebum secretion. In men the decrease is minimal, but in women there is a gradual diminution in sebum secretion after menopause with no significant changes after the seventh decade. There are fewer sebaceous glands in older people, which appears related to the loss of hair follicles. The decrease in sebum secretion and in the number of sebaceous glands results in the dryer, coarser skin associated with aging.

Sweat glands generally decrease in size, number, and function with age. In the eccrine glands, the secretory epithelial cells become uneven in size, ranging from normal to small, and there is a progressive accumulation of lipofuscin in the cytoplasm. In the very old, the secretory coils of many eccrine glands are replaced by fibrous tissue, which drastically diminishes their capacity to produce sweat. The thermal threshold for sweating is raised, so that the amount of sweat output at a body temperature of 38 degrees centigrade decreases. This may be due to the fact that there are fewer blood vessels and nerve cells around the glands that enable the body to respond to temperature changes. Apocrine glands do not decrease in number or size, but they do decrease in function. An accumulation of lipofuscin has also been noted in apocrine glands. The diminished functioning of sweat glands in the elderly greatly impairs the ability to maintain body temperature homeostasis.

Comprehending?   Yes ____   No ____

• CUES FOR DETERMINING WHAT IS IMPORTANT

During the course of the lecture, your instructor will directly and indirectly give you cues that indicate what is important to write down. Being able to recognize these cues is critical to taking good notes. Below are some cues you should watch for in the lecture.

• Ideas Written on the Board

Whatever information your instructor writes on the board, make sure you copy it accurately in your notes. Most instructors take the time and make the effort to write on the board only those facts they feel are most important. After you have copied what was on the board, write a "B" for board in your handwritten margin by these notes.

• Verbal Tips

Sometimes your instructors will tell you what is important. They may use such words as important, chief, significant, essential, or key. Make sure you have written in your notes any facts that follow these or similar cues.

Your instructors may say that the information they are presenting will appear on a test. Make sure these concepts are written accurately in your notes and indicate that you must know this for the test. The easiest way to do this is by writing "T" for test in the handwritten margin by these notes.

• Reading from a Text

At some point in the lecture your instructor may read aloud from a text or other sources. This added reference is a cue that your instructor believes that the information is important. Copy as much information as you believe significant and write an "R" for "read aloud" in the handwritten margin by these notes.

• Enumerations and Terminology

Any ideas that are presented in numerical order should be considered important. For example, if your instructor presents information saying "first," "second," "third," and so on, make sure you have written down all these components. Also, include in your notes any new terms presented orally or written on the board.

• Subtle Cues

Watch your instructor carefully to catch any indirect cues that indicate important information. A louder voice emphasizing a point, repeating an idea, pausing for you to write, and overt hand gesturing are all indications that what is being said is significant. Sit close to your instructor and pay attention to these indirect cues.

• End of Lecture

As the class comes to an end, you may be tempted to stop listening and taking notes and to start packing up books. This may not be wise, since many instructors take these final moments to summarize their main points. You should be listening and taking notes right up to the last word. Don't cheat yourself out of critical information just to get a jump start in leaving the classroom.

• EXERCISE 14–7 •

Directions.   In your next nursing lecture, practice taking notes using the suggestions described above. Pay attention to the direct and indirect cues given by your instructor. Make sure you annotate the relevant information in the handwritten margin with a "B" for facts copied from the board, "T" for items that will appear on tests, and "R" for what the instructor read aloud. Write down all enumerations and terms. Keep taking notes until your instructor is finished.

• REVIEWING YOUR NOTES

Soon after the lecture, review your notes for completeness. If you feel that you have left out something important, you may have to ask to see another student's notes. Make sure that person is there to explain the notes because one person's personalized note-taking style may not be clear to someone else. It makes no sense to copy something you do not understand.

• TAPING THE LECTURE

A way to verify the completeness of your lecture notes is to tape the lecture. This method has many advantages. First, you will have the opportunity on your own, during your study period, to replay and hear the entire lecture again. This is wonderful reinforcement. Second, you can review your notes and fill in any blanks without having to rely on anyone else. Third, you can prepare for your exam by listening to the tape of the lecture when you are at home, driving, or commuting to school.

Before you tape, make sure you get permission from your instructor. Use a portable battery-operated recorder. Make sure the casettes are long playing and that you have extra batteries in case the power begins to run out. Sit as close to the lecturer as possible, so the recording will be clear and the speaker's words distinct.

• STUDYING YOUR NOTES

The purpose of note taking is to have a permanent record of the information you will need to learn in order to pass exams in nursing school. The note taking is just the first part of the procedure. You also need a good system for studying your notes.

• HEADINGS IN NOTES

Just as sections in your nursing textbooks are divided by headings, so should your notes be divided by headings. Read over your notes and decide where one topic ends and a new one begins. This is the most natural place for a heading. Ask yourself, "What is the section mostly about?" The answer will be the topic, and this should be used as the heading. Write the heading in a different color ink than you used for note taking. See the example below, in which an excerpt from a nursing book is used to represent your lecture notes.

• EXAMPLE 14–3 •

<u>Psychotherapy</u> is practiced by persons with advanced training: psychiatric nurses, psychiatric social workers, psychologists, and psychiatrists. Therapeutic experiences permit the child to explore his or her feelings and make corrective changes. A child crippled by ambivalent, negative, and confused feelings is unable to grow into a happy, confident, and fulfilled adult.

Since children often have difficulty identifying or discussing painful feelings, alternative modes of therapy are often successful. Play therapy and art therapy are frequently used modalities to help children explore their feelings. For children, especially those children who have been sexually abused, expression through art, in contrast to verbalization, is often a less threatening way to communicate confusing and painful emotions (Varcarolis, p. 240).

What is this passage mostly about?
Child psychotherapy = topic = heading

• EXERCISE 14–8 •

Directions. Take a page from your nursing lecture notes. Decide on the appropriate places for headings. Ask, "What is this section mostly about?" (The brief answer will be the topic, which can be used for the heading.) Write these headings where you think they belong.

Comprehending? Yes ____ No ____

• QUESTIONS

Once you have written headings for the different topics in your lecture notes, turn these headings into questions. Use 5 W types of questions (who, what, when, where, why or how). Referring back to Example 14–3, you see the heading is "child psychotherapy." You can turn this into a question by asking, "What is child psychotherapy?" Once you have turned all the headings in your notes into questions, you will read and remember the facts in your notes that answer the questions. This will keep you focused on your studying and help you distinguish the more important information from the less important. Underline or highlight all facts in your notes that answer the heading question.

• EXERCISE 14–9 •

Directions. Below are headings. In the space provided, turn these headings into questions.

HEADING	QUESTION
Perceptual processes related to <u>self-concept</u>	_____ _____
Engagement phase	_____
Using physical and nonverbal behavioral cues	_____ _____
Creating personal space in hospital situations	_____ _____
Computer-assisted <u>charting</u>	_____

Comprehending? Yes ___ No ___

• EXERCISE 14–10 •

Directions. Using your notes from Exercise 14–8, turn all the headings you have made into questions. Then underline all the information that directly answers these questions.

• OTHER WAYS OF STUDYING FROM YOUR NOTES

When studying from your notes, be creative. Don't just read over the same words with the hope of memorizing them. In addition to the heading and questions method of studying from notes, other activities can keep you actively involved in the studying task:

- Write out quizzes based on your notes.
- Take these quizzes at the beginning of each of your study sessions.
- Make a chart covering the main points from your notes. Then fill in the details without looking at your notes.
- Dictate into your cassette recorder the main points from your lecture notes and listen to it at some later time.
- Create flashcards of the important terms from your notes and practice learning these words with them.

- Create your own ideas for making studying your notes exciting.

You have learned new techniques for organizing, taking, and studying lecture notes. Use these methods conscientiously in your upcoming lectures. Eventually you will see rewards for your efforts—improved grades.

• EXERCISE 14–11 •

Directions.   After a few weeks of practicing your new note-taking system, re-read the checklist at the beginning of this chapter. See if your responses have improved.

• VOCABULARY CHECK

Directions.   Below are 10 words taken from the key words section of this chapter. Circle the letter of the best definition from the four choices.

1 Concepts
    a thoughts
    b feelings
    c suspicions
    d fears

2 Anatomy
    a science dealing with fetal development
    b science dealing with organ structures
    c science dealing with physical processes
    d science dealing with the form and structure of living organisms

3 Streamlined
    a a rough finish
    b functioning at top speed
    c stripped of nonessentials
    d gauge of water depth

4 Pulmonary
    a pertaining to the brain
    b pertaining to the lungs
    c pertaining to the kidney
    d pertaining to the spinal cord

5 Dilemma
    a a heated discussion
    b an abrasive response
    c an unattainable goal
    d difficult or persistent problem

6 Coagulability

    a ability to fend off microorganisms

    b ability to form clots

    c ability to conceal

    d ability to bond

7 Conversely

    a reacting in a negative way

    b acting in anger

    c reversed in order, action

    d responding in like manner

8 Ambulatory care

    a care of patient in the ambulance

    b care of patient outdoors

    c care of patient confined to bed or chair

    d care of patient who is not confined to bed

9 Regardless

    a despite everything

    b not noticing

    c not caring

    d not usual

10 Self-concept

    a one's own fears

    b one's reaction to other people

    c when someone perceives another to be similar to herself or himself

    d the way someone views himself or herself

• SUMMARY

In this chapter you learned a new system for organizing, taking, and studying lecture notes. You were shown the value of reading before the lecture and being organized. You were taught not only how to assess how much information to write, but also how to determine which ideas are important. Suggestions were given on how to take notes more efficiently and how to differentiate major concepts from minor ones. You were then given suggestions for studying your notes.

• Chapter 15 •

Test-Taking Strategies

OBJECTIVE

KEY WORDS

PREPARING FOR EXAMINATIONS

STUDYING FOR OBJECTIVE TESTS

THE MAIN IDEA QUESTION

ELIMINATING ANSWERS TO THE MAIN
IDEA QUESTION

DETAIL QUESTION

INFERENCE QUESTION

VOCABULARY IN CONTEXT QUESTION

STUDYING FOR ESSAY TESTS

TACKLING TEST-TAKING ANXIETY

VOCABULARY CHECK

SUMMARY

• OBJECTIVE

To learn the strategies that will help you to improve your scores on both objective and essay examinations.

• KEY WORDS

Pay attention to the following key words, which are underscored the first time they appear in this chapter. Try to determine the meaning of these words from the surrounding words in the passage. If you need further help, use your dictionary or the glossary in the back of this book.

Look up the medical terminology in your medical dictionary or the glossary. As you read the exercises in this chapter, write additional words that you need to learn in the space provided.

MEDICAL TERMINOLOGY	GENERAL VOCABULARY
anorexia	allegations
arthritis	deficits
hallucinations	deviation
malnutrition	exotic
mobility	haphazard
obesity	impairments
paralysis	ingrained
resuscitate	intricate
scoliosis	myths
sensory	revisions
_____	_____
_____	_____
_____	_____

• PREPARING FOR EXAMINATIONS

You have learned the strategies for reading the textbook, active listening, and note taking in previous chapters of this textbook. These study skills will help you to learn the material in your liberal arts and nursing textbooks and nursing lectures as you keep up with your weekly assignments. To do well on tests, however, you must do more than keep up with your assignments. You have to prepare for doing well on your nursing class exams. Test preparation is a planned series of steps. It is not haphazard. If you want to be successful, you should develop a plan that works for you and then follow it.

Successful students use their calendars to plan ahead for study time. Even if you feel you already know the information that will be on the test, you will forget a certain amount of material by the time you have the exam. That is why a review is essential.

• STEPS FOR TEST PREPARATION

The first step for test preparation is to know what material will be covered on the exam. You should know which of the text assignments and lecture information will be included in the test. The second step is to look at your calendar and schedule enough time to study. Be realistic. Allow time for sleeping and meals. You have to be physically fit to concentrate on your notes and underlined text material. The third step is to find out whether the exam will be objective or essay. You will then be better prepared to study for the test.

• STUDYING FOR OBJECTIVE TESTS

Objective tests—those with multiple-choice, short answer, matching, and true-false questions—require you to know both details and main ideas. You have to retain facts as well as understand general concepts.

To study for objective tests:
- Review class notes carefully.
- Review all underlined material, outlines, and summaries from your text.
- Take practice tests:
  Go over any end of chapter questions.
  Try to predict the test questions. Then prepare answers to your own questions.

• LEARNING HOW TO ANSWER MULTIPLE-CHOICE QUESTIONS

Practicing how to answer the specific types of questions on multiple-choice tests will help you improve your grades in your nursing and liberal arts courses. When answering multiple-choice questions, you select one answer from several choices. The following strategies will help you select the correct answer:
- If two choices are the same, they are both incorrect. Therefore you eliminate both these choices.
- When "all of the above" is given as a choice, it is usually correct unless you determine that one of the choices is obviously wrong.
- Be aware of directional words such as but, except, and however, since they signal opposite meanings.
- Read all answer choices before making your decision.
  To answer multiple-choice questions you need to know how to:
- Find main ideas
- Locate and retain the details that support the main idea
- Make inferences
- Learn vocabulary meanings through context
  The following techniques will help you to answer questions on each of these skills.

• Main Idea Question

The answer to a main idea question will be:
- Who or what is the selection about?
- What is the main point being made about the selection?
  The following are examples of questions that require you to find the main idea:
- The primary concern is:
- The major purpose is:
- The idea primarily discussed is:
- The main point is:
- What is the most important _____?

ELIMINATING ANSWERS TO THE MAIN IDEA QUESTION

Learning how to eliminate answers is an important test-taking strategy in multiple-choice tests. When answering main idea questions, you should eliminate any answers that are:
- *Too general.* The answer covers more information than is discussed in the passage.

- *Too specific.* The answer covers just a detail from the selection, not the main idea.
- *Not mentioned.* The answer is an idea not discussed in the passage.

• EXAMPLE 15–1 •

Directions.   Read the following excerpt from a nursing textbook (Iyer et al., p. 152) and the explanation of the answer to the main idea question based on the selection.

Age also affects ability to learn. The very young child may have difficulty in grasping concepts unless they are presented in very concrete terms. Some elderly clients may have <u>ingrained</u> ideas or "<u>myths</u>" that affect their ability to accept new changes. Additionally, they may have physiological <u>deficits</u> that interfere with their ability to learn (e.g., vision or hearing problems).

The main point of this passage is:
a learning disabilities in children
b age affects learning
c physiological deficits interfere with learning
d ability to learn

The correct answer to this passage is (b) age affects learning. Choice (a) is not mentioned in the passage. Choice (c) is too specific; it is just a detail from the selection. Choice (d) is too general; the answer covers more information than is discussed in the passage.

• EXERCISE 15–1 •

Directions.   Read the following excerpt from a nursing textbook (Sorensen and Luckmann, pp. 583–584). Then answer the five multiple-choice main idea questions based on this selection. Use the test-taking strategy of eliminating any answers that are too general, too specific, or not mentioned before you choose the correct answer.

• HALLUCINATIONS, ILLUSIONS, AND DELUSIONAL THINKING

<u>Hallucinations</u>, illusions, and delusional thinking are other examples of disorganized thought and behavior patterns.

• Hallucinations

Hallucinations are sensory impressions occurring in the absence of external stimuli whether the person is aware of the unreal nature or not. Any of the senses can be affected. Hallucinating people may believe they see, hear, smell, feel, or taste stimuli that are not actually present in the physical world. Hallucinated stimuli have no source in the external environment. They are sensations arising from within the person.

Visual hallucinations often suggest organic brain disease. They typically occur with acute infectious diseases or toxic psychosis and with acute, reversible organic brain disorders. Some drugs may cause visual hallucinations. These include not only exotic drugs such as mescaline but also regularly prescribed medications, e.g., amphetamines and medication for Parkinson's disease.

Additional causes of visual hallucinations include the following.

- Brain tumors and other space-occupying lesions
- The aura of an epileptic attack or migraine headache
- Metabolic disorders such as adrenal insufficiency, dehydration, hypoparathyroidism, pernicious or addisonian anemia, hypoglycemia, anorexia, and uremia
- Trauma
- Collagen diseases
- Cerebrovascular accidents (strokes)
- Degenerative diseases, e.g., Pick's and Alzheimer's diseases

- Mental illness such as acute psychosis (auditory hallucinations are associated with chronic psychosis)
- Sensory deprivation

- **Illusions**

Illusions differ from hallucinations. With an illusion there is a real stimulus but the person misinterprets it. For example, a shadow may be present on a wall but the person thinks it is a person standing near the wall. Whenever possible, identify the stimulus the person is responding to and then control, reduce, or remove the stimulus. A person's overresponsiveness may be controlled by reducing environmental stimuli.

- **Delusional Thinking**

Delusional thinking is thoughts and beliefs that are false. For example, a person may believe he/she is being persecuted by the police when it is not true.

1 Hallucinations, illusions, and delusional thinking are examples of:
a physical diseases of the elderly
b organized group behavior
c patterns of organized behavior
d disorganized thought and behavior patterns

2 Hallucinations are:
a always present in the physical world
b external stimuli found in the material world
c sensory impressions occurring in the absence of external stimuli
d created by the absence of taste or other sensory stimuli

3 Visual hallucinations:
a can have more than one cause
b are always caused by organic brain disease
c are caused only by exotic drugs
d cause brain tumors

4 Illusions are:
a the same as hallucinations
b correctly interpreted stimuli
c a misinterpretation of a real stimulus
d caused by reduction of environmental stimuli

5 Delusional thinking:
a is caused by persecution
b is the result of persecution
c is based on reality
d is false thoughts and beliefs

• Detail Question

When you are reading for details, concentrate on reading accurately. The most minor misinterpretation of a fact can cause you to choose an incorrect answer. When you study, try to retain facts. A helpful study strategy is to try to classify facts under main ideas. Retaining organized information is easier than remembering random facts. When answering detail questions:

- Read the question carefully. Are you asked to know when, why, or how? You must understand the question before you can choose an answer.
- Be careful of such words as all, only, always, every, and never. These words are too general. Their presence in a multiple-choice response often means the response is incorrect.

• EXAMPLE 15–2 •

Read the following excerpt from a nursing textbook (Sorenson and Luckmann, p. 585) and the explanation of the answer to the detail question based on the selection.

The ability to move is something that most of us take for granted. We seldom think about the numerous complex and intricate bodily movements that are involved in every activity. As a result, we often fail to realize how vital mobility is to our physical, psychologic, emotional and economic well-being. Indeed, active healthy people may fail to appreciate just how threatening immobility can be to their life styles.

Immobility is:

a   vital to our physical, psychologic, emotional, and economic well being
b   linked to numerous bodily movements
c   threatening to people's life styles
d   underestimated by everyone

The correct answer is choice (c), which is stated in the last sentence of the passage. A careful reading of the passage will eliminate choices (a) and (b) because those statements are true of mobility, not immobility. Choice (d) is incorrect because the word "everyone" is too general.

• EXERCISE 15–2 •

Directions.   Read the following excerpt from a nursing textbook (Sorensen and Luckmann, pp. 589–590). Then answer the five detail questions based on this selection. Concentrate on reading and understanding the questions before you choose your answers.

Despite our efforts to maintain physical fitness and activity, *immobility* can strike suddenly or gradually. It can be *partial* (e.g., the person with a broken leg who can still hobble around on crutches) or *total,* as with the totally paralyzed person or the unconscious individual. The goals for nursing care differ according to the type and the permanence of the immobility. In general, however, nursing intervention aims at (a) promoting activity within the limits of the person's ability and (b) preventing complications arising from immobility. Nursing assessment precedes intervention and begins by identifying individuals who are at *risk* for mobility problems.

• IDENTIFYING THE CAUSES OF IMMOBILITY

Many conditions and diseases can immobilize an individual. Common *causes* of immobility include:
- *Pain* severe enough to seriously limit motion and activity. For example, people with diseases such as rheumatoid arthritis may be able to move joints, but severe pain causes them to limit movement. *Chronic* pain increases the risk of complications due to immobility.
- *Impairments of motor nervous function* that seriously and sometimes permanently decrease body movements. Examples of conditions in this category include progressive degenerative disorders such as muscular dystrophy, myasthenia gravis, and amyotrophic lateral sclerosis. Paralysis from a stroke and spinal cord injury are other examples.
- *Structural problems,* e.g., scoliosis (lateral deviation of the spine), or joint contractures.
- *Generalized weakness* from chronic illness (e.g., cancer), anorexia and malnutrition, or profound obesity.
- *Psychologic problems* such as severe depression and certain psychoses.
- *Medical and nursing treatments* that decrease activity. If a person needs to be restrained, for example, movement is greatly limited. *Orthopedic* problems treated by immobilization of a limb (e.g., casts and the application of traction) also restrict activity. *Bed rest* is another important example of a therapy that results in immobility. Because bed rest is a part of many treatment regimens, we discuss it in detail.

1 The risk of complications from immobility is increased by:
   a severe pain   c only arthritis
   b chronic pain   d the lack of pain

2 Impairments of motor nervous function:
   a decrease pain
   b decrease all body movements
   c inhibit movements
   d sometimes permanently decrease body movements

3 Scoliosis is a:
   a joint contracture   c cause of structural problems
   b deviation of the spine d cause of paralysis

4 Immobility can be:
   a caused only by a physical disease
   b caused only by psychological problems
   c caused by severe depression
   d cured by improved nutrition

5 Immobility is the result of:
   a bed rest   c new medical and nursing treatments
   b removal of a cast d all orthopedic problems

• Inference Question

An inference question requires you to understand unstated meanings. When you are answering inference questions, choose an answer that is based on information you have studied in your nursing and liberal arts courses. Do not choose an answer that is not related to ideas or facts in the material.

The following are examples of statements that require you to make inferences:

- You can conclude . . .
- It is implied that . . .
- One can infer . . .
- Which is most probably . . .

• EXAMPLE 15–3 •

Directions.   Read the following excerpt from a nursing textbook (Iyer et al., p. 252) and the explanation of the answer to the inference question based on the selection.

During an attempt to <u>resuscitate</u> a woman in the intensive care unit the client opened her eyes. She said to the nurse, "Let me go. Leave me alone." The physician, who was standing by her side, verified that the client wanted no further treatment. The resuscitation effort ended and the client was allowed to die.

You can conclude that the resuscitation effort ended because:
- **a** the nurse had no hope for the patient's recovery
- **b** the doctor failed to save the patient's life
- **c** the patient has the right to refuse care
- **d** the patient had only a few hours to live

Choice (a) is not based on any statement in the passage. The nurse's feelings about the patient's chances for recovery are not mentioned. Choice (b) is incorrect because the doctor was not involved in the resuscitation effort and merely was a witness to the patient's request to end treatment. Choice (c) is correct based on the third sentence, in which the physician verified that the client wanted no further treatment. Choice (d) is incorrect because the reader is not given any information on the life expectancy of the patient.

• **EXERCISE 15–3** •

Directions. Read the following excerpt from a nursing textbook (Iyer et al., p. 253). Then answer the five inference questions based on the selection. Remember to use the test-taking strategy of basing your answer on information stated in the selection.

• **Nurse's Rights**

Under this principle of law the nurse has rights and responsibilities as an employee and professional. For example, required testing for AIDS as a condition of employment violates a nurse's privacy and confidentiality and may lead to charges of discrimination. The nurse has a right to a safe working environment according to the Occupational Safety and Health Administration (OSHA) laws. The regulations permit a nurse to refuse to work in proven unsafe conditions. The employer is obligated to provide the nurse with safety equipment. The nurse has a responsibility to use the equipment. For example, the nurse is expected to wear gloves when handling blood and body fluids. If the nurse does not utilize gloves when drawing blood and contracts hepatitis, the nurse would not be entitled to compensation from the employer.

Working with inadequate staffing is a controversial issue that affects the nurse's rights and responsibilities. "Prevention of litigation is a simple matter of providing a standard of nursing care equivalent to that which should be available to patients under ordinary circumstances. Extraordinary circumstances do not minimize the obligation to provide safe, professional care. Thus, the fact that there is a nursing shortage and hospital units must be staffed by tired or inexperienced nurses is not a defense. The institution's first legal responsibility is to the provision of safe and adequate care. Should staffing shortages make provision of safe and adequate care questionable, the hospital has an obligation not to offer care."

Accrediting agencies, such as JCAHO, reinforce the agency's legal obligation to provide appropriate numbers of nurses. "There are sufficient qualified nursing staff members to meet the nursing care needs of patients throughout the hospital." When a patient is injured, staffing issues may be a factor in an ensuing lawsuit.

1 Occupational Safety and Health Administration laws are designed:
   a to discharge nurses with AIDS
   b to encourage litigation
   c to protect only the patients
   d to establish standards of hospital safety controls

2 One can infer that staffing shortages:
   a create safety problems
   b always prevent adequate care of patients
   c may interfere with safe care
   d injure all patients and nurses

3 A nurse can sue a hospital if an injury results:
   a while refusing to use safety equipment
   b while using safety equipment
   c while drawing blood without gloves
   d outside hospital grounds

4 It is implied that hospitals have adequate nursing staffs:
    a to prevent lawsuits
    b to keep nurses employed
    c to avoid trouble with the union
    d to improve hospital-patient relations

5 According to this article, testing for AIDS:
    a is required of all nurses
    b is a safety control for patients
    c should not be required of all nurses
    d is a safety hazard

• Vocabulary in Context Question

Follow these three steps when you are asked to define a word in context, that is, to define an unknown word by looking at surrounding words:
- Decide on the part of speech of the unknown word.
- Use clues in the surrounding words to find the meaning.
- Check your answer choice by placing it in the original sentence and reading to see if it makes sense.

• EXAMPLE 15–4 •

Note how the word *resuscitation*, is used in the following sentence. "The *resuscitation* effort ended and the client was allowed to die" (Iyer et al., p. 252).

Resuscitation means:
a life-saving
b life saver
c failed
d resentful

Choice (a) is the correct answer. Since the effort ended, resuscitation had to have a meaning opposite of "to die." Choice (b) is incorrect because a lifesaver is a person and therefore a noun while resuscitation is used as an adjective. Choice (c) is incorrect because the phrase "allowed to die" lets the reader know that the effort was stopped; it didn't fail. Choice (d) is incorrect because there is no basis in the sentence for the negative word "resentful."

• EXERCISE 15–4 •

Directions. Read the following five sentences. Use the three-step plan learned in this chapter to define each boldface word (Iyer et al., p. 252).

1   This **principle** applies to families who are seeking detailed information.
    a   administrator of a school
    b   to theorize
    c   pressure point
    d   question

2   Prevention of **litigation,** or lawsuits, is of concern to all nurses and health care professionals.
    a   disease-like
    b   lawsuits
    c   lawyers
    d   safety problems

3   There are guidelines for a nurse's conduct and mechanisms for **enforcing** those rules (Iyer et al., p. 255).
    a   procedures
    b   putting into action
    c   arresting
    d   changing

4   For instance, the board may be asked to rule on whether licensed practical nurses may **insert** intravenous needles (Iyer et al., p. 255).
    a   remove   c   stick in
    b   an order   d   request

5   The board is expected to take disciplinary action when a nurse has a physical, mental, or substance abuse **impairment** (Iyer et al., p. 255).
    a   weakness   c   habit
    b   disease   d   license

Comprehending? Yes ____ No ____

• Answering Other Types of Objective Test Questions

In your nursing classes most objective test questions will be multiple choice. However, in your liberal arts classes some objective test questions will be in other forms. Therefore you should learn how to answer the other types of objective test questions, such as:

- *Short answers.* Short answer questions ask you to fill in the blank. Since you will be completing sentences, make sure that your answer choice fits grammatically and contextually.
- *Matching.* When matching items, keep track of the answers you've already used. In this way you monitor your progress.
- *True-false.* When answering true-false questions, focus on the part of the statement that makes it either true or false. Usually, close attention to detail is needed in reading true-false questions. The entire statement has to be correct for the answer choice to be true. If a part of the statement is incorrect, the answer is false.

Directions.　Read the following excerpts from a nursing textbook (Iyer et al., pp. 254–256). Study the material, then answer the objective test questions based on the selection.

• Law is Based on a Concern for Fairness and Justice

The third principle of law seeks to protect the rights of one party from infringement by the actions of another party. It serves to set guidelines for conduct and mechanisms for the enforcement of those guidelines. The rights of individuals are protected by the legal system. The laws are designed to achieve a fair outcome in legal disputes, and to provide structure for managing the complexities of the health care system.

There are guidelines for a nurse's conduct and mechanisms for enforcing those rules. The expectations of professional conduct are defined by the American Nurses Association and other specialty organizations, by standards published by the Joint Commission, and by the state board of nursing in the nurse practice act. The state board of nursing consists of a group of nurses and, in some states, non-nurses who are appointed by the governor. The board is charged with a number of responsibilities:

1　Approval of the curriculum of schools of nursing located in the state.

2　Inspection of employer records to be sure the nursing employees are credentialed and complying with professional standards.

3　Rulings on questions which are submitted to it. These questions clarify the scope of nursing practice. For instance, the board may be asked to rule on whether licensed practical nurses may insert intravenous needles.

4　Determining who is competent to be licensed as a nurse and the granting of licenses.

5　Disciplining of nurses who are found to be unfit or incompetent to practice nursing.

A nursing license is a legal document that permits the nurse to offer certain skills and knowledge to the public of the state, where such practice would otherwise be unlawful without a license. Nurses are required to hold a current license issued by their state in order to practice. A nurse must be in good health to apply for an initial license, a license renewal, or to receive a license in another state (licensure by endorsement). Schools of nursing are expected to screen out those individuals who have physical and mental disabilities that would prevent them from practicing safely. Those with physical or mental disabilities who are applying for a license renewal or by endorsement are required to present evidence that they are able to practice nursing in a safe and competent manner in spite of their disability. Physical disabilities which have led to concern about safe practice include legal blindness, severe hearing impairment, and the loss of motor skills and normal speech.

The board is expected to take disciplinary action when a nurse has a physical, mental, or substance abuse impairment. Through surveys of state boards of nursing [it was] found that:

99 percent of the boards had dealt with cases of illegal substance abuse
76 percent with alcohol abuse
70 percent with legal substance abuse that impaired practice
20 percent with cases of mental impairment
5 percent with cases of physical impairment.

Murphy and Connell studied 100 records of Arizona nurses who had violated the state's nurse practice act and discovered that 60 percent of the nurses had been disciplined for substance abuse and 40 percent for incompetence.

Nurses have also been disciplined or lost their licenses for failure to file tax returns and pay taxes, allowing the daughter of a nurse to pose as a nurse, and failing to comply with regulations for nurse midwives. Advanced nursing practice was the basis of a Missouri case on the role of nurse practitioners. An Idaho nurse named Jolene Tuma provided a client with information on alternative cancer therapies and retained her license after the Idaho board sought to remove it for unprofessional conduct. The Idaho court ruled that the nurse practice act was sufficiently vague on what constituted unprofessional conduct.

A Colorado nurse lost her license after being charged with seventeen <u>allegations</u> of failure to administer medication, treatment, and feedings to patients; fourteen allegations of making false or incorrect entries in patients' records regarding the administration of medication, treatment, and feedings; numerous allegations of sleeping on duty; three allegations of removing patients' call bells during the night; two allegations of leaving open the door of the medicine storage room; several allegations of patient abuse, including the forced feeding of one patient and hitting the stumps of two amputees against their bed rails; four allegations of failure to check on patients who were reportedly experiencing difficulties; one allegation of failure to recognize that a patient was not dead and could be resuscitated; numerous allegations of failure to make rounds; and charges of permitting unlicensed nurse's aides to administer medication. When the nurse appealed the revocation of her license, the Colorado Supreme Court upheld the decision.

Objective Test

Part I. After reading this selection, fill in the blanks.

1 The _____ principle of law seeks to protect the rights of one party from infringement by the actions of another party.

2 The rights of individuals are protected by _____.

3 The state board of nursing is appointed by the _____.

4 A nursing license is issued by the _____.

5 The expectations of professional conduct are defined by the _____ and other organizations.

Part II. Match the letters in column B with the numbers in column A.

A		B	
1	Murphy and Connell study	a	Reason for discipline
2	Nursing license	b	Responsibility of state board of nursing
3	Failure to pay taxes	c	Requirements to apply for license
4	Good health	d	Legal document
5	Approval of nursing school curriculum	e	100 records of Arizona nurses

Part III. Answer the multiple-choice questions based on the passage you have read.

1 A nursing license is
   a unlawful
   b required for practice
   c automatically renewed
   d issued upon request

2 A practicing nurse must
   a have her initial license
   b apply for a new license each year
   c reapply for nursing school each year
   d have a current license

3 If a nurse has an impairment, disciplinary action is taken by
 a the national board
 b the physicians
 c the state board
 d the local board

4 Nursing boards have dealt with 70% of cases of
 a alcohol abuse
 b legal substance abuse that impaired practice
 c illegal substance abuse
 d mental impairment

5 The percentage of cases of alcohol abuse dealt with by state boards was
 a 20%
 b 99%
 c 76%
 d 70%

6 In Murphy and Connell's study the percent of Arizona nurses disciplined for incompetence was
 a 40%
 b 60%
 c 100%
 d 76%

7 The basis of a Missouri case was
 a tax fraud
 b substance abuse
 c alternative cancer therapies
 d advanced nursing practice

8 The nurse who was charged with seventeen allegations of failure to administer medicine was from
 a Arizona
 b Colorado
 c Idaho
 d Missouri

9 The number of responsibilities listed for the state board is
 a five
 b one
 c two
 d ten

10 Competency for nurses is determined by
 a the state board
 b the hospital administration
 c patients
 d physicians

Part IV. Read the following statements. In the space provided write "T" if the statement is true or "F" if the statement is false.

1 State boards of nurses consist only of nurses. _____

2 Nurses are required to hold state licenses in order to practice. _____

3 The board of nurses takes disciplinary action when a nurse has a drug problem. _____

4 Eighty-nine percent of the boards have dealt with illegal substance abuse. _____

5 Nurses can lose their licenses for not filing tax returns. _____

• EXERCISE 15–6 •

Directions.   Read the following excerpt from a nursing textbook (Iyer et al., pp. 256–257). Create your own objective test based on the selection. Create five short answers, five matching, five true-false, and ten multiple-choice questions.

A Nurse's Actions are Judged on the Basis of What a Similarly Educated Reasonable and Prudent Person Would Have Done in a Similar Situation

This fourth principle refers to the concepts that are applied in nursing malpractice cases. In a society that has increasingly turned to the courts for resolution of disputes, standards are needed to judge nursing performance. The number of lawsuits being filed against nurses is increasing, although physicians are sued with greater frequency. According to the American Nurses Association, 6.2 nurses per 10,000 are sued each year. This is in contrast to 1,800 physicians per 10,000. Despite the relatively small number of nurses who are sued each year, nurses need to continue to be concerned with the legal aspects of nursing practice. Lawsuits against nurses are on the increase for a number of reasons:

1 The consumer has become better educated on what to expect from the health care system and nursing care.

2 Plaintiff's attorneys (who represent the client) are becoming more able to identify the case that has merit.

3 Plaintiff's attorneys are likely to name as many people as possible when filing a lawsuit. This allows them to potentially tap the pocket of the hospital and the nurse's insurance companies, as well as the physician's insurance carrier.

4 Plaintiff's lawyers are more aware that nurses are professionals and accountable for their own actions.

5 Many nurses are providing increasingly specialized and complex care that exposes the client and the nurse to greater risk.

6 The nursing shortage has had an impact on the quality of nursing care.

The terms negligence and malpractice are often used interchangeably. *Negligence* is a general term referring to a deviation from the standard of care that a reasonably prudent person would use in a particular set of circumstances. *Malpractice* is a specific type of negligence that refers to deviations from a professional standard of care. Nurses, doctors, lawyers, and accountants are some of the types of professionals that may be liable for malpractice.

Insurance studies show that of all medical malpractice cases filed, half are dropped, one third are settled out of court, and the remainder go to trial. The third that settle out of court represent those cases that the team defending the nurse or physician believes would result in a verdict in favor of the plaintiff. The cases chosen for trial are either the ones that the defense believes it can win, or those that cannot be settled out of court because the plaintiff will not accept the dollar amount offered by the defense. The defense is successful in winning approximately 90 percent of the cases that get into court, although this varies from state to state [of 1,886 malpractice cases in various geographical areas that were studied, there was a 68 percent defense success rate].

Under the law each nurse is held accountable for his or her actions. A nurse cannot evade this responsibility by explaining that a physician or nursing supervisor ordered the nurse to commit the actions which injured the client. It is expected that the nurse will use judgment to question the orders that are inappropriate or likely to result in harm to the client.

Student nurses are expected to provide nursing care as would a competent registered nurse. If the nursing student fails to possess or use the degree of knowledge and skill that a registered nurse would have, the student would still be found liable for any harm to a client. While lawsuits against students are rare, the client could sue the student, instructor, facility, physician, and RN staff.

If a jury decides that a nurse is guilty of malpractice the nurse has a legally enforceable responsibility for compensating the client for the harm done. In addition, the state board of nursing may discipline the nurse.

It is now recommended that nurses carry their own malpractice insurance policies in addition to whatever coverage may be provided by their employer. One of the reasons for having personal insurance includes needing coverage for actions outside of the employment setting, such as private duty nursing and giving advice to neighbors.

Comprehending?   Yes ___   No ___

• STUDYING FOR ESSAY TESTS

You can improve your grades on essay tests by learning the test-taking strategies for writing and revising essays. The first step in preparing for an essay test is to review your class notes and underlined material, outlines, and summaries of textbooks. Then you should organize all information into topics, main ideas, and major details. Organizing your information will help you to retain the material.

Writing strategies can help you to learn the information. These strategies, such as taking notes, composing questions, and writing summaries and outlines, will help you to prepare for your test.

• ANSWERING ESSAY QUESTIONS

• Before Writing

- Read the entire test, paying special attention to the directions.
- Find out how many questions you are required to answer.
- Notice the points given for each question. You will want to spend more time on a 30-point question than a 10-point question.
- Read the question carefully.
- Determine how you should organize your information. Is the question asking you to *list*, *explain*, *compare*, *contrast*, or *sequence* information?
- Think about approaches and construct an outline.

• While Writing

- State main ideas in clear topic sentences.
- Support main ideas with relevant major details.
- Make sure you are answering the question that was asked.

• After Writing

- Make necessary <u>revisions</u> in organization, word choice, and mechanics.
- Check to make sure that you have answered all the parts of each question.

• EXAMPLE 15–5 •

Directions.   Read the following excerpt from a nursing text (Sorensen and Luck-mann, p. 163–164). Review the sample essay question and answer based on the selection.

• TRENDS IN HEALTH CARE DELIVERY

Health care delivery is intimately connected to the society within which it operates, and it generally reflects the social, political, and economic climates of the times. Ideally the delivery of health care addresses current societal needs and resources. For example, appropriate health care services for a developing nation like Ethiopia would focus on increasing the food supply, preventing malnutrition, and improving sanitation. On the other hand, health care delivery goals in Canada or the United States might center on controlling costs.

Some major trends in the American health care industry include: (1) an increase in community, ambulatory, and home health care services; (2) attempts to establish more comprehensive health care programs aimed at health promotion and disease prevention; (3) a shift toward self-care; (4) changes in the numbers and types of health care workers; and (5) changes in government involve-ment in the health care industry.

Increase in Ambulatory, Community, and Home Health Care

The trend toward *disease prevention* coupled with the concern over *rising health costs* has re-sulted in the proliferation of *ambulatory* health care services, e.g., neighborhood clinics, day care cen-ters, birthing clinics, and free-standing emergency centers that provide 24-hour health services for mi-nor trauma and illness. Also, minor surgery is being performed on an outpatient or "same-day" basis more frequently; i.e., the person is not admitted to a hospital but instead undergoes surgery, stabilizes in a recovery room, and goes home, all in the same day. This is also called *ambulatory surgery.* Spur-ring this trend toward ambulatory surgery is the refusal of health insurance companies to cover costs for minor surgical procedures when they are performed in inpatient hospital settings.

The increase in *chronic disorders* accompa-nying an expanding older population has also shifted health care from the hospital and long-term care facility to the community. Home health care agencies and hospices are more common now. These services maintain the ill person in a home setting, thus decreasing costs and allowing the per-son to escape the impersonal hospital or long-term facility environment. In addition, many chronically ill older people do not require the sophisticated nursing and medical services provided by in-patient facilities but need only supportive home care, e.g., visiting nurse service or "meals on wheels" dietary service.

Which of the health care services mentioned in the article do you think is most important? Why?

Sample Answer

NOTE: In the following paragraph the first sentence introduces the topic of the paragraph; the next three sentences provide the supporting details; and the final sentence supplies the conclusions.

An increase in home health care services is the most important trend in health care today. Many people cannot afford the staggering cost of hospitalization. In-surance companies and government funding for hospital care are being cut back. Some individuals respond better to home treatment because they are uncomfortable in the institutional setting of the hospital. If home care services were increased, health care costs would be reduced and patients would have the added comfort of their familiar home environment.

• EXERCISE 15–7 •

Directions. Read the following excerpt from a nursing textbook (Iyer et al., p. 252). Answer the following essay question based on the selection.

A maternity nurse told her teenage daughter that a 17 year old classmate had given birth and planned to give her baby for adoption. The nurse didn't realize that the teenage mother has been out of school for months to conceal her pregnancy. The teenage mother returned to school to find out that every-one knew of her pregnancy. Tracing the information to the nurse's daughter, she filed a complaint with the hospital. The nurse was fired.

Question: Do you think the nurse should have been fired? Why or why not?

• EXERCISE 15–8 •

Directions. Read the following excerpt from a nursing text (Iyer et al., p. 252). Create your own essay question based on the selection. Answer your question.

Right to Expect that all Communications and Records Pertaining to Care Will be Kept Confidential. The ethical aspects of this issue will be discussed later in this chapter. Nurses are prohibited from sharing information about a client with anyone other than health care professionals directly responsible for the client's care. This principle applies to families who are seeking detailed information. It is best to ask the client's permission before giving information to friends and family.

Example. A nurse was on duty one night when a client's son asked about his mother's condition. The nurse answered his questions and the client protested to the hospital that her health was her own business. The nurse was officially reprimanded and a copy was placed in her personnel record.

The nurse should be sure to determine the procedure to follow if a family member wants to see the client's record. Most facilities require the client to give written permission and expect the nurse to notify the physician of the request.

Nurses should not discuss the client's condition in public areas. The elevator is one such place in which a casual comment could be overheard by a family member or friend. Additionally nurses should not talk about their clients outside of the hospital or agency.

Comprehending? Yes _____ No _____

• TACKLING TEST-TAKING ANXIETY

Test-taking anxiety occurs because of worrying about not learning the information or worrying about time.

Research in study skills indicates that *overpreparation* is the best cure for test-taking anxiety. Keep up with your assignments. Take notes, underline, write summaries and outlines, and review, and you will go into a test feeling confident. This preparation can be done either alone or in study groups with other students.

Students worry that they will not finish their exam, whether objective or essay, in the allotted time. For both objective and essay tests, the following strategies will help you to finish the test:

- Be aware of time. Do not spend too much time on any one question.
- Answer the questions you are sure of first. You can return to the more difficult questions.
- On essay tests, if you run out of time, construct an outline of the remaining main points and major details you would have included in your answer. You may then get partial credit.

• VALUE OF PRACTICE TESTS

Take timed practice tests when you have completed your review. Use the questions at the end of the chapter or create your own test questions. This type of rehearsal before the performance helps you go into your test feeling prepared and positive. Remember, nothing succeeds like success.

• VOCABULARY CHECK

Directions. Below are 10 words taken from the key words section of this chapter. Circle the letter of the best definition from the four choices.

1 Hallucinations
   a mind reading or other extrasensory perception
   b psychosis, especially that which occurs after adolescence
   c accurate sensory impressions based on external stimuli
   d sensory impressions that have no basis in external stimuli

2 Haphazard
   a backwards
   b slanted
   c wrong direction
   d lack of plan

3 Scoliosis
   a lateral deviation of the spine
   b a normally straight spine
   c a ruptured disc
   d a fracture of the spine

4 Deficit
   a lacking interest
   b unplanned
   c leaning toward an idea
   d impairment in functional capacity

5 Resuscitate
   a to restore health
   b to rehabilitate
   c to restore to life
   d to regain strength

6 Allegations
   a false statements
   b statements of proof
   c days in court
   d illegalities

7 Sensory
   a pertaining to sight
   b pertaining to sensations
   c extremely sensitive
   d referring to clotting

8 Myths
   a mystery stories
   b false notions
   c nightmares
   d intentional lies

9 Malnutrition
- **a** loss in weight
- **b** poor nourishment
- **c** using food properly
- **d** diet control

10 Exotic
- **a** strikingly different
- **b** extremely beautiful
- **c** highly dangerous
- **d** very mysterious

• SUMMARY

Test-taking strategies will help you improve your grades on both objective and essay tests in nursing school. Schedule your study time, keep up with weekly assignments, and review all notes and underlined material, summaries, and outlines from tests.

Find out whether the test will be objective or essay. Take practice tests from end-of-chapter questions or create your own questions. Carefully read all directions on the exam before starting. Check over your paper to make necessary revisions. A positive attitude, careful preparation, and practice will ensure your success.

• U N I T •

V

READING SELECTIONS

In Unit V, "Reading Selections," you will have the opportunity to apply the strategies for reading nursing textbooks that you have learned in Units I through IV.

Each of the 15 reading selections is an excerpt taken from an actual chapter in a nursing text. The reading selections are designed to give you practice in prereading strategies, improving your comprehension through active reading, and monitoring comprehension through summarizing and answering multiple-choice questions.

These reading selections can be used on a weekly basis or as a culmination of your studies at the end of the semester.

With the successful completion of Unit V, "Reading Selections," you should be able to read your nursing textbook assignments confidently, with improved concentration, comprehension, and retention. Reading your nursing texts with competency will ensure your success in nursing school.

• Reading Selection 1 •

• PREVIEW QUESTION

Considering your own experiences, what do you know about people's reactions to their own dying?

• VOCABULARY

Underline any medical terminology or general vocabulary words you may need to learn in order to understand the ideas in the reading selection.

• CONCEPTUALIZATIONS OF LOSS, DYING, AND DEATH

The conceptual systems that we use in discussing loss, dying, and death have been derived through research. These formulations are not meant to be prescriptive. Rather, they serve as general guides to sensitize the nurse to what may occur and, therefore, what to look for and how to proceed when a response is indicated. Using these findings to help guide care is similar to using the systematic protocols of signs and symptoms of disease that help guide all nursing observations. For example, not all persons with a myocardial infarction show all of its possible clinical manifestations, nor do they all follow the same clinical course. Knowing what can occur helps us make observations and devise √ early interventions to prevent complications.

• Responses to Dying

In 1969, Elisabeth Kübler-Ross, a psychiatrist, described a series of stages through which people pass in response to their living through the dying process. She described the first stage as *shock and disbelief.* People could not believe that they were dying. The second stage was described as *denial.* People might say, "Yes, most people with this disease are dying, but not me!" The third stage was called *anger,* often characterized by the questions "Why me?" or "What did I do to deserve this?" The fourth stage was termed *bargaining.* In this stage, characteristic responses were, "I'll do any-

thing if . . . " or just let me live until my son gets married . . . or my daughter graduates." The next stage, when the person's deteriorating physical condition led to the realization that death was inevitable, was identified as *depression.* The final stage was termed *acceptance.* Acceptance according to Kübler-Ross was a stage of self-actualization, of feeling at peace with one's self, with one's imminent death, and with the cosmos.

• Patterns of Living-Dying

When death from a known fatal illness is preceded by several years of life, the use of the term dying from the time of diagnosis until the moment of death is paradoxical. These people frequently not only look robust, but enjoy full activity for prolonged periods. We say that they are living yet dying, and in these cases the living-dying period has the characteristics of a chronic illness.

Nursing research (Martocchio, 1982) has described four patterns of living-dying that are useful for understanding the uncertainties of living with life-threatening illness. These patterns (Table V–1), all having a general downward course concluding in death, reflect the natural history of various diseases, such as some cancers and many cardiovascular, renal, and hepatic conditions. They also describe the effects of specific therapeutic regimens. The categories remain consistent regardless of type of disease or treatment. The patterns are termed peaks and valleys, descending plateaus, downward slopes, and gradual slants.

The *peaks and valleys* pattern is characterized

From Ignatavicius and Bayne, pp. 199–200.

TABLE V–1   Characteristics of the Four
Patterns of Living-Dying

PATTERN	MAIN CHARACTERISTICS
Peaks and valleys	Hopeful highs/terrible lows
Descending plateaus	Rehabilitation/loss/ rehabilitation
Downward slope	No time to prepare
Gradual slant	Barely living/place- ment problems

by a series of peaks and valleys, or remissions and exacerbations. The peaks represent periods of well-being and the valleys, loss of well-being. Clients describe "hopeful highs" and "terrible lows." They see past highs as indicators of hope that they can rally one more time. They see the lows as threats to any hope of recovery.

The *descending plateaus* pattern is a series of steps. Each downward step represents a tangible reduction in functional ability and each plateau, a leveling-off or stable period. The plateaus and drop-offs can last for an indeterminate period and may occur any number of times. This pattern creates marked frustration as dying people and their families try, again and again, to take part in rehabili-

tation programs to maintain a level of function that is relentlessly but unpredictably declining.

The third pattern of living-dying is the *downward slope.* This pattern, frequently seen in intensive care units, is represented by a continuous and usually rapid downward course. In these cases, when there are relatively short-term illnesses or unexpected deaths, clients and family members have little time to prepare for the death.

The *gradual slant* pattern is characterized by a gradual decline over time. Toward the end, it is difficult to know whether these people are alive or dead. In this dying pattern, difficulties regarding quality of life and definitions of death become issues of concern. Family members and caregivers begin to see the unresponsive individual as a biologically living creature but also as a nonexistent person. As there is less meaningful interaction, the client is considered to be socially dead.

Regardless of the pattern, the direction is down. As the dying person declines and draws nearer to death, all involved with him or her undergo losses. For each person, the loss is different: The mother loses her son; the wife, her husband; the children, their father; the business partner, his colleague. Each person manifests the loss both in a universally recognized pattern and in his or her unique way.

• SUMMARY

Directions.   In the space provided, rewrite the above selection in your own words, focusing on the main idea and major details.

• COMPREHENSION QUESTIONS

Directions.   Below are 10 multiple-choice questions. Circle the letter of the best answer from the four choices.

1 In 1969, Kübler-Ross described:
   a what it is like to die
   b nurse's responses to dying
   c stages of the dying process
   d ways to aid a dying patient

2 Stage one of Kübler-Ross' theory is characterized by:
   a disbelief
   b anger
   c withdrawal
   d defiance

3 According to Kübler-Ross, another response to dying is:
   a confrontation
   b excessive talking on the subject
   c seeking vengeance
   d denial

4 As the patient moves closer to death, Kübler-Ross says the patient asks:
   a Can you help me?
   b Why me?
   c Would you help me die quicker?
   d How can I stop dying?

5 The final stage of Kübler-Ross' theory is:
   a bargaining
   b concern for relatives
   c continuous denial
   d acceptance

6 The purpose of Kübler-Ross' theory is to:
   a help the nurse to observe and devise interventions if necessary
   b allow the nurse to educate the patient about his dying
   c provide prescriptive formulations for nurses
   d none of the above

7 The title of the table in this selection is:
   a patterns of death and dying
   b responses to the four stages of living-dying
   c characteristics of the four patterns of living-dying
   d stages of living-dying

8 In Martocchio's research the peaks and valleys pattern is characterized by:
   a highs and lows
   b acceptance and denial
   c rehabilitation and deterioration
   d gains and losses

9 The four patterns of living-dying describe:
   a when death is preceded by many years of life
   b the ways of dying from a long illness
   c the uncertainties of living with a chronic illness
   d all of the above

10 The four patterns of living-dying:
   a sometimes lead to death
   b always lead to death
   c can be reversed
   d allow family members to have a lot of time to prepare for the death

Comprehending?   Yes ____   No ____

• Reading Selection 2 •

• PREVIEW QUESTION

What questions can you create from the boldface headings?

• VOCABULARY

Underline any medical terminology or general vocabulary words you may need to learn in order to understand the ideas in the reading selection.

• IMPAIRED SKIN INTEGRITY

• Planning: Client Goals

The primary goal for this nursing diagnosis is that the client will experience minimal skin impairment and contamination as a result of surgery.

• Interventions

Surgery is an invasive procedure that places the client at risk for complications related to the surgical wound, such as incisional tears and lacerations, bacterial contamination, and loss of body fluids from the wound during and after surgery. Sterile surgical technique and the use of protective drapes, skin closures, and dressings help to minimize complications and promote wound healing.

PLASTIC ADHESIVE DRAPE

The scrub nurse helps the surgical assistant apply a sterile plastic adhesive drape after the surgical site has been cleaned and dried. The plastic drape is applied directly to dry skin to prevent tearing of the surgical incision. The surgeon makes the incision through the plastic drape; the cut edge remains adherent to the skin and keeps the surgical incision sealed from tears and the migration of bacteria into the wound. After closure of the surgical incision, the drape is carefully removed by the nurse and the surgical assistant. The nurse pays special attention to the elderly and clients with fragile skin to prevent denuding of the skin during removal of the adhesive drape.

From Ignativicius and Bayne, pp. 468–470.

SKIN CLOSURES

Skin closures, such as sutures and clamps, are used to approximate wound edges until wound healing is complete; occlude the lumen of blood vessels, preventing hemorrhage and loss of body fluids; and prevent wound contamination. The quality of the approximated tissue and the type of closure material are two factors that determine the strength of the closure. Suture material, when used, ensures wound integrity immediately after closure. To facilitate proper healing, the wound is usually closed in layers to maintain tissue integrity and promote healing with minimal scarring. The surgeon selects the method and type of closures to be used on the basis of the surgical site, the size and depth of the surgical wound, and the age and medical history of the client. A combination of sutures and clamps is commonly used for closure of internal layers of the wound. Staples, stay and retention sutures, and skin closure tapes (Steri-Strips) are used for closure of superficial wounds or the epidermis. Figure V–1 illustrates commonly used wound closures.

There are two classifications of suture material: absorbable and nonabsorbable. These are categorized according to diameter and tensile strength. A suture consists of one or more strands of material that are designated by size or gauge of the suture material. The designation sequence is in descending order from number 5 to 0, then 2-0, 3-0, and so forth, to 11-0. Size 5 is the heaviest material and is used to close the deep layers of an abdominal wound; 11-0 is the smallest-diameter suture and is used for plastic surgery.

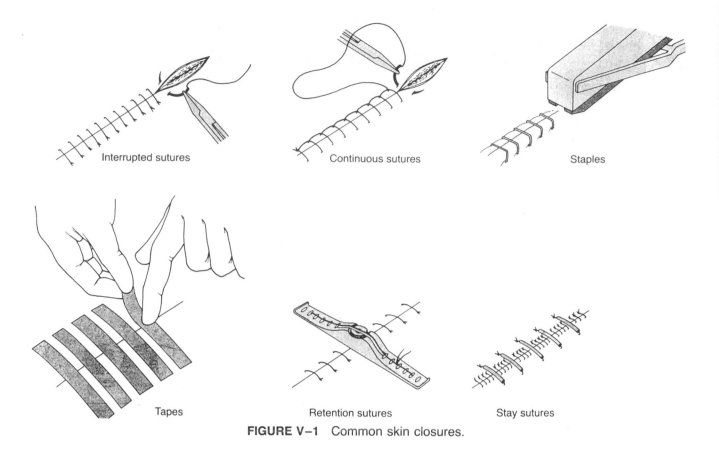

Interrupted sutures

Continuous sutures

Staples

Tapes

Retention sutures

Stay sutures

FIGURE V–1 Common skin closures.

Absorbable sutures are digested by body enzymes. These sutures first lose strength and then gradually disappear from the tissue. Catgut is a common type of absorbable suture material. The rate of absorption is influenced by the client's physical status, the presence of inflammation, and the type of catgut used.

Nonabsorbable sutures are not affected by enzymes or inflammation. Nonabsorbable sutures become encapsulated in the tissue during the healing process and remain embedded in the tissue unless they are removed. Nonabsorbable sutures are used to secure orthopedic prosthetic devices in place and to close external wounds. The surgeon may use a double or interlocking stitch to increase the integrity of the closure. Figure V–1 shows retention and stay sutures, which are frequently used in addition to standard suture material for high-risk clients, such as those having major abdominal surgery, obese clients, diabetic individuals, and clients taking steroids that inhibit wound healing.

After the incision is closed, a dressing is applied to protect it from contamination, absorb drainage, and provide support to the incision. A pressure dressing may be applied to prevent or stop a vascular area from bleeding postoperatively.

After the dressing is secure, the nurse coordinates the surgical team in repositioning and transferring the client. A roller board or a lift sheet is used to transfer the client safely from the operating room table to a stretcher or bed. The circulating nurse accompanies the client and anesthesiologist to the postanesthesia area or recovery room and gives a report of the client's intraoperative experience to the PAR nurse. Important information to be relayed includes the client's level of anxiety before anesthesia, the type and length of the surgical procedure, the location of incisions, previous reactions to anesthesia, respiratory dysfunctions, joint or limb immobility, primary language, and any special requests the client may have verbalized.

• **Evaluation**

On the basis of the identified common nursing diagnoses, the nurse evaluates the care of the intraoperative client. Expected outcomes for the client in the intraoperative phase of the perioperative experience include that the client

1 Describes the anesthesia to be used

2 Is safely anesthetized

3 Does not experience any injury related to positioning or electrical equipment

---

• SUMMARY

Directions. In the space provided, rewrite the above selection in your own words, focusing on the main idea and major details.

• COMPREHENSION QUESTIONS

Directions. Below are 10 multiple-choice questions. Circle the letter of the best answer from the four choices.

1 During surgery, which of the following helps minimize complications?
 a protective drapes
 b skin closures
 c sterile surgical techniques
 d all of the above

2 The nurse helps to apply the adhesive drape:
 a after surgical site has been cleaned and dried
 b before the surgical site has a chance to dry
 c immediately before cleaning surgical site
 d none of the above

3 The purpose of skin closures is to:
 a allow the surgeon to inspect the surgery site
 b to approximate wound edges until the wound is healed
 c keep the surgery site flexible
 d allow for gradual loss of body fluids

4 The strength of the closure is determined by:
  a the size of the surgery site
  b the age and skin condition of the patient
  c the age and weight of the patient
  d the quality of the approximated tissue

5 The two classifications of suture material are:
  a reusable and nonreusable
  b flexible and nonflexible
  c absorbable and nonabsorbable
  d strong and delicate

6 To facilitate proper healing, the wound is:
  a inspected hourly
  b usually closed in layers
  c always closed with clamps
  d never closed with clamps

7 Some types of sutures:
  a are digested by body enzymes
  b become encapsulated in the tissue
  c a but not b
  d both a and b

8 The reason a dressing is not applied to a closed incision is:
  a to protect it from contamination
  b to allow quicker ambulation
  c to provide support to the incision
  d to absorb drainage

9 Right after the dressing is in place, the nurse's responsibility is to:
  a coordinate the surgical team in repositioning and transferring the patient
  b examine the surgical site frequently
  c remain with the patient in the operating room before transfer
  d reposition and transfer client himself or herself

10 The primary nursing goal for patients with impaired skin integrity is:
  a the patient will experience minimal skin contamination
  b the patient will experience minimal skin impairment
  c neither a nor b
  d both a and b

Comprehending? Yes ___ No ___

• Reading Selection 3 •

• PREVIEW QUESTION

Name the three stages of inflammatory responses.

• VOCABULARY

Underline any medical terminology or general vocabulary words you may need to learn in order to understand the ideas in this reading selection.

• INFLAMMATORY RESPONSES

Inflammatory responses for protecting the body against side effects of tissue injury or invasion by foreign proteins occur in a predictable sequence. The sequence is the same regardless of the initiating stimulus. Responses at the tissue level are responsible for the five cardinal physical manifestations of inflammation: increased warmth, redness, swelling, altered sensations (usually pain), and altered function (usually decreased). Tissue and cellular events that cause these manifestations are described as part of the different stages of inflammation. The responses of inflammation can be divided into three distinct functional stages, although the timing of the stages may overlap.

• Stage I

This stage is called the *vascular stage* because most of the early effects of this response involve physiologic changes at the vascular level. When inflammation occurs as a result of tissue injury, this stage has two phases.

The first phase is an immediate but short-term vasoconstriction of arterioles and venules as a direct result of physical trauma to vascular smooth muscle. This phase lasts only seconds to minutes and may be so short that the individual undergoing the response is unaware of the vasoconstriction. Usually, this phase does not occur when inflammation is purely a response to invasion of the body.

The second phase is characterized by hyperemia and swelling (edema formation) at the site of injury or invasion. Injured tissues and the leuko-

cytes in this area secrete vasoactive amines (histamine, serotonin, and kinins) that cause constriction of the venules and dilation of the arterioles in the immediate area. The effects of these changes in blood vessel dilation cause the symptoms of redness and increased warmth of the tissues. The purpose of this response is to increase the supply of nutrients at the tissue level by increasing the blood flow.

Some of these same vasoactive amines increase capillary permeability, which allows blood plasma to leak into the interstitial space. This response causes the symptoms of swelling as fluid collects and pain as both the pressure of an increased amount of fluid in the area and caustic chemicals in the fluid stimulate local sensory nerve endings. Pain, although an uncomfortable sensation, is somewhat beneficial to the individual experiencing inflammation. Pain increases the individual's awareness that a problem exists and encourages the individual to take actions that avoid further injury or alter the conditions that caused the inflammation. Edema formation at the site of injury or invasion is an overall helpful event. This swelling can protect the area from further injury by creating a cushion of fluid. The extra fluid can also dilute the concentration of any toxins or microorganisms that entered the area. The plasma that leaked into the interstitial space contains fibrin and other protein factors that can cause the interstitial fluid in the area of injury or invasion to clot, which isolates the site and confines the effects largely to the immediate area. The duration of these responses depends on the severity of the initiating event.

The major leukocyte that is involved in this

From Ignatavicius and Bayne, pp. 538–539.

229

stage of inflammation is the tissue macrophage. The response of the tissue macrophages is immediate because they are already in place at the site of injury or invasion. However, this response is limited because the number of such macrophages is so small. In addition to functioning in phagocytosis, the tissue macrophages secrete several substances to enhance the inflammatory response. One substance is colony-stimulating factor, which stimulates the bone marrow to reduce leukocyte production time from 14 days to a matter of hours. In addition, tissue macrophages secrete substances that increase the release of neutrophils from the bone marrow and attract them to the site of injury or invasion, which leads to the next stage of inflammation.

- **Stage II**

This stage of inflammation is also called the *cellular exudate stage.* It is characterized by neutrophilia (increase in the percentage and number of circulating neutrophils), secretion of many factors into the interstitial fluid, and formation of exudate.

The most prominent leukocyte in this stage is the neutrophil. Under the influence of chemotactic agents and substances that increase the number and rate of maturation of neutrophils, the actual neutrophil count can increase up to fivefold within 12 hours of the onset of inflammation. The purposes of the neutrophils at the site of inflammation are to (1) attack and destroy foreign materials and (2) remove dead and dying tissue. Both of these functions are accomplished through phagocytosis.

During acute inflammatory responses that are short, the otherwise healthy individual can synthesize enough mature neutrophils to keep pace with the side effects of injury and invasion and to eventually overcome the ability of invaders to multiply. At the same time, these leukocytes secrete factors that permit reproduction of tissue macrophages and increase bone marrow production of monocytes. Although this reaction is slower to start, its effects are relatively long-lasting.

When infectious processes stimulating inflammation are longer or chronic, the bone marrow cannot synthesize and release enough mature neutrophils into the blood to keep pace with the ability of microorganisms to multiply. In this situation, the bone marrow begins to release immature neutrophils, many of which cannot phagocytose or complete maturation. Such a reduction in the number of functional phagocytic neutrophils limits the effectiveness of the inflammatory response and dramatically increases the susceptibility of the individual to new and recurring microbial infections.

- **Stage III**

This stage of inflammation is also called the *tissue repair and replacement stage.* Although this stage is completed last, it begins at the time of injury and is critical to the ultimate function of the inflamed area.

Some of the leukocytes involved in inflammation are capable of stimulating repair of lost or damaged tissues by inducing the remaining healthy tissue to divide. In tissues that are not mitotically active (nondividing tissues), leukocytes stimulate revascularization and the laying down of different types of collagen to form scar tissue. Because scar tissue does not behave in the same manner as normal differentiated tissue, some functional loss occurs in areas where damaged tissues are replaced with scar tissue. The extent of the functional loss is determined by the percentage of tissue that is replaced by scar tissue.

Inflammation provides immediate protection against the side effects of tissue injury and invading foreign proteins. Although inflammatory responses are usually beneficial, some are accompanied by unpleasant and even tissue-damaging actions. The capacity of an individual to generate an inflammatory response is a critical component to the overall health and well-being of an individual. Alone, inflammation cannot confer immunity; however, the interaction of specific components of inflammation with other leukocytes and tissues assists in providing long-lasting immunity against re-exposure to the same microorganisms.

• SUMMARY

Directions.   In the space provided, rewrite the preceding selection in your own words, focusing on the main ideas and major details.

• COMPREHENSION QUESTIONS

Directions.   Below are 10 multiple-choice questions. Circle the letter of the best answer from the four choices.

1 In the inflammatory response:
   a the sequence is the same regardless of cause
   b the sequence is determined by the initiating stimulus
   c there is no set sequence
   d there is sometimes a set sequence and sometimes not

2 The vascular stage is characterized by:
   a one phase
   b two phases
   c three phases
   d four phases

3 The purpose of changes in blood vessel dilation in stage I is to:
   a stop bleeding
   b fight invading foreign protein
   c make the individual aware of injury
   d increase the supply of nutrients

4 Edema in stage I is helpful because:
   a it prevents further injury
   b it dilutes concentration of toxins
   c neither a nor b
   d both a and b

5 Pain, as part of the inflammatory response:
a increases the individual's awareness of injury
b exacerbates the healing process
c is not yet understood
d none of the above

6 The function of neutrophils is to:
a evoke the pain response
b cause the dilation of the vascular system
c promote formation of scar tissue
d none of the above

7 One problem with chronic infections is that:
a tissue microphages are produced
b too many neutrophils are released
c the bone marrow releases immature neutrophils
d the bone marrow production of monocytes is increased

8 Stage III:
a begins at the time of injury
b begins after stage I
c begins after stage II
d is not always a part of the inflammatory response

9 Scar tissue is formed:
a in mitotically active tissue
b in nondividing tissue
c only in dividing tissues
d before the inflammatory response

10 Inflammatory responses are:
a sometimes accompanied by unpleasant actions
b always beneficial
c able to confer immunity
d independent of the individual's overall health

Comprehending? Yes ____ No ____

• Reading Selection 4 •

• PREVIEW QUESTION

An assessment of the skeletal system consists of assessing which parts of the body?

• VOCABULARY

Underline any medical terminology or general vocabulary words you may need to learn in order to understand the ideas in this reading selection.

• PHYSICAL ASSESSMENT

Although bones, joints, and muscles are usually assessed simultaneously utilizing a head-to-toe approach, each subsystem is described separately for emphasis and understanding.

• Assessment of the Skeletal System

GENERAL INSPECTION

The nurse observes the client's posture, gait, and mobility for gross deformities and impairment. *Posture* includes the individual's body build and alignment when standing and walking. Curvature of the spine and the length, shape, and symmetry of extremities are inspected. Figure V–2 shows common musculoskeletal deformities. *Muscle mass* is inspected for size and symmetry. The client's *gait* is evaluated for balance and steadiness, and ease and length of stride; a limp or other asymmetric leg movement or deformity is noted. The nurse observes the client's need for ambulatory devices during transfer from bed to chair and while walking and climbing stairs. *Mobility* is also assessed by asking the client to perform simple activities of daily living (ADL), such as donning shoes. Pain and deformity may limit physical mobility.

After a general evaluation is performed, the nurse assesses major bones, joints, and muscles by inspection, palpation, and determination of function. As shown in Figure V–3, a *goniometer,* used commonly by physical therapists and clinical specialists, provides an exact measurement for joint

From Ignatavicius and Bayne, pp. 722–723.

range of motion (ROM), but the nurse can estimate the degree of joint mobility by putting each joint through its respective ROM. For each anatomic location, the nurse observes the skin for color, elasticity, and lesions that may relate to musculoskeletal dysfunction.

ASSESSMENT OF THE HEAD AND NECK

The nurse inspects and palpates the skull for *shape, symmetry, tenderness, and masses.* The temporomandibular joints (TMJs) are best evaluated by asking the client to open her/his mouth while the nurse palpates the TMJs. Common abnormal findings are tenderness or pain, crepitus (a grating sound), and a spongy swelling caused by excess synovium and fluid, which can be palpated.

Each vertebra of the spine in the neck is observed and palpated. Clinical findings may include malalignment, tenderness, and inability to flex, extend, and rotate the neck as expected.

ASSESSMENT OF THE VERTEBRAL SPINE

The thoracic spine, lumbar spine, and sacral spine are evaluated in the same manner as the neck. In addition, the nurse places both hands over the lumbosacral area and applies pressure with his/her thumbs to elicit tenderness. Clients often do not complain of discomfort until the area is palpated.

ASSESSMENT OF THE UPPER EXTREMITIES

The nurse assesses both extremities concurrently. For example, both shoulders are inspected and palpated for *size, swelling, deformity, malalignment, tenderness or pain,* and *mobility.* A shoul-

233

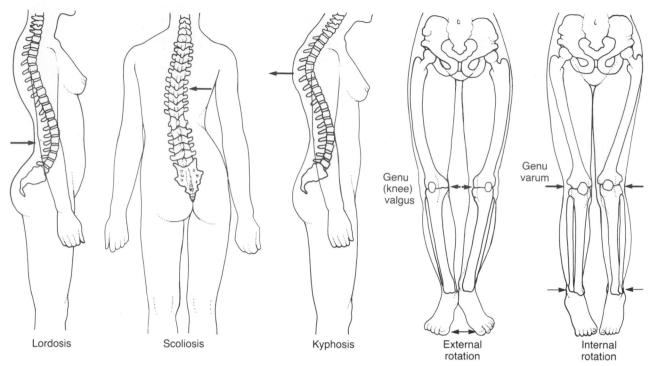

FIGURE V–2 Common musculoskeletal deformities.

Lordosis   Scoliosis   Kyphosis   Genu (knee) valgus   Genu varum   External rotation   Internal rotation

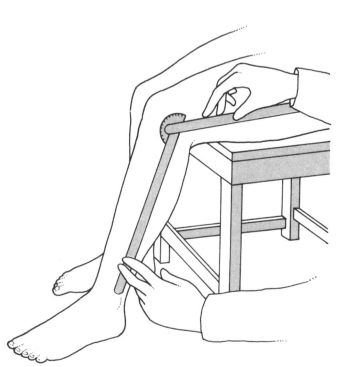

FIGURE V–3 Goniometric measurement of the knee joint.

der injury may prevent the client from combing his/her hair with the affected arm, but severe arthritis may inhibit movement in both arms. Similarly, the elbows and wrists are assessed.

Assessment of hand function is perhaps the most critical part of the examination, as the hand has multiple joints in a single digit. The nurse inspects and palpates the metacarpophalangeal (MCP), proximal interphalangeal (PIP), and distal interphalangeal (DIP) joints, comparing the same digits on right and left hands. ROM for each joint is also determined using active movement if possible.

ASSESSMENT OF THE LOWER EXTREMITIES

Evaluation of the hip joint relies primarily on determining its degree of *mobility,* as the joint is deep and thereby difficult to inspect or palpate. On the other hand, the knee is readily accessible for nursing assessment, particularly when the client is sitting and the knee is flexed. Fluid accumulation, or effusion, is easily detected in the knee joint, and limitations in movement with accompanying pain are common findings. The ankles and feet are often neglected in the physical examination, yet they contain multiple bones and joints that can be affected by disease and injury. Each joint should be observed, palpated, and tested for ROM.

• SUMMARY

Directions.   In the space provided, rewrite the preceding selection in your own words, focusing on the main ideas and major details.

• COMPREHENSION QUESTIONS

Directions.   Below are 10 multiple-choice questions. Circle the letter of the best answer from the four choices.

1   Figure V–2 shows:
   a   common difficulties of the vertebral spine
   b   common musculoskeletal deformities
   c   lower and upper extremities deformations
   d   assessment of the head and neck

2   Figure V–3 shows goniometric measurement of the:
   a   skeletal system
   b   spine
   c   head and neck
   d   knee joint

3   Posture refers to:
   a   curvature of the spine
   b   an individual's body build and alignment
   c   only how you stand
   d   only how you walk

4   Muscle mass is inspected for:
   a   strength and size
   b   size and symmetry
   c   strength and symmetry
   d   strength and flexibility

5 Gait is evaluated for all but:
a endurance
b balance
c ease and length of stride
d steadiness

6 The function of the goniometer is to provide measurement of:
a bone strength
b bone length
c joint range of motion
d spinal alignment

7 The nurse inspects the skull for:
a smoothness, rotation, and misalignment
b deformity, swelling, size, mobility
c rotation, shape, mass, mobility
d shape, symmetry, tenderness, masses

8 The nurse needs to apply pressure to the lumbosacral area because:
a the nurse needs to assess for swelling
b the patient does not complain of discomfort until pressure is applied
c the nurse needs to assess for flexibility
d the patient has complained of tenderness

9 In an assessment of the upper extremities, the most critical part is the assessment of:
a hand function
b shoulder flexibility
c elbow function
d wrist function

10 Evaluation of the hip joint relies on determining hip:
a strength
b density
c injury
d mobility

Comprehending? Yes ____ No ____

• Reading Selection 5 •

• PREVIEW QUESTION

What is the purpose of assessing the cranial nerves?

• VOCABULARY

Underline any medical terminology or general vocabulary words you may need to learn in order to understand the ideas in this reading selection.

• ASSESSMENT OF CRANIAL NERVES

• Cranial Nerve I: Olfactory

With the client's eyes closed, one nostril at a time is tested (the client occludes the other with a finger). The nurse has the client identify familiar *odors,* such as coffee, tobacco, mint, or soap. Alcohol sponges and ammonia are not used, as these stimulate the trigeminal nerve, not the olfactory. Lack of or decreased smell sensation may not be significant, as loss or decrease occurs with age, smoking, colds, and allergies. The client's report that smell was suddenly lost without a predisposing factor or that odors are distorted is more significant.

• Cranial Nerve II: Optic

Each eye is tested alone with the other eye covered but open. *Central* vision is tested by the Snellen chart, asking the client to read out loud from a pocket reader card, a magazine, or a newspaper. The test should be done with glasses if the client uses glasses for far or near vision. *Peripheral* vision can be tested by asking the client to focus his/her eye on the examiner's nose. The nurse wiggles one finger of each hand in the superior visual field, asking the client to indicate where the movement is. He/she should see movement on both sides. The nurse then repeats in the inferior visual field. To begin testing the second eye, the nurse wiggles the finger of only one hand to prevent the client from repeating the previous answers. The nurse then tests the superior and inferior fields using a finger

of each hand. If the client cannot see the fingers in one or more of the fields, further testing is required. The *fundus,* or internal eye, is inspected with the ophthalmoscope to check for vascular problems, retinal disease, papilledema, or optic atrophy. Special training is required for the nurse to operate the ophthalmoscope.

• Cranial Nerve III: Oculomotor

Eye movement (medial, superior and medial, superior and lateral, and inferior and lateral) is tested with the assessment of cranial nerve VI. *Pupil constriction* is tested with the room darkened, if possible. The nurse brings the penlight in from the side or from above or below and shines the light in the client's eye. The pupil should constrict and stay constricted. The nurse repeats with the other eye and watches for *consensual* (involuntary) constriction in the eye not being tested (consensual response will be less than direct response). Pupils should be equal in size, round, regular, and react to light and accommodation (PERRLA). The pupils should react to light with the *same rate* of speed and to the *same degree.* Glaucoma, cataract surgery, and iridectomy may influence the shape and size of the pupil, as well as its reaction to light. A pupil may dilate slightly after constricting with the light stimulus still present (Gunn's pupil sign); this reaction may be normal. However, if the dilation is marked, it may represent optic nerve or retinal pathologic changes. A few people have one pupil larger than the other (Adie's pupil); this may also be normal, if there are no other eye symptoms. The client is usually aware of the size difference. Adie's

---

From Ignatavicius and Bayne, pp. 850–852.

pupil is slow to react to light and constricts only a little. *Accommodation* is tested by bringing an object from far to near the client's eyes. The pupils should constrict and the eyes converge (turn in to focus on the object). Accommodation need not be tested if constriction to light is normal. Some medications may affect constriction and dilation. To assess for *lid elevation,* the upper eyelid should rest approximately at the top or slightly below the top of the pupil. Strength and closure of the lid are a function of cranial nerve VII, but can be tested with the eye examination.

- ### Cranial Nerve IV: Trochlear

Eye movement (inferior and medial) is tested with assessment of cranial nerve VI.

- ### Cranial Nerve V: Trigeminal

The client's eyes are closed for the *sensory* portion of the testing. The nurse asks the client to indicate when touched by saying "now." By stroking a piece of cotton over the client's skin *(light touch),* the nurse tests all three branches of the trigeminal nerve (ophthalmic—forehead, maxillary—cheek, mandibular—jaw), alternating sides for comparison. Next, the nurse asks the client to indicate whether the sensation is sharp or dull while using an object that has sharp and dull components (e.g., a safety pin) and then repeats the process. The *motor* aspect can be done with the client's eyes open. The nurse palpates the temporal and masseter (jaw) muscles (with one hand on each side) for strength and equality while the client clenches her/his teeth. The *corneal reflex* has traditionally been tested by using a wisp of cotton and touching the edge of the cornea, which normally causes blinking. However, that procedure can cause abrasion to the cornea. In a routine examination, blinking will be seen by the examiner and the corneal reflex need not be tested. If there is concern that the corneal reflex is absent, there are two safer ways to test. One is to bring a fist quickly toward the client's face in a threatening motion. If the client has vision, this will cause blinking. Alternatively, the nurse can use a syringe full of air and expel it toward the eyes. Blinking will result if the reflex is intact.

- ### Cranial Nerve VI: Abducens

Eye movement, a function of cranial nerves of III, IV, and VI, is tested by checking the *six cardinal positions of gaze.* The nurse asks the client to follow the examiner's finger or a held object while keeping his/her head still. The nurse starts at 1 o'clock position and moves clockwise through the six positions shown in Figure V–4. The nurse pauses in the horizontal and vertical positions to check for *nystagmus* (involuntary oscillation of the eyes) or deviation. Some nystagmus in the extreme lateral position is normal. Severe lateral nystagmus or nystagmus in any other position is abnormal. If there is weakness or paralysis of a particular muscle, the eye will not turn in that direction.

- ### Cranial Nerve VII: Facial

Only the *motor* aspect is tested. Testing of taste on the anterior portion of the tongue is done with cranial nerve IX testing. The nurse asks the client to *frown, smile, wrinkle the forehead,* and *puff out the cheeks,* while looking for symmetry of both sides. *Eyelid closure and strength* are tested by asking the client to close the eyes tightly and keep them closed while the examiner tries to pry them open.

- ### Cranial Nerve VIII: Vestibulocochlear (Acoustic)

Hearing is tested initially with the client's eyes closed. The nurse rubs a thumb and finger together next to the client's ear and asks where sound is heard and then repeats this maneuver for the other ear. A watch can also be used, or the examiner can whisper close to each ear. The Weber and Rinne tests (with the client's eyes open) are done to check for conductive or sensorineural hearing loss. *Conductive* hearing loss occurs because of external-ear and middle-ear problems (e.g., excessive cerumen, presence of pus, ossicle fusion, or a damaged eardrum). *Sensorineural* loss occurs because of cochlear or nerve damage. In the *Weber* test, in which a vibrating tuning fork is placed on top of the head or the forehead, the client should hear sound equally in both ears. (Touching the fork tines will stop the vibration; therefore, the fork must be held by the handle only.) With conductive loss, the sound is heard louder in the ear with the deficit because the sound bypasses the obstruction. The

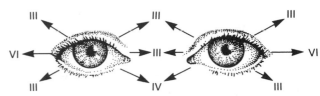

FIGURE V–4 Checking extraocular movements in the six cardinal positions indicates the functioning of cranial nerves III, IV, and VI.

sound will be louder in the better ear in sensori-neural loss. The *Rinne* test, in which a vibrating tuning fork is placed on the mastoid bone until sound is no longer heard and then moved near the external ear canal, measures the difference between bone and air conduction. Normal, or *positive,* results occur when the client hears the sound about twice as long by air conduction as by bone. In conductive hearing loss, the client hears the sound longer through bone (*negative* Rinne's test). The sound is heard longer by air than by bone (positive) in sensorineural loss. *Equilibrium,* although controlled by cranial nerve VIII, is generally tested with cerebellar testing at the end of the examination to avoid having the client stand and sit excessively.

• Cranial Nerve IX: Glossopharyngeal

The *motor* portion is tested with cranial nerve X assessment. *Taste* (posterior one-third of tongue) is often not tested unless the client reports loss of taste. When testing taste, it is important to remember the tongue must be rinsed in between the sweet, sour, bitter, and salt samples. Taste only occurs when the substance is in solution, so the tongue must be moist for a true test result.

• Cranial Nerve X: Vagus

The *motor* portion is tested by asking the client to say "Ah" when the examiner looks into the throat.

The uvula and palate should rise bilaterally and equally. Stimulating the gag reflex with a tongue blade reflects sensitivity to a stimulus. Ability to *swallow* and *normal phonation* also imply intact nerves IX and X.

• Cranial Nerve XI: Spinal Accessory

The *strength* of the sternocleidomastoid and trapezius muscles is tested by having the client turn his/her head against the resistance (provided by the examiner's hand on the side of the face toward the turn) and then repeat in the other direction. The second test requires the client to shrug his/her shoulders upward against the resistance of the examiner's hands placed on the client's shoulders.

• Cranial Nerve XII: Hypoglossal

Motor innervation to the tongue is tested by asking the client to stick out her/his tongue. The nurse checks for deviation to one side or the other. The tongue deviates toward the same side where the lesion has occurred in the brain. *Strength* may be tested by asking the client to push against a tongue blade held at one side of the tongue and then repeat on the other side.

• SUMMARY

Directions. In the space provided, rewrite the above selection in your own words, focusing on the main ideas and major details.

• COMPREHENSION QUESTIONS

Directions.   Below are 10 multiple-choice questions. Circle the letter of the best answer from the four choices.

1 When assessing for smell, it is permissible to use all of the following familiar odors except:
   a mint
   b ammonia
   c soap
   d coffee

2 When assessing the optic nerve, the nurse checks:
   a central vision only
   b peripheral vision only
   c both central and peripheral vision
   d neither central nor peripheral vision

3 Light touch perception is the function of the:
   a trochlear nerve
   b oculomotor nerve
   c abducens nerve
   d trigeminal nerve

4 When the facial nerve is assessed, the aspect tested is:
   a motor
   b sensory
   c parasympathetic motor
   d none of the above

5 Hearing is the property of the:
   a facial nerve
   b vagus nerve
   c abducens nerve
   d vestibulocochlear nerve

6 The Weber test uses a:
   a syringe full of air
   b piece of cotton
   c tuning fork
   d tongue blade

7 The nerve assessed for taste is the:
   a glossopharyngeal
   b facial
   c hypoglossal
   d vagus

8 The nerve responsible for the gag reflex is the:
  a glossopharyngeal
  b facial
  c hypoglossal
  d vagus

9 When assessing the hypoglossal, the nurse is checking for:
  a ability to swallow
  b motor innervation of the tongue
  c strength of the sternocleidomastoid
  d normal phonation

10 The purpose of the nurse assessing the 12 cranial nerves is to:
  a judge reflex activity
  b judge cerebellar function
  c judge motor and sensory functioning
  d none of the above

Comprehending? Yes ___ No ___

• Reading Selection 6 •

• PREVIEW QUESTION

This selection is about uveitis, an eye disease. What, as a nursing student, do you think you need to know about uveitis?

• VOCABULARY

Underline any medical terminology or general vocabulary words you may need to learn in order to understand the ideas in this reading selection.

• UVEAL TRACT DISORDERS

The uveal tract is composed of three separate but interrelated parts, the iris, the ciliary body, and the choroid. All of these structures contribute to the ability of the eye to focus an image in the proper area of the retina. Problems with any or all of these structures result in some degree of visual impairment. The most common problem associated with these structures is inflammation. Inflammatory diseases of the uveal tract are characterized by location and extent. They can be acute or chronic.

• Uveitis

OVERVIEW

Uveitis is a general term for inflammatory diseases of the uveal tract. One or more segments of the eye may be involved at any given time because a common blood supply nourishes these areas.

Anterior uveitis includes iritis, which is inflammation of the iris; iridocyclitis, which is inflammation of both the iris and the ciliary body; and cyclitis. The etiology of anterior uveitis is unknown but may be related to exposure to allergens, fungi, bacteria, viruses, or chemicals; anterior uveitis can also follow surgical or accidental trauma. Systemic diseases such as rheumatoid arthritis, ankylosing spondylitis, herpes simplex, and herpes zoster may predispose an individual to development of anterior uveitis.

Symptoms of anterior uveitis include moderate periorbital aching, tearing, blurred vision, and photophobia, which is due to the pain that accompanies contraction of the inflamed iris in bright lights. A small, irregular, nonreactive pupil is caused by the adhesions that form between the iris and the lens during inflammation. Engorgement of the episcleral vessels near the corneal-scleral limbus creates a purplish discoloration called *ciliary flush* (Boyd-Monk & Steinmetz, 1987). Fibrinous material or a hypopyon, which is an accumulation of purulent matter in the anterior chamber, may be noted in severe cases.

Posterior uveitis is the common term for retinitis, which is inflammation of the retina, and chorioretinitis, which is inflammation of both the choroid and the retina. Posterior uveitis is usually associated with infectious processes such as tuberculosis, syphilis, and toxoplasmosis. The onset of symptoms is slow and insidious. Visual impairment in the affected eye is the primary symptom. It results from the exudation of protein-rich fluid, fibrin, and cells into the vitreous cavity (Newell, 1986). The location and extent of visual impairment depend on the size and site of inflammation. The vision loss appears to be more severe than the amount of choroid or retina involved.

On examination, the pupil is seen to be small, nonreactive, and irregularly shaped because of the adhesions that bind the iris to the lens. Vitreous opacities composed of fibrin and inflammatory cells are seen as black dots against the red background of the fundus. Chorioretinal lesions are seen as grayish-yellow, defined patches on the retinal surface.

From Ignatavicius and Bayne, pp. 1052–1053.

COLLABORATIVE MANAGEMENT

Treatment of anterior and posterior uveitis is largely symptomatic because the etiology is difficult to determine. The treatment plan includes putting the ciliary body to rest with a cycloplegic agent such as atropine. The pupil is dilated to prevent adhesions between the iris and the lens. Steroid drops, e.g., prednisolone acetate (Pred-Forte), are administered every hour to decrease the inflammatory response of the eye and to prevent adhesions of the iris to the cornea and lens. Ointments such as dexamethasone phosphate (Maxidex) are also used. Subconjunctival injections of steroids may be used in posterior uveitis or when topical steroids have been ineffective. If inflammation causes intraocular pressure to increase, the use of timolol (Timoptic) may be initiated. Treatment is also aimed at controlling the causative systemic disease. If the iritis is due to tuberculosis, appropriate drug therapy for the infection is instituted. Early syphilitic lesions respond well to antibiotics. Analgesics such as acetaminophen (Tylenol or Tylenol with Codeine) are ordered for pain. Antibiotics may be initiated for the client with posterior uveitis (Boyd-Monk & Steinmetz, 1987).

Any client who complains of reduced or blurred vision should be thoroughly questioned, and a baseline visual acuity should be measured before further evaluation of the eye. The client presenting with blurred vision or visual impairment may be anxious about the actual change and may fear that they may not regain useful vision. Careful and sensitive listening by the nurse to these concerns can allay much anxiety. Warm compresses may be used for complaints of ocular pain. Darkening the room and encouraging the client to wear sunglasses reduce the complaints of photophobia. Because vision will be blurred from the use of cycloplegic drops, the client should be advised not to drive or to operate machinery. Signs and symptoms of bacterial and fungal ulcers, for which steroid eyedrops have been prescribed, must be reviewed with the client. Eyedrop instillation by the client should be observed by the nurse before the client leaves the health care facility. Indications of increased intraocular pressure should be reviewed with the client.

The client may become irritable and restless because of sleep deprivation associated with frequent eyedrop administration. The nurse should facilitate the client's resting whenever possible.

• SUMMARY

Directions. In the space provided, rewrite the above selection in your own words, focusing on the main ideas and major details.

• COMPREHENSION QUESTIONS

Directions. Below are 10 multiple-choice questions. Circle the letter of the best answer from the four choices.

1   The uveal tract is composed of:
    a   iris, ciliary body, and choroid
    b   the vitreous, iris, and ciliary bodies
    c   optic nerve, iris, and the vitreous
    d   lens, iris, and the choroid

2   The purpose of the uveal tract is to:
    a   provide the eye's shape
    b   help the eye focus an image in the retina
    c   provide a sheath for the optic nerve
    d   transmit light

3   One or more segments of the eye may be involved with uveitis because:
    a   of their close proximity
    b   of the infectious nature of uveitis
    c   of the difficulty in diagnosing and treating uveitis
    d   a common blood supply nourishes these segments

4   The two types of uveitis are:
    a   right eye and left eye
    b   interior and exterior
    c   anterior and posterior
    d   dorsal and ventral

5   One possible cause of uveitis is:
    a   aging
    b   bacteria
    c   poor nutrition
    d   heredity

6   One symptom of uveitis is:
    a   hemorrhaging
    b   photophobia
    c   headaches
    d   bleeding

7   Treatment of uveitis is mostly symptomatic because:
    a   the cause is difficult to determine
    b   of the time of onset of symptoms
    c   of previous or other existing eye problems
    d   none of the above

8 A common treatment of uveitis is:
 a laser therapy
 b surgery
 c steroids
 d agents that enhance pupillary constriction

9 When an individual complains of ocular pain relating to uveitis, the nurse should:
 a darken the patient's room
 b validate the patient's concerns
 c advise the patient to avoid driving
 d use warm compresses

10 Before the client leaves the health facility, the nurse should:
 a make sure the client can instill eye drops
 b identify for the patient those activities that cause uveitis
 c remind the patient to wear an ocular shield
 d encourage the patient to change eyeglass prescriptions

Comprehending? Yes ＿＿ No ＿＿

• Reading Selection 7 •

• PREVIEW QUESTIONS

What features of the ear does this selection discuss? What do you already know about these features?

• VOCABULARY

Underline any medical terminology or general vocabulary words you may need to learn in order to understand the ideas in this reading selection.

The ear is a sensory organ whose function includes both hearing and the sense of balance. Nurses who work with clients who have ear disorders need a thorough understanding of the normal anatomy and physiology of the external ear, middle ear, and inner ear, as well as the process and nature of hearing. Auditory screening is conducted from the neonatal period throughout life. If problems with the ear or with hearing are suspected, the nurse refers clients to a physician and/or audiologist for specialized diagnostic assessments. An audiologist is a health care professional who is educated in the science of hearing, including the treatment and rehabilitation of persons with impaired hearing.

• ANATOMY AND PHYSIOLOGY REVIEW

• Structure

The ear consists of three structural parts: external, middle, and inner. Each of these structures and their functions are significant and integral parts of the process of hearing.

EXTERNAL EAR

The external ear is developed in embryonic life at the same time that the kidneys and urinary tract are developed. Hence, defects of the external ear may be present in conjunction with congenital renal anomalies.

The external ear is embedded in the temporal bone bilaterally at the level of the eyes, at approx-

imately a 10-degree angle with the head. Cartilage and skin attach the external ear to the head. The external ear extends from the visible auricle, or pinna, through the external canal to the lateral side of the tympanic membrane, or eardrum. The *pinna* is composed of the helix, antihelix, tragus, concha, external canal opening, and lobule (Fig. V–5). The external ear canal is slightly S shaped and is lined with cerumen (wax)-producing glands, sebaceous glands, and hair follicles. The hair follicles and cerumen serve to protect the tympanic membrane and the middle ear. The length of the external canal varies with age. In the adult, the distance from the opening of the external canal to the tympanic membrane is approximately 2.5 to 3.75 cm (1 to 1½ in). In addition, the external ear includes the *mastoid*

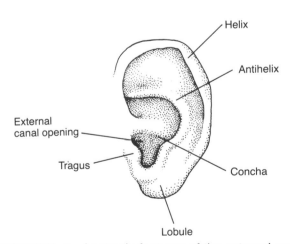

FIGURE V–5 Anatomic features of the external ear.

From Ignatavicius and Bayne, pp. 1076–1078.

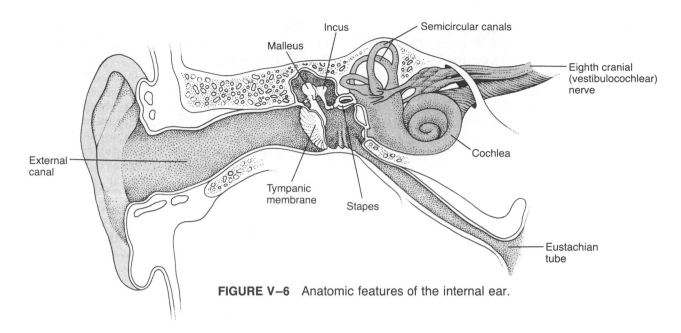

FIGURE V–6 Anatomic features of the internal ear.

process, the bony ridge located over the temporal bone behind the pinna, which covers the mastoid air cells.

MIDDLE EAR

The middle ear consists of the medial side of the tympanic membrane and a compartment called the *epitympanum,* or attic, which contains the three bony *ossicles:* malleus, incus, and stapes (Fig. V–6). In addition, the proximal end of the eustachian tube opens in the middle ear. The *tympanic membrane* is a thick, transparent sheet of tissue, 9 mm (0.35 in) in diameter, that provides a barrier between the external ear and the middle ear. The entire tympanic membrane is embedded in the temporal bone surrounded by the mastoid air cells. The landmarks on the tympanic membrane include the annulus, pars flaccida, and pars tensa (Fig. V–7). The *annulus* is the site where the tympanic membrane attaches itself to the external canal; it cannot be visualized directly as it is embedded in the temporal bone. The *pars flaccida* is that portion of the tympanic membrane above the short process of the malleus, which is usually less transparent and less mobile than the pars tensa portion of the tympanic membrane. The *pars tensa* is that portion of the tympanic membrane surrounding the long process of the malleus. It is usually referred to as transparent, opaque, or pearly gray and is mobile when air is injected into the external canal. The tympanic membrane is attached to the first bony ossicle, the *malleus,* at a site designated the *umbo* (see Fig. V–7). The umbo is seen through the tympanic membrane as a white dot at the end of the long

process of the malleus. The short process of the malleus, the long process of the malleus, and the umbo are structures that can be seen *through* the transparent tympanic membrane. The pars flaccida and pars tensa are sites on the tympanic membrane itself. The bony ossicles behind the tympanic membrane are joined together, although not rigidly, which allows vibratory movement.

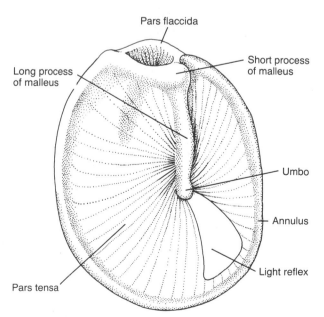

FIGURE V–7 Landmarks on the tympanic membrane.

The middle ear is protected from the inner ear by the round and the oval window membranes. The eustachian tube originates from the floor of the middle ear at the proximal end and opens at the distal end in the nasopharynx. The distal opening in the nasopharynx is surrounded by adenoid lymphatic tissue (Fig. V–8). The eustachian tube allows for equalization of pressure on both sides of the tympanic membrane.

INNER EAR

The inner ear, lying on the other side of the oval window, contains the semicircular canals, the cochlea, and the distal end of the eighth cranial nerve, the vestibulocochlear nerve (see Fig. V–6). The *semicircular canals* are structures containing fluid and hair cells, which are connected to the sensory nerve fibers of the vestibular portion of the eighth cranial nerve. They help to maintain a person's sense of balance, or equilibrium. Separating the semicircular canals from the cochlea are the utricle and saccule, which are vestibular receptors that respond to the position of the head.

The *cochlea* is the spiral-shaped organ of hearing that is divided into two parts, the scala tympani and the scala vestibuli. Reissner's membrane stretches across the scala vestibuli and forms the duct of the cochlea, or the scala media. The scala media is filled with *endolymph,* a fluid that is similar to intracellular fluid. The scala tympani and scala vestibuli are filled with *perilymph.* These fluids are important in the protection of the cochlea and the semicircular canals because these structures literally float in the fluids, which cushion against abrupt movements of the head. The cochlea's basilar membrane is approximately 30 mm long and is composed of thousands of fibers. The *organ of Corti,* the receptor end organ of hearing, is found on this membrane and contains hair cells resting on the fibers of the basilar membrane, which are surrounded by the cochlear division of the eighth cranial nerve. The *eighth cranial nerve* has two branches: the cochlear and the vestibular. The cochlear branch transmits neural impulses from the cochlea to the brain, where they are interpreted as sound.

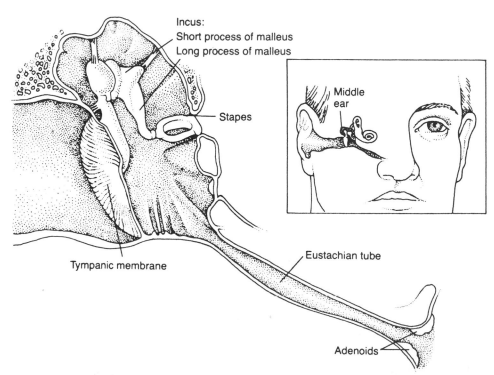

Incus:
Short process of malleus
Long process of malleus

Stapes

Middle ear

Tympanic membrane

Eustachian tube

Adenoids

FIGURE V–8 Anatomic features and attached structures of the middle ear.

• SUMMARY

Directions. In the space provided, rewrite the above selection in your own words, focusing on the main ideas and major details.

• COMPREHENSION QUESTIONS

Directions. Below are 10 multiple-choice questions. Circle the letter of the best answer from the four choices.

1 The external ear is located:
   a   bilaterally at the level of the eyes
   b   at a 25-degree angle with the head
   c   bilaterally at the level of the nose
   d   at a 20-degree angle with the head

2 The shape of the external canal is:
   a   slightly V shaped
   b   slightly L shaped
   c   slightly T shaped
   d   slightly S shaped

3 The common name for the tympanic membrane is:
   a   hair follicle
   b   ear drum
   c   ear lobe
   d   ear canal

4 The tube that opens in the middle ear is the:
   a   incus
   b   malleus
   c   eustachian
   d   stapes

5 The function of the tympanic membrane is to:
  a provide a barrier between the external and the middle ear
  b cover the mastoid air cells
  c produce cerumen
  d equalize pressure

6 Four major features of the middle ear are:
  a tragus, concha, lobule, helix
  b stapes, incus, helix, tragus
  c lobule, concha, malleus, incus
  d malleus, incus, tympanic membrane, stapes

7 The pars flaccida is a feature of the:
  a external ear
  b tympanic membrane
  c inner ear
  d middle ear

8 The eustachian tube:
  a maintains balance
  b allows vibratory movement
  c equalizes pressure on both sides of the tympanic membrane
  d is connected to sensory nerve fibers

9 The part of the ear closest to the adenoids is the:
  a eustachian tube
  b tympanic membrane
  c stapes
  d incus

10 The inner ear contains:
  a semicircular canals
  b cochlea
  c the eighth cranial nerve
  d all of the above

Comprehending? Yes ___ No ___

• Reading Selection 8 •

• PREVIEW QUESTION

What is Figure V-9 on p. 252 illustrating?

• VOCABULARY

Underline any medical terminology or general vocabulary words you may need to learn in order to understand the ideas in this reading selection.

• SUMMARY

In the space provided, rewrite the main features of Figure V–9 in your own words.

• COMPREHENSION QUESTIONS

Directions.   Below are 10 multiple-choice questions. Circle the letter of the best answer from the four choices.

1 In the diagram unoxygenated blood is represented by a:
  a black dotted line   **c** black arrow
  b white dotted line   **d** white arrow

2 In this diagram oxygenated blood is represented by a:
  a black dotted line   **c** black arrow
  b white dotted line   **d** white arrow

3 Blood from the upper body enters the heart via the:
  a superior vena cava   **c** left pulmonary artery
  b inferior vena cava   **d** right pulmonary artery

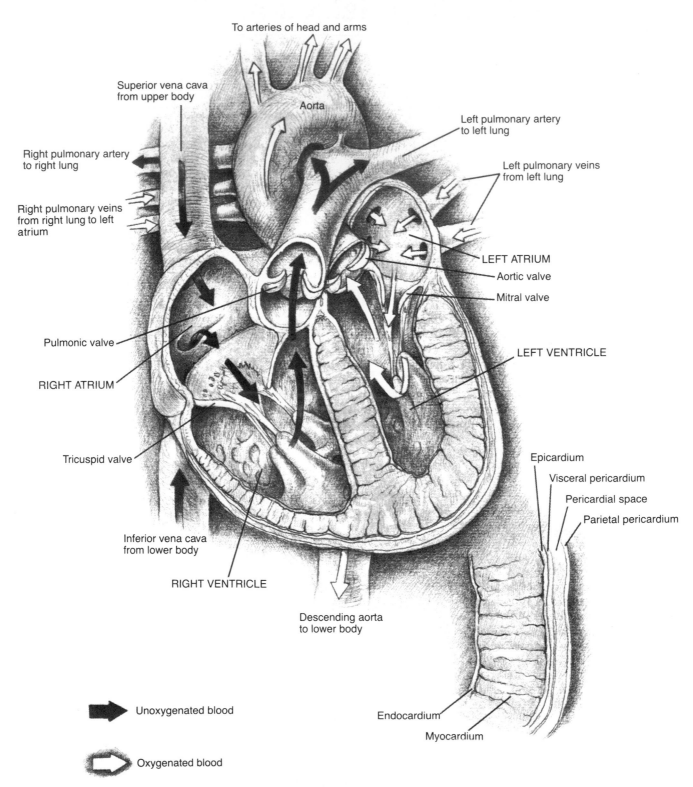

To arteries of head and arms

Superior vena cava
from upper body

Aorta

Left pulmonary artery
to left lung

Right pulmonary artery
to right lung

Left pulmonary veins
from left lung

Right pulmonary veins
from right lung to left
atrium

LEFT ATRIUM

Aortic valve

Mitral valve

Pulmonic valve

LEFT VENTRICLE

RIGHT ATRIUM

Tricuspid valve

Epicardium

Visceral pericardium

Pericardial space

Parietal pericardium

Inferior vena cava
from lower body

RIGHT VENTRICLE

Descending aorta
to lower body

Endocardium

Myocardium

➤ Unoxygenated blood

⇨ Oxygenated blood

FIGURE V–9 How blood flows through the heart. (From
Ignatavicius and Bayne, p. 2071)

4 The first valve the unoxygenated blood flows through is the:
  a aortic valve
  b tricuspid valve
  c mitral valve
  d bicuspid valve

5 In the diagram the left ventricle is located in the:
  a bottom right portion of the heart
  b upper right portion of the heart
  c bottom left portion of the heart
  d upper left portion of the heart

6 The first part of the heart the newly oxygenated blood flows through is the:
  a right ventricle
  b aorta
  c pulmonary artery
  d pulmonary veins

7 The first valve the oxygenated blood flows through is the:
  a aortic valve
  b mitral valve
  c tricuspid valve
  d bicuspid valve

8 After leaving the left ventricle, the blood flows into the:
  a aorta
  b aortic valve
  c arteries to head and arms
  d right ventricle

9 Blood in the aorta flows into arteries in the:
  a upper and lower body
  b left pulmonary artery
  c right pulmonary artery
  d lungs

10 The blood enters the lungs through the right and left:
  a atriums
  b ventricle
  c pulmonary arteries
  d pulmonary veins.

Comprehending? Yes ____ No ____

• Reading Selection 9 •

• PREVIEW QUESTION

Primary head injuries include injuries to which three areas?

• VOCABULARY

Underline any medical terminology or general vocabulary words you may need to learn in order to understand the ideas in this reading selection.

Injuries may also be classified according to the *structure damaged* (e.g., brain stem) and whether they are primary or secondary. *Primary head injury* refers to *impact* damage, the severity of which is estimated by initial signs and symptoms. *Secondary* or *delayed* events following head injury include edema, hemorrhage, or infection. These processes can significantly impede recovery or even cause death from what initially appeared to be a mild injury.

• PRIMARY HEAD INJURIES

Primary head injuries include injuries to the scalp, skull, or brain, or all of these. The injuries result from the original *impact*.

• Scalp Injuries

Scalp injuries can cause lacerations, hematomas, and contusions or abrasions to the skin. These injuries may be unsightly and bleed profusely. Scalp injuries not accompanied by damage to other areas are minor and do not require hospitalization. The person needs instruction about appropriate wound care. Infants, small children, and hypovolemic adults are especially prone to shock and may require observation in a health care facility until their condition stabilizes.

Cover open head wounds and apply pressure to bleeding scalp wounds *unless there appears to be underlying depressed or compound skull fracture.* Do not attempt to remove foreign objects or any penetrating objects from the wound. Uncom-

TABLE V–2 Primary Head Injury Sites: Summary

- *Scalp,* injury may be disfiguring but is usually not serious and is easily treated.
- *Skull,* injury is usually a fracture that may or may not produce brain damage.
- *Brain tissue.* (a) *Concussions* injure brain tissue but cause no long-term effects or only minimal ones. (b) *Contusions* significantly injure brain tissue, causing permanent disability or death.
- *Other structures,* including the meninges and major arteries, may be damaged.

---

plicated scalp wounds (that do not lie over depressed or compound skull fractures) are anesthetized locally, cleansed, and sutured.

• Skull Injuries

Skull fractures are often caused by a force sufficient to cause both fracture and brain injury. The fractures in themselves *do not* mean brain injury is also present. However, skull fractures are often present in people with serious brain damage. *Depressed skull fractures* injure the brain by bruising it (abrasion) or by driving bone fragments into it (lacerations). The site of a fracture and the extent of brain injury may not correlate.

There are three *types of skull fractures:*
- *Linear skull fractures* appear as thin lines on x-ray and do not require treatment. They are important only if there is significant underlying brain damage.

From Luckmann and Sorensen, pp. 507–508.

- *Depressed skull fractures* may be palpated and are seen on x-ray. Surgery may be required within the first 24 hours after injury if the depression is as deep as the skull thickness. Depressed fractures may be associated with bone fragments penetrating into brain tissue. When this occurs, the area is usually surgically explored and debrided.
- *Basilar skull fractures* occur in bones over the base of the frontal and temporal lobes. They are rarely seen on x-ray. Clinical signs include (a) CSF or other drainage from the ear or nose, (b) various cranial nerve injuries, (c) blood behind the eardrum, (d) periorbital ecchymosis (bruise around the eyes), and (e) later, a bruise over the mastoid *(Battle's sign).*

Indications of cranial nerve damage may occur at the time of the initial injury or may develop later. They include

- Vision loss, e.g., blindness, blurred vision, from *optic nerve damage*
- Hearing loss with postural vertigo and nystagmus from *auditory nerve damage*
- Loss of the sense of smell (bilaterally or unilaterally) from *olfactory nerve damage*
- Squint and/or fixed dilated pupil and loss of some of the eye movements from *oculomotor nerve damage*
- Facial paresis/paralysis (unilateral) from *facial nerve damage*

Basilar skull fractures, depressed fractures, and other open (compound) fractures all allow communication between the exterior environment and the brain. *Infection* is therefore a possible complication. Some physicians prescribe prophylactic antibiotics, although this is controversial.

CSF leakage from the nose or ear is indicative of *intracranial cerebrospinal fluid fistula.* It is not always easy to detect CSF leakage because it is frequently mixed with blood. If a CSF fistula persists longer than 24 hours, the head of the bed is kept elevated. Diamox may be prescribed to decrease CSF formation. A lumbar drain may be inserted to divert CSF to the spinal cord and allow the fistula to close. Surgery to close such a fistula is rarely necessary.

Simple skull depressions are *electively* treated by surgically elevating the depressed bone fragment and repairing the dura if it is lacerated. All bone fragments are removed. *Compound depressed skull fractures* are *immediately* treated surgically. The scalp, skull, and devitalized brain are debrided and the wound cleansed thoroughly. Unless all foreign material is removed, a brain abscess develops. Debridement of a penetrating wound or depressed skull fracture frequently leaves a cranial defect that is cosmetically unsightly. The defect is surgically corrected by *cranioplasty.*

- ### Brain Injuries

There is a wide variety of brain injuries (see mechanisms of injury). A single classification for brain injuries does not exist. However, the terms *open, closed, contusion,* and *concussion* are often applied to brain injuries.

CONCUSSIONS

A *concussion* is head trauma producing a brief loss of consciousness, immediately followed by confusion or memory loss (i.e., amnesia). Usually, there are no other abnormal neurologic findings. Concussions may cause brain damage. The severity of a concussion apparently correlates with the duration of "post-traumatic amnesia" (i.e., from the time of injury to when the person is completely oriented to the environment).

TABLE V–3   When to Go to a Health Care Facility Following Head Injury

SHOULD GO TO HEALTH CARE FACILITY	CAN BE WATCHED AT HOME
1 Any loss of consciousness	1 No loss of consciousness
2 Pupils grossly unequal or do not constrict to light	2 Pupils equal and constrict to light
3 Evidence of weakness or loss of sensation in any extremity	3 No loss of coordination or sensation in extremities
4 Bizarre behavior, increased irritability, or any decrease in level of consciousness	4 Normal behavior, no change in awareness or attention span
5 Injuries in addition to head injuries	5 No evidence of additional injuries
6 Blow to head sufficient to suspect skull fracture	6 Impact of injury was not excessive
7 Pain or stiffness of neck or any suspicion of spine injury	7 No evidence of scalp laceration
8 Any bleeding or drainage of fluid from nose or ears	
9 Seizure activity	

From Rudy, E.B.: *Advanced neurological and neurosurgical nursing,* St. Louis: C.V. Mosby Co., 1984.

People with concussions are frequently seen in emergency rooms. They require close observation for possible complications.

Systematic, frequent assessment of a head-injured person's neurologic status is essential. Steady worsening of level of consciousness (LOC) is significant and probably indicates the development of secondary events.

Be sure that (a) a reliable person will observe the injured person closely at home, (b) this observer is aware of indications of change in the injured person's condition, (c) subsequent medical intervention is available if needed, and (d) the injured person and "observer" know how to obtain such care if it is necessary.

CONTUSIONS

Contusions cause more extensive damage than concussions. Contusions damage the brain substance itself, causing multiple areas of petechial and punctate hemorrhage and bruised areas. Microscopic nerve fiber lesions also occur. Abnormalities may be mainly in one area of the brain, but other areas may also be *injured.* This is particularly true of brain stem contusions, which are a very serious type of lesion.

There are various *assessment findings* in people with contusions. This is partly because of the numerous areas of damage. Contusions are often associated with other serious injuries, including cervical fractures. Secondary effects, e.g., brain swelling and edema, accompany serious contusions. Increased ICP and herniation syndromes may result.

Contusions may be divided into *cerebral contusions* and *brain stem contusions.*

Cerebral Contusions

These contusions can only be diagnosed if the person is alert, although they may be present in comatose people. *Assessment findings* vary, depending on which areas of the cerebral hemispheres are damaged. An agitated, confused head-injured person who remains alert may have a *temporal lobe contusion.* Hemiparesis in an alert head-injured person may indicate a *frontal contusion.* An aphasic head-injured person may have a *frontal-temporal contusion.* Other findings indicate contusions in other areas. Remember that while these findings correlate with cerebral contusion, they do not rule out other abnormalities such as a developing mass or lesion. Adverse changes in the person's condition require immediate medical attention. They may indicate treatable complications.

Brain Stem Contusions

Brain stem contusions render a person immediately unresponsive or partially comatose because of significant brain stem disruption. Typically, an altered LOC continues for at least several hours and usually days or weeks. The person may regain partial consciousness within hours or remain in a coma. Other neurologic abnormalities are present and are usually symmetric (i.e., on both sides of the body). Some may be lateralized (asymmetric, on one side of the body only), indicating development of a secondary event such as a hematoma.

In addition to the altered LOC that is always present with brain stem contusion, respiratory, pupillary, eye movement, and motor abnormalities may occur.

- *Respirations* may be normal, ataxic, periodic, or very rapid.
- *Pupils* are usually small, equal, and reactive. Damage to the upper brain stem (third cranial nerve) may cause pupillary abnormalities.
- *Loss of normal eye movements* may occur since pathways controlling eye movements traverse the midbrain and pons.
- The person may respond to light or noxious stimuli by *purposeful movements* pushing the stimulus away. Or the person may have *no response to stimuli,* i.e., may be flaccid. In the presence of profound LOC alterations, flexion and extension posturing may be elicited with or without noxious stimuli.

Assessment findings (see above) often vary from one observation to another (whereas findings indicating a developing hematoma are more consistent). Careful documentation of assessment findings is important to identify *patterns* or *trends* in the person's condition.

Brain stem contusions do not usually injure the brain stem alone. Swelling or direct injury to the hypothalamus may produce *autonomic nervous system* effects. The person has a high temperature, rapid pulse and respiration, and perspires profusely. These *effects* may wax and wane but if sustained can lead to serious complications.

• SECONDARY EVENTS IN HEAD INJURIES

Secondary events after head injury (problems occurring soon after the primary injury) often cause rapid deterioration in the injured person's condition. Among these *secondary events* are (a) *hemor-rhage,* with hematoma formation (epidural, sub-dural, and intracerebral); (b) *infections,* including meningitis and brain abscess; (c) *secondary brain swelling* and *edema;* and (d) *carotid artery occlusion.* All may turn a relatively "benign" head injury into a disastrous event.

• SUMMARY

Directions.   In the space provided, rewrite the above selection in your own words, focusing on the main ideas and major details.

• COMPREHENSION QUESTIONS

Directions.   Below are 10 multiple-choice questions. Circle the letter of the best answer from the four choices.

1   A skull fracture:
   a   always is an indication of brain injury
   b   is often accompanied with brain injury
   c   does not cause brain injury
   d   is caused by an insufficient force

2   Blindness may occur from damage to the:
   a   frontal lobe
   b   scalp
   c   optic nerve
   d   auditory nerve

3 Oculomotor nerve damage causes loss of:
  a smell
  b hearing
  c eye movements
  d touch

4 Simple skull depressions are treated by:
  a mandatory surgery
  b observation
  c medicine
  d elective surgery

5 Contusions cause:
  a more extensive damage than concussions
  b less extensive damage than concussions
  c no damage
  d the same damage as concussions

6 Amnesia means:
  a loss of consciousness
  b confusion
  c brain damage
  d memory loss

7 A fracture that does not require treatment is a:
  a depressed skull fracture
  b linear skull fracture
  c cranial nerve damage
  d contusion

8 Table V–3 indicates:
  a when to go to a health care facility
  b when head injuries can be watched at home
  c both a and b
  d none of the above

9 Primary head injury sites include the:
  a skull and scalp
  b scalp and brain
  c skull and brain
  d arteries and tissues

10 A person has to be alert to diagnose a:
  a concussion
  b vision loss
  c linear skull fracture
  d cerebral contusion

Comprehending? Yes ___ No ___

• Reading Selection 10 •

• PREVIEW QUESTIONS

Are dementias part of the normal aging process? Why or why not?

• VOCABULARY

Underline any medical terminology or general vocabulary words you may need to learn in order to understand the ideas in this reading selection.

• ALZHEIMER'S DISEASE

Alzheimer's disease is the most common, irreversible dementia. About half of all admissions, to long-term care facilities in the United States are due to Alzheimer's disease. This disease may soon be the fourth or fifth leading cause of death in the U.S.

Dementias are a broad diagnostic category in which the main *assessment finding* is deterioration in intellectual functioning due to pathologic changes. Dementias are pathologic. They are not part of the normal aging process. Dementias can be caused by more than 50 diseases. However, more than half of all people who have dementias have Alzheimer's disease. (Senile dementia of the Alzheimer's type is abbreviated SDAT.) Cerebrovascular disease is the second most frequent cause of dementia, causing about one-fourth of instances. The remaining one-fourth of all dementias are caused by various degenerative, infectious, inflammatory, toxic, or metabolic diseases. Familiar neurologic disorders among these are Parkinson's, Pick's and Huntington's disease.

Alzheimer's disease is a severe disorder of cognition and widespread brain atrophy that is receiving increasing attention. This disease is a gradual, progressive disorder with high mortality. Death usually occurs 2 to 4 years after diagnosis.

Although the *etiology* of Alzheimer's disease is unknown, it seems likely that a profound reduc-

tion occurs in neurotransmitters in the hippocampus and cortex, especially somatostatin and choline acetyltransferase. This accounts for *memory loss,* the disease's primary feature. *Predisposing factors* to Alzheimer's disease may include genetic and unknown environmental factors. Many *pathologic changes* occur in the brain of a person with Alzheimer's disease. These include enlarged ventricles, loss of brain weight and loss of neurons in the basal ganglia, substantia nigra and cortex (neurons responsible for higher cerebral functions such as memory, cognition and thought). Microscopically, neurofibrillary tangles are present in the neocortex and senile plaques in the hippocampus and neocortex.

• Assessment Findings

Indications of Alzheimer's disease typically appear in people after late middle age. Differentiating between neurologic changes associated with normal aging and pathologic changes is important. *Diagnosis* is based on (a) history, (b), type of symptoms and their progression, and (c) a process of elimination. Assessment findings may suggest various medical and psychiatric conditions that may be treatable in their early stages (e.g., depression, head injury, vitamin deficiencies, drug intoxication, or brain tumor).

People experiencing the early stages of Alzheimer's disease may look well but (a) have difficulty concentrating at times, and have subtle short-term memory problems and some inappropriate behavior, and (b) may be somewhat depressed, withdrawn, and a little forgetful. Also, abstract thinking and decision making gradually become more dif-

From Luckman and Sorensen, pp. 489–491.

259

ficult. However, all of these symptoms may not seriously interfere with the person's ability to function independently. Neurologic deficits are probably not present.

Problems of memory, reasoning, judgment, and social interaction become more pronounced as the second stage of Alzheimer's disease progresses. This usually takes several years. Areas of the cerebral cortex involved with memory and motor function are largely affected. The frontal and temporal lobes become smaller than normal. The person becomes lost, loses coordination and the ability to speak and write and may begin frequent motion and pacing and roaming about with slow, shuffling steps. Balance is unsteady and stooped posture develops. Hyperorality may develop (i.e., a desire to take everything into the mouth to suck, chew, or taste). Swallowing may become difficult. Smoking may increase. Severe memory loss causes the person to become lost and forget to eat, drink, etc. Personality changes include depression, irritability, and disorientation to time and place. Wakefulness at night is common. The person may be *incontinent of feces* and urine.

Physically and mentally disabled individuals with Alzheimer's disease are at risk for accidents and infection. They may require residency in a long-term care facility or hospitalization for health-related problems, including malnutrition and dehydration as their illness makes them unable to care for themselves, and gradually they become unmanageable at home. Aspiration pneumonia is the usual cause of death.

- ## Nursing Intervention (Table V-4)

People with Alzheimer's disease and their significant others need a lot of support to safely manage the person at home for as long as possible.

NURSING DIAGNOSIS: ALTERATION IN THOUGHT PROCESSES DUE TO NEURONAL DEGENERATION

Address a person who has Alzheimer's disease by name. Approach the person in a quiet, calm, and kind manner. Face the person when speaking and speak slowly, using simple sentences. Give clear, simple directions, one at a time. Give the person direct attention. Listen carefully, respond to meaningful statements, and focus on the person's appropriate behavior. Avoid negative experiences (e.g., arguments, criticism, confrontation). Help the person find lost objects. Use kind, inclusive humor in interactions with the person. Encourage the person to interact with others. Help the

person with telephone numbers. Allow the person to have personal belongings and help to keep track of them. Reorient the person as necessary. Place calendar and clock in obvious places and keep them accurate. Allow the person to reminisce. The person should wear an identification bracelet stating name, address, and telephone number. Provide care for pets or other dependents as *necessary.* The person often forgets to provide them with food, water, and health care.

NURSING DIAGNOSIS: DEFICIT IN DIVERSIONAL ACTIVITY DUE TO DECREASED ATTENTION SPAN, RESTLESSNESS, AND BOREDOM

Arrange simple outings (e.g., short walks, short car rides). Plan activities within the person's interests and capabilities and pace them according to the person's speed.

NURSING DIAGNOSIS: POTENTIAL FOR INJURY DUE TO IMPAIRED JUDGMENT AND FORGETFULNESS

The person has a slowed metabolic rate and therefore feels the cold more. Assist with adequate clothing and bedding for warmth. Pneumonia is a major cause of death in the presence of Alzheimer's disease. Observe carefully for nonverbal physiologic signs (e.g., the person may be in pain but not say so). Listen carefully to what the person says. Sometimes the person may ask a question that is really a personal statement (e.g., Are you hungry? meaning, I am hungry.) Minimize environmental hazards (e.g., use "child-proof" locks; lock away medications and poisons; avoid throw rugs).

NURSING DIAGNOSIS: SELF-CARE DEFICIT DUE TO INABILITY TO PERFORM ACTIVITIES OF DAILY LIVING, FORGETFULNESS, FRUSTRATION

Encourage a person with Alzheimer's to do as much as possible independently and to dress attractively. Assist as necessary to prevent frustration. Carefully balance helping the person with allowing autonomy. Anticipate hygiene needs (e.g., nail, hair, and oral care). Allow plenty of time with self-help activities. Take one task at a time.

NURSING DIAGNOSIS: POTENTIAL ALTERATION IN NUTRITION DUE TO FORGETFULNESS AND REGRESSED HABITS

A person with Alzheimer's may overeat or undereat owing to impaired memory. Help the person responsible for meal planning to provide adequate nutrition. Frequent snacks may be appropriate for

TABLE V–4 Nursing Guidelines for the Care of a Person with Alzheimer's Disease

Admission to the Nursing Unit

- Keep admission interview short; do not appear hurried
- Utilize significant others for details; however, don't discuss or assess the person in his/her presence
- Explain every intervention carefully and patiently—repeat as often as necessary
- Use a calm and reassuring tone of voice
- Do not react to person's panic behavior

Location on Nursing Unit

- Admit to a single room near the nurse's desk accessible to an area that allows safe or secured space for walking
- Avoid placing the person near noise makers such as telephones and paging systems
- Avoid placing person near stairways and outside doors, especially if she/he has a tendency to roam

Stabilizing Environment

- Establish *definite routines* for care, patterned after home care if possible
- Have same staff provide care each time
- Give explanations for care
- Provide person with list of things to do and give specific times
- Display familiar objects from home such as pictures of significant others
- A calendar and clock should be in the room to keep the person oriented
- Label articles, door to bathroom, etc.

Hygiene and Dressing

- Encourage independence
- Assist and supervise only when necessary, i.e., baths or showers
- Suggest clothing that slips on easily; avoid zippers, buttons, and ties
- Label clothing, drawers, personal items

Meals and Nutrition

- Allow person to select food
- Observe difficulty in swallowing

- Avoid hot foods. Cut solid foods, such as meat, into small portions. Finger foods or those that require little hand coordination may encourage better eating
- Suggest supplements if nutritional intake is inadequate

Sleep and Rest

- Allow to rest and sleep at will; except irregular patterns. Things that may facilitate rest and sleep include food, warm baths, or exercise prior to bedtime
- Mild tranquilizers and hypnotics may help, but use cautiously
- Expect increased agitation from some medications

Exercise and Activity

- Allow enough space for safe walking activities
- Encourage walks with an attendant
- Provide passive exercise for those confined to bed

Elimination

- Monitor intake and output record
- Encourage fluids, fiber in the diet, and exercise to avoid constipation
- Label urinals and bathroom door
- Expect confused people to use any convenient container or the floor for elimination purposes

Medications

- Avoid large capsules or pills
- Observe that medications are taken and swallowed without difficulty
- Crush pills or order liquid preparation
- Observe for reaction or effectiveness
- Do not leave medications at bedside

Love and Belonging

- Person may withdraw and become isolated early in disease
- Although person may not be able to express feelings, he/she usually can respond to touch and kindness
- Many continue sexual activities until late stage of disease

Modified from Dodson, J.: The slow death: Alzheimer's disease. *Journal of Neurosurgical Nursing,* 14(5):270-275, 1985.

reducing food intake. Allow plenty of time with meals. Assist with eating as necessary.

NURSING DIAGNOSIS: POTENTIAL ALTERATION IN ELIMINATION PATTERNS DUE TO FORGETFULNESS, LOSS OF NEUROLOGIC FUNCTION

A person with Alzheimer's may become incontinent or constipated. This may be due to an inability to locate the bathroom or forgetfulness about elim-

ination habits. Make clear, bright signs showing the person where the bathroom is and regularly take the person there. Provide adequate lighting, especially at night. Encourage the person to take increased fluids early in the day and limit fluids in the evening. Watch for nonverbal signs of the need to eliminate (e.g., restlessness, holding self, picking at clothes). Stool softeners and increased dietary fiber help prevent constipation.

NURSING DIAGNOSIS: POTENTIAL INEFFECTIVE FAMILY COPING DUE TO CHANGE IN PERSONALITY, BEHAVIOR, AND SOCIAL ROLES

Significant others need a lot of support and understanding. Provide learning/teaching opportunities for them to learn as much as possible about Alzheimer's disease. Information about support facilities is helpful. These may include adult day care, Alzheimer's Disease and Related Disorders Association (ADRDA) or the Alzheimer's Support Group (ASIST). Various books written for the lay public help significant others understand and cope with a person who has Alzheimer's disease. If the person needs placement in a long-term care facility, significant others need considerable support and understanding with this decision. Help them examine all options and provide information but do not make their decision for them. Unlimited visiting by significant others is important in such a facility.

• SUMMARY

Directions. In the space provided, rewrite the above selection in your own words, focusing on the main ideas and major details.

• COMPREHENSION QUESTIONS

Directions. Below are 10 multiple-choice questions. Circle the letter of the best answer from the four choices.

1 The primary feature of Alzheimer's disease is:
   a appetite loss
   b memory loss
   c weight loss
   d aging

2 Alzheimer's disease is:
   a reversible
   b irreversible
   c cured by environmental factors
   d the leading cause of death in the United States

3 Dementia is:

   a a deterioration in intellectual functioning

   b an increase in intellectual functioning

   c unrelated to intellect

   d always caused by infection

4 Dementias are:

   a part of the normal aging process

   b always caused by toxic disease

   c pathologic

   d unrelated to Alzheimer's disease

5 Indications of Alzheimer's disease often appear during:

   a young adult years

   b old age

   c middle age

   d late middle age

6 The usual cause of death for patients with Alzheimer's disease is:

   a aspiration pneumonia

   b environmental hazards

   c dehydration

   d depression

7 Alzheimer's disease is:

   a a sudden decline

   b a progressive disorder

   c stable

   d not life threatening

8 The patient can usually function independently:

   a during the first stage of Alzheimer's disease

   b during the second stage of Alzheimer's disease

   c during both stages of Alzheimer's disease

   d after recovering from Alzheimer's disease

9 Table V–4 gives guidelines for the care of patients with Alzheimer's disease to:

   a physicians

   b family members

   c nurses

   d hospital administrators

10 The information about medications in Table V–4 indicates that the patient with Alzheimer's disease:

   a can self-administer medication

   b requires supervision of medication

   c is unable to take medicine

   d will have serious side effects from the medication

Comprehending? Yes ____ No ____

• Reading Selection 11 •

• PREVIEW QUESTION

What is an advantage of open heart surgery?

• VOCABULARY

Underline any medical terminology or general vocabulary words you may need to learn in order to understand the ideas in this reading selection.

• OPEN HEART SURGERY

The greatest advantage of open heart surgery is that it allows the surgeon to *directly visualize* the heart during the operation. However, before open heart procedures could be developed, surgeons had to discover how to (a) slow or halt the person's circulation without causing brain anoxia (using hypothermia) and (b) detour the blood that would normally enter the heart and lungs through an artificial heart-lung machine (ECC).

Hypothermia was the first technique to make open heart surgery possible. Two purposes of hypothermia are to (a) *decrease* the person's *metabolic needs,* thereby lowering the rate at which the body uses oxygen, and (b) provide the surgeon with a *bloodless field* in which to operate. The person's reduced need for oxygen allows the surgeon to clamp off the venae cavae and azygos veins, thereby halting circulation through the heart for a time.

How long circulation can be stopped depends on the *depth* of hypothermia. At normal body temperature, circulation can stop for only two to three minutes without tissue damage from anoxia. However, at 28° C (82.4° F) (moderate hypothermia), circulation can be interrupted for 15 to 20 minutes—adequate time to complete certain simple procedures. At 10° C (50° F) (profound hypothermia), circulation can be stopped for about one hour.

To induce hypothermia, the person must be anesthetized. The body is cooled by a hypothermia

blanket that reduces body temperature to the desired level. The major danger of hypothermia is *ventricular fibrillation,* which occurs when the temperature drops to around 26° C (78.6° F). Other complications are cardiac arrest and cardiac failure. Today, some surgeons continue to use hypothermia in combination with ECC.

The heart-lung machine (pump-oxygenator), more than any other apparatus, has made sophisticated open heart surgery possible. The first pump-oxygenator was used for a human in 1951 in an unsuccessful attempt at ECC. Two years later, the machine was used again in the successful repair of an atrial septal defect. The person remained on cardiopulmonary bypass for 30 minutes. Since 1955, improved versions of the machine have been built, and surgeons now use ECC routinely throughout the world for open heart surgery.

Four purposes of the heart-lung machine are to: (1) divert circulation from the heart and lungs, providing the surgeon with a bloodless operative field; (2) perform all gas exchange functions for the body while the person's cardiopulmonary system is at rest; (3) filter, rewarm, or cool the blood; and (4) circulate oxygenated, filtered blood back into the arterial system.

Briefly, the procedure for ECC is as follows:

The machine is primed (filled) with 3 or 4 liters of either heparinized blood or a blood substitute such as low molecular weight dextran (Rheomacrodex) or Ringer's lactate solution. After opening the person's chest, the surgeon inserts two large-bore cannulas through the right atrium into the su-

From Luckmann and Sorensen, pp. 1001–1002.

perior and inferior venae cavae and suction catheters into the thoracic cavity and ventricles. Blood is next pumped from the venae cavae, the thoracic cavity, and the ventricles into the heart-lung machine (Fig. V–10). In the machine, a heat exchanger rewarms (or cools, if the surgeon desired hypothermia) the blood. An oxygenator then removes CO_2 from the blood and adds oxygen. Finally, the blood passes through a filter that removes air bubbles and other emboli before returning to the body via either the aorta or the femoral artery.

Despite its beneficial effects, the heart-lung machine does have *risks.* The pump can crush and

destroy blood cells, sludging of cells can lead to thrombus formation, or air emboli can form. Other complications related to ECC are shock, hemorrhage, hemolysis, and kidney or lung damage.

Currently the extracorporeal membrane oxygenator (ECMO) is a more expensive method of ECC. Advantages include decreased trauma to blood cells and prolonged pump time (up to days). Unlike the current bubbling oxygenators that force O_2 into the blood, membrane oxygenators, like the lungs themselves, oxygenate the blood across a membrane.

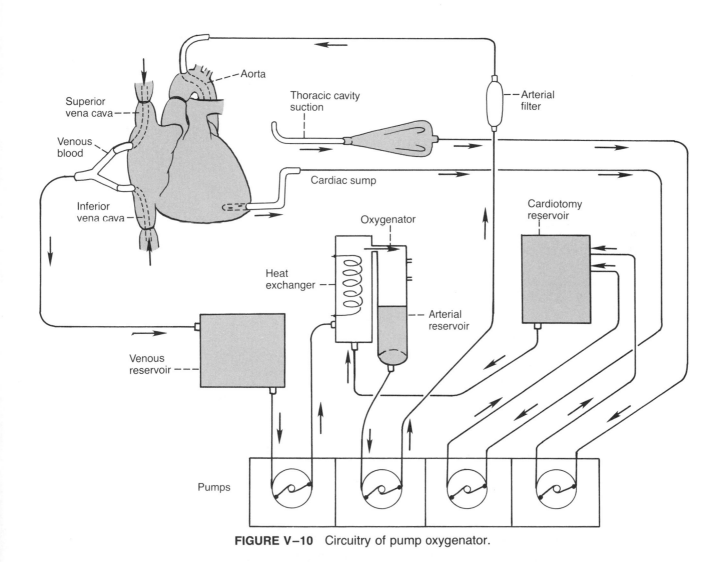

FIGURE V–10 Circuitry of pump oxygenator.

• SUMMARY

Directions.   In the space provided, rewrite the above selection in your own words, focusing on the main ideas and major details.

• COMPREHENSION QUESTIONS

Directions.   Below are 10 multiple-choice questions. Circle the letter of the best answer from the four choices.

1   Open heart surgery allows the surgeon to:
   a   always cure the patient's heart problems
   b   prevent any recurrence of heart disease
   c   prevent the spread of disease
   d   directly visualize the heart during the operation

2   The first technique to make open heart surgery possible was:
   a   visualization
   b   hypothermia
   c   increasing the patient's need for oxygen
   d   maintaining the patient's normal body temperature

3   ECC is:
   a   open heart surgery
   b   a treatment for reversing hypothermia
   c   a method for detouring the blood through a machine
   d   an anesthetic used only during heart surgery

4 The heart lung machine is called:
  a ECC
  b a pump-oxygenator
  c a hypothermia blanket
  d the cardiopulmonary system

5 The danger of hypothermia occurs when the temperature drops to:
  a 26° C
  b 26° F
  c 78.6° C
  d 78.6° F

6 Sophisticated open heart surgery has been made possible by the:
  a correct anesthetic
  b patient's uninterrupted circulation
  c patient's uncomplicated health history
  d pump-oxygenator

7 The first time that the pump-oxygenator was used successfully on a human was:
  a 1951
  b 1953
  c 1955
  d 1957

8 The heart lung machine:
  a has risks
  b always destroys blood cells
  c is risk free
  d causes immediate kidney failure

9 Figure V–10 depicts the:
  a risks of the heart-lung machine
  b advantages of the heart-lung machine
  c advantages of ECMO over ECC
  d circuitry of the pump-oxygenator

10 The blood returns to the body through the:
  a aorta
  b thoracic cavity
  c ventricles
  d heat exchanges

Comprehending? Yes ____ No ____

• Reading Selection 12 •

• PREVIEW QUESTION

Who would be especially prone to hip fractures?

• VOCABULARY

Underline any medical terminology or general vocabulary words you may need to learn in order to understand the ideas in this reading selection.

• FRACTURES OF THE PROXIMAL END OF THE FEMUR ("FRACTURED HIP")

Fractures of the proximal end of the femur (i.e., the end that engages with the acetabulum in the innominate bone to form the "hip joint") are classified as intracapsular or extracapsular.

- *Intracapsular* fractures occur within the "hip" joint and capsule (a) through the head of the femur (capital fracture), (b) just below the head of the femur (subcapital), or (c) through the neck of the femur (transcervical).
- *Extracapsular* fractures occur outside of the joint and capsule, through the femur's greater or lesser trochanter or in the intertrochanteric area (i.e., pertrochanteric and intertrochanteric fractures). Extracapsular fractures occur distal to the neck of the femur but not more than 2 inches below the lesser trochanter (Fig. V–11).

> Elderly women with osteoporosis are especially prone to fractures of the proximal end of the femur if they fall.

• Assessment

Even accidents that appear relatively minor can cause a fractured hip in an elderly person. Therefore, x-ray films of the hip are routinely taken of older people after falls or other accidents. If a hip fracture is impacted, the injured person may be able to weight-bear and perhaps even walk for a short time after injury. More typically a fractured hip causes displacement and immediately incapacitates the person. Typically a person with a fractured hip lies with a painful, injured leg that is shortened, adducted, and in a position of external rotation. The greater trochanter may be felt, displaced in the buttock. Nursing and medical interventions for elderly people with hip fractures are often complicated by other problems, e.g., diabetes or cardiac, peripheral vascular, or neurologic disorders. Thorough assessment is essential.

• Intervention

Treatment programs for a person with a fractured hip vary, depending on (a) the person's condition, (b) time since the injury, and (c) type of fracture. Sometimes traction is used temporarily before open reduction. Open reduction eliminates long-term immobilization, which is often difficult for elderly people to tolerate.

Internal fixation is often used, including (a) insertion of pins or nails, (b) fixation of screw plates, or (c) implantation of a prosthesis to replace the head and neck of the femur. Internal fixation usually allows mobilization soon after surgery. A fixation device is chosen that securely holds the fractured fragments. Pins and nails are inserted through the trochanter and femoral neck into the head of the femur. Plates may be fixed with screws to the femur shaft. A *hip prosthesis* may be used for intracapsular fractures that are difficult to reduce, are comminuted, or are prone to nonunion or in the presence of aseptic necrosis (see below). During surgery, while internal fixation is being performed, x-ray films or fluoroscopy may be used to guide the

---

From Luckmann and Sorensen, pp. 1536–1538.

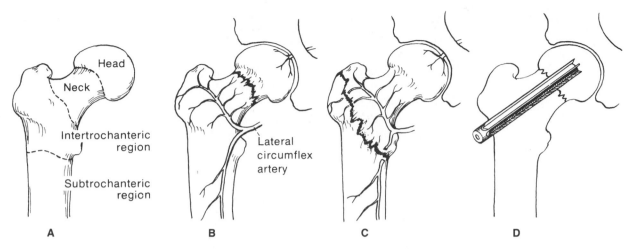

FIGURE V–11   *A,* Normal proximal end of femur. *B,* Intracapsular fracture of proximal end of femur. Note blood supply. *C,* Extracapsular intertrochanteric fracture. Note effect of fracture on blood supply. *D,* Intracapsular fracture with nail inserted for reduction.

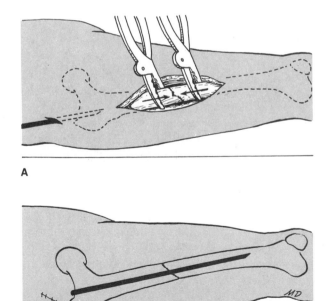

FIGURE V–12   Open reduction and internal fixation of a fractured shaft of femur. *A,* Fractured bone ends are realigned by open reduction. Intramedullary nail is inserted through the proximal end of femur. *B,* Fractured bone ends secured in correct position with intramedullary nail.

placement of fixating devices. Sometimes bone grafts are placed around the fracture line in an attempt to facilitate healing by stimulating bone growth. These grafts may be taken from the person's tibia or iliac bones.

- **Complications**

    Possible complications of proximal femur fractures include
    - *Shock and hemorrhage.* At the time of injury or early postoperatively.
    - *Complications of immobility.* Especially in elderly people, e.g., pneumonia, thrombophlebitis, pulmonary embolus.
    - *Delayed healing, nonunion.* Often intracapsular fractures heal more slowly than do extracapsular fractures because they may have an impaired blood supply.
    - *Aseptic necrosis of head of femur.* Complication of fractures of proximal femur and traumatic dislocation of hip.
    - *Deformities, malposition of the femur, secondary arthritis.* Displacement of fragments can produce deformities and trauma can predispose to arthritis.
    - *Postoperative problems with the internal fixation devices.* Internal fixation devices may weaken and break or migrate out of position, causing soft tissue damage. Repeat surgery may be necessary.

• Postoperative Care

Assess for indications of *complications* such as shock, hemorrhage, infection, paralytic ileus, confusion, fat embolism, thrombosis, hip dislocation, aseptic necrosis, and nonunion. Document and promptly report assessment findings indicating problems. Observe for indications of *hip dislocation,* i.e., sharp hip pain or "abnormal" positioning of the affected leg (leg shortened and externally rotated). If dislocation has occurred (confirmed by x-ray and physical examination), further surgery is needed. An *excessive temperature elevation* may indicate wound infection, urinary tract infection, pneumonia, or other complications. Lower quadrant pain or calf pain and/or tenderness may indicate *thrombophlebitis. Inadequate reduction* or *avascular necrosis of the head of the femur* may produce pain or muscle spasm during the postoperative period. *Avascular (aseptic) necrosis* following hip pinning causes pain, muscle spasm, and limping. Continued weight-bearing can crumble the bone. Early intervention is important. The person may be taken to surgery where the pins and *head of the femur* are removed and replaced with a prosthesis. *Nonunion* may be treated by bone grafts.

Following hip surgery, carefully check the physician's instructions about position and activity. It is usually important to prevent acute hip flexion and adduction and external leg rotation.

NURSING DIAGNOSIS: IMPAIRED PHYSICAL MOBILITY DUE TO POSTOPERATIVE POSITION REQUIREMENT

Handle the operated leg gently following hip surgery. Before moving the person, explain what you are going to do and how the person can help. An overbed trapeze helps with moving. Teach the person how to use the trapeze. Avoid extremes of position following hip surgery. *Keep the leg abducted,* i.e., out to the side, at all times. Never adduct the leg past the body's midline (e.g., over the other leg), or the head of the femur (or prosthesis) may dislocate out of the acetabulum. Place a pillow between the person's legs to help maintain abduction and to remind the person not to cross the legs.

Avoid acute flexion of the operated hip. This can be caused by excessive elevation of the head

TABLE V–5 After a Fracture Has Been Treated

- Elevate an injured arm or leg to reduce swelling and pain.
- Exercise joints above and below a cast as your physician instructs to prevent their getting stiff.
- Keep a cast dry.
- Do not walk on a leg or foot cast without your physician's permission. You may be able to walk immediately on a fiberglass cast, but wait 48 hours to allow a plaster cast to dry and harden.
- Contact your physician immediately about severe pain, whiteness or blueness, coldness, numbing ("pins and needles"), or inability to move the toes or fingers of your injured leg or arm. These may indicate circulation problems.
- If you have a future appointment, be sure to keep it. Severe breaks need close professional attention.

of the bed. Check the physician's instructions about how high the head of the bed can be safely elevated. Some people can have the head of the bed raised 35° to 40°. If the head of the bed can be somewhat elevated, instruct the person not to lean farther forward, e.g., to reach for something, since this further flexes the hip and may cause dislocation.

Prevent external rotation of the leg on the operated side by placing a trochanter roll beside the external aspect of the thigh. Without this intervention, the operated leg may tend to lie slightly externally rotated when the person is supine.

Turn the person only with the physician's order following hip surgery. Commonly after hip surgery the person can be turned to the unoperated side. Following hip pinning some people are permitted to turn to either side. However, after other types of hip surgery, e.g., total hip replacement, turning is not permitted for several days. When helping a person to turn following internal fixation, (a) avoid adduction of the operated leg and excessive movement, (b) prevent strain on the hip, and (c) keep the leg and hip in proper alignment. If the person is permitted to turn onto the operated side, roll the person gently toward you after placing pillows between the legs. The bed acts as a splint for the injured leg. If not permitted to turn to either side, the person may be able to lift straight up off the bed by using a trapeze for back care and linen changes.

> Postoperative instructions about positioning following the insertion of a hip prosthesis usually depend on the operative approach taken through the joint capsule. Positioning must prevent straining the incision line.

Strain on a joint capsule's incision can cause a hip prosthesis to dislocate and push out through the weakened capsule. Commonly following an *anterior* surgical approach the operated limb is positioned so it is rotated internally and is maintained either in a neutral or an abducted position. The individual may be permitted to sit up unless the capsule was removed. With a *posterior* approach the operated leg is positioned in slight abduction and *external rotation* (a change from "typical" positioning) and the person lies fairly flat.

Do not position the bed too low when a person is getting up after hip surgery. Less hip strain and bending occur if the bed is somewhat elevated. Be sure the bed's casters are locked so it will not move while the person is getting up. For the same reasons, elevated toilet seats are needed following hip surgery once the person can go to the bathroom.

Usually when a person first gets up in a chair following hip surgery, the operated leg is kept extended, well supported, and elevated. Once the operated leg may be lowered, the person should sit with hips even with knees. Tell the person not to cross legs but to *keep both feet on the floor.* Crossing the legs adducts the operated leg and can dislocate the hip. The first few times the leg is lowered, assess for swelling and discoloration.

Assist with *exercises* as soon as they are prescribed. These may include quadriceps setting, gluteal setting, breathing exercises, exercises for the upper extremities (to prepare the person for crutch walking), and exercises for the unoperated extremities. Most exercises begin on the first postoperative day. Exercises to flex and dorsiflex the foot on the operated leg and to move the knee on the operated leg may be ordered.

Periodic x-ray examination determines when enough healing has occurred to allow *ambulation.* Further assessment determines when weight-bearing on the injured leg is prescribed. Parallel bars and a walker may be used before crutches. Walkers especially help elderly people, who are not strong or coordinated enough to use crutches safely. After *discharge* from the health care facility, follow-up care is important. The physician continues to assess progress. Visiting nurse services provide valuable home services for people living alone until they are able to move easily again.

NURSING DIAGNOSIS: ANXIETY DUE TO PROLONGED INCAPACITATION

The person and significant others may become discouraged at what seems slow healing following hip surgery. Carefully planned learning/teaching opportunities help them understand what to expect and so reduce anxiety. Referrals to community agencies for assistance during rehabilitation are important. Encouragement, emotional support, diversion, and self-care can help through periods of discouragement. Elderly people may think they will not recover. These deep, real concerns should be discussed if the individual wishes to do so.

NURSING DIAGNOSIS: POWERLESSNESS

A person experiencing a fractured hip is very likely to have a sense of loss of control or powerlessness. This is especially true for elderly people who may have to consider whether they are able to continue in their preinjury life style. They may be

---

> **LEARNING/TEACHING GUIDE ABOUT FRACTURES FOR INJURED PEOPLE AND SIGNIFICANT OTHERS**
>
> A *fracture* is a break in a bone. A fracture usually shows on an x-ray film. However, sometimes a crack may be so small that it does not show until healing begins. This is why an x-ray film taken after a week or two may show a fracture that was not seen immediately after an injury. Most fractures need support so that proper bone healing can occur. This support may be provided by a cast, splint, or brace. Sometimes fractured bones are fixed with metal pieces placed inside them during surgery. Before support can be applied a fracture may need reduction (setting). This means putting the broken bones back in the correct position. Fractures need time and support to heal properly. Healing usually takes longer (a) for big or long bones, (b) if a bone is severely shattered, or (c) if the person is elderly. Following the instructions listed below improves healing. Failing to follow these instructions can cause improper healing, resulting in deformity and/or disability.

afraid that they will no longer be able to be independent. This may or may not be true, but if the person experiences it, it is a real concern for that time. Reduce feelings of powerlessness by allowing the person to control as many decisions as possible, e.g., regarding treatment plans, food, clothing, television. Encourage as much self-care as possible, e.g., washing face, dressing upper body. As the person's condition improves, encourage increasing self-care. Coordinate with the person and significant others in planning rehabilitation so it will allow a gradual return to independence.

• SUMMARY

Directions. In the space provided, rewrite the above selection in your own words, focusing on the main ideas and major details.

• COMPREHENSION QUESTIONS

Directions. Below are 10 multiple-choice questions. Circle the letter of the best answer from the four choices.

1 Fractures that occur within the hip joint and capsule are called:
   a extracapsular
   b intracapsular
   c femur
   d trochanter

2 Even minor accidents can cause a fractured hip in:
   a babies
   b teenagers
   c elderly people
   d women of all ages

3 Letter D in Figure V–II depicts:
   a anatomic regions
   b osteoporosis
   c complications of surgery
   d internal fixation

4 Repeat surgery might be necessary if:
   a pneumonia develops
   b internal fixation devices break
   c there is delayed healing
   d arthritis develops

5 Thrombophlebitis may be indicated by:
   a urinary tract infection
   b sharp hip pain
   c lower calf pain
   d dislocation

6 A wound infection may be indicated by:
   a a slight rise in temperature
   b an excessive temperature elevation
   c immobility
   d muscle spasm

7 Following hip surgery a patient should be turned:
   a routinely
   b every few days
   c only at the patient's request
   d only with the doctor's orders

8 In Figure V–12, the fractural bone ends are secured in the correct position with a:
   a nail
   b plate
   c graft
   d hip prosthesis

9 The patient may become discouraged after hip surgery because of:
   a swelling of the lower leg
   b difficult exercises
   c slow healing
   d foot pain

10 After surgery the hip may become dislocated by:
   a staying in bed
   b acute hip flexion
   c placing a pillow between the patient's legs
   d using an overbed trapeze

Comprehending? Yes ___   No ___

• Reading Selection 13 •

• PREVIEW QUESTION

What are possible side effects of strong analgesics?

• VOCABULARY

Underline any medical terminology or general vocabulary words you may need to learn in order to understand the ideas in this reading selection.

• COMPLICATIONS WITH STRONG ANALGESICS

Narcotics and other analgesics may produce pain relief. However, problems can arise in both short- and long-term administration of analgesics. Narcotics must be used cautiously and with an understanding of possible side effects and how these may be avoided or reversed.

• Respiratory Depression

A common complication of narcotic analgesic therapy, respiratory depression is caused by diminished sensitivity of the respiratory center to carbon dioxide. This is usually dose related and accompanies the administration of all potent narcotic analgesics, and to a somewhat lesser extent of the agonist-antagonist analgesics. The potential for respiratory depression is particularly significant in elderly people and individuals with respiratory impairment.

Deaths that are secondary to narcotic overdose (narcotic poisoning) are usually due to respiratory depression. Maximal respiratory depression usually occurs within seven minutes of intravenous administration, 30 minutes after intramuscular injection, and up to 90 minutes after subcutaneous administration.[65] Hence, these are important times to remember in assessing a person's respiratory status following administration of narcotics.

Intervention for respiratory depression includes establishing a patent airway, artificial ventilation as necessary, and possible administration of an opiate antagonist (e.g., naloxone).

• Circulatory Depression

In a supine individual, therapeutic dosages of morphine or synthetic opioids have very little effect on blood pressure and cardiac rate or rhythm. However, some people experience orthostatic hypotension when moving from a supine position to a head-up or standing position. This hypotension is secondary to a direct dilating action on peripheral blood vessels, reducing the capacity of the cardiovascular system to respond to gravitational shifts. Avoid abrupt body position changes in people who have received narcotics. Narcotics are used very cautiously in people with decreased blood volume.

• Nausea and Vomiting

Narcotics may precipitate nausea and vomiting owing to their action on the brain stem centers. Morphine-like drugs also affect the vestibular system, which can also produce these symptoms. Changing the type of narcotic used may stop the side effect, or the addition of an antiemetic agent may help.

• Constipation

Morphine and other narcotics increase smooth muscle tone and decrease the motility of the gastrointestinal tract. Narcotics diminish the propulsive peristaltic contractions in the small and large intestine, and delay the passage of gastric contents through the duodenum. People taking narcotic analgesics need to be on some type of bowel regimen

---

From Luckmann and Sorensen, pp. 202–203.

to prevent constipation. A high roughage diet with plenty of fluids and stool-softening medications is common prophylactic treatment. It is better to prevent constipation than to begin treatment after it develops.

- ## Paresthesia

The intramuscular injection of analgesic agents is generally not irritating to the local tissues. However, two exceptions are meperidine and methadone. Subcutaneous methadone may cause local tissue irritation. Both subcutaneous and intramuscular meperidine cause local tissue irritation and induration, and frequent administration can lead to severe fibrosis of muscle tissue.[55]

If any analgesic is deposited in the region of a nerve when injected intramuscularly, paresthesia and paresis may result along the course of the nerve.

Proper injection techniques prevent nerve injury.

- ## Physical Dependence

This is an altered physiologic state produced by repeated administration of a drug. Continued administration of the drug is necessary to prevent withdrawal syndrome. Physical dependence on opioids can develop as well as on other substances such as alcohol, barbiturates, and nicotine.

Physical dependence does not imply addiction, but that a stereotypical withdrawal syndrome will occur if the individual ceases to take a particular drug.

Individuals who receive a therapeutic dose of morphine several times a day will develop some physical dependence in approximately two weeks.[43] This means that if morphine were suddenly discontinued a withdrawal syndrome would occur. *Assessment findings* indicating a withdrawal syndrome include diarrhea, lacrimation, sweating, dilated pupils, restlessness, tremor, and anorexia. Most symptoms, if untreated, subside in five to ten days. Withdrawal symptoms can be avoided by gradually (over one to two weeks) reducing and finally discontinuing an individual's opiate intake.[38]

- ## Tolerance

Opioid tolerance is characterized by a shortened duration of pain relief, a decrease in peak analgesic effect, and an increase in the amount of narcotic needed to produce a lethal respiratory depression. An example of tolerance is when pain has been adequately controlled by a particular dosage of a narcotic, but the narcotic begins to be less effective for the same period of time. A higher dosage is needed to obtain the desired effects. The usual treatment for tolerance when pain relief is necessary is to increase the analgesic dose or decrease the interval between doses.

- ## Addiction

Addiction is a behavioral pattern of drug use characterized by (a) overwhelming involvement with the use of a drug (compulsive use) and securing a supply of it and (b) a high tendency to relapse after withdrawal from the drug, i.e., to begin taking it again. The vast majority of individuals who take narcotic analgesic medication for pain are not "addicted."

• SUMMARY

Directions. In the space provided, rewrite the above selection in your own words, focusing on the main ideas and major details.

• COMPREHENSION QUESTIONS

Directions. Below are 10 multiple-choice questions. Circle the letter of the best answer from the four choices.

1 Respiratory depression is caused by:
   a increased sensitivity of the respiratory center to carbon dioxide
   b decreased sensitivity of the respiratory center to carbon dioxide
   c diminished insensitivity of the respiratory center to carbon dioxide
   d rejection by the respiratory system of carbon dioxide

2 Another term for narcotic overdose is:
   a narcotic poisoning
   b respiratory depression
   c narcotic intervention
   d artificial ventilation

3 A supine position is:
   a standing up
   b sitting
   c lying down
   d a change in position

4 Morphine:
   a increases smooth muscle tone
   b increases motility
   c decreases smooth muscle tone
   d decreases motility

5 If a patient receives a therapeutic dose of morphine several times a day, a physical dependence will develop in about:
  a 2 hours
  b 2 days
  c 2 weeks
  d 2 months

6 Nerve injury is prevented by:
  a all injection techniques
  b proper injection techniques
  c intramuscular injection
  d paresis

7 The usual treatment for tolerance when pain relief is necessary is to:
  a increase the analgesic dose
  b decrease the analgesic dose
  c increase the time between doses
  d eliminate the interval between doses

8 If withdrawal symptoms are untreated, they:
  a continue at least 10 days
  b disappear in 1 week
  c last over 2 weeks
  d subside in 5 to 10 days

9 Physical dependence is implied by:
  a a withdrawal syndrome
  b addiction
  c tolerance
  d overdose

10 Addiction is characterized by:
  a taking narcotics
  b requiring analgesic medicine for pain
  c compulsive drug use
  d opioid tolerance

Comprehending?   Yes ___   No ___

• Reading Selection 14 •

• PREVIEW QUESTION

What does the gate-control model of pain explain?

• VOCABULARY

Underline any medical terminology or general vocabulary words you may need to learn in order to understand the ideas in this reading selection.

• GATE-CONTROL MODEL OF PAIN

The *physiology* of pain transmission and perception is less well understood than the underlying *physical structure* (anatomy). There are various theoretical models attempting to explain how neural units interact during the experience of pain. One such model is the gate-control theory, produced over 20 years ago and periodically revised. It explains many aspects of pain and how pain may be controlled by thoughts, emotions, and action.

In 1965, Melzack and Wall presented the first version of the gate-control theory. They suggested the existence of a "gate" that could either facilitate or inhibit the transmission of pain signals. The gate is controlled by the dynamic function of certain cells in the spinal cord's dorsal horn. The fibers bringing information about pain from tissue synapse for the first time in laminae (layers) of the dorsal horn. Laminae II is known as the *substantia gelatinosa* (SG). The SG is visually distinct from other laminae when the spinal cord is inspected in cross section. Melzack and Wall proposed that the SG is the anatomic location of the gate. Both small fibers (carrying information about pain) and large fibers (carrying information such as touch) converge in SG. Also, fibers sending their pain-inhibitory information down from the brain act here. They come from areas such as the periaqueductal gray matter, the hypothalamus, the raphe nucleus, and the locus ceruleus.

Melzack and Wall propose that a *spinal cord transmission cell (T cell)* exits in the SG. Depending on its input from other cells, the T cell either facilitates pain transmission (opens the gate) or inhibits pain transmission (closes the gate). The gate can be influenced (opened or closed) by information from various sources. Activity from large-diameter fibers (carrying such information as touch) can inhibit pain transmission (close the gate). Small fiber activity (pain) tends to open the gate. Whether the gate is open or closed, it can be influenced by fibers carrying information from many different brain centers down to the T cells. According to this theory, information from nonpain fibers or information from the brain can reduce or totally block pain information before it is experienced. When the gate is open, pain information influences multiple centers in the brain. When working together, these centers produce the complex but integrated responses that occur in a person experiencing pain. The model suggests, however, that the brain can also influence whether or not the gate is open. Thus, factors such as attention, memory, thinking, and emotion may either inhibit or enhance the transmission of pain signals.

A recent version of the gate-control theory (called *Mark II* by Melzack and Wall[58]) is presented in Figure V–14. The newer model emphasizes the probability that there is an inhibitory system within the brain stem that also acts as a "gate" inhibiting pain transmission. This brain-stem inhibitory circuit

---

From Luckmann and Sorensen, pp. 176–177.

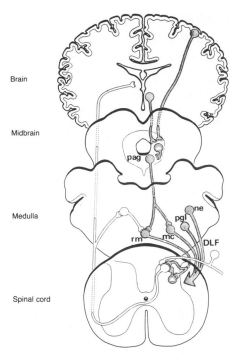

FIGURE V–13 Pain modulating network. Diagram of critical structures that contribute to control of pain-transmission neurons. The network includes connections from midbrain periaqueductal grey (pag) to medullary nucleus raphe magnus (rm)/recticularis magnocellularis (mc) and, via the dorsolateral funiculus (DLF), to the spinal cord dorsal horn. Additional bulbospinal pathways potentially relevant to analgesia arise from the nucleus paragigantocellularis (pgl) which also receives input from pag and the noradrenergic medullary cell groups (ne) lateral to pgl. (From Fields, H., and Bosbaum, A.: Endogenous pain control mechanisms. *In:* Wall, P., and Melzack, R.: *Textbook of Pain.* New York: Churchill Livingstone, 1984.)

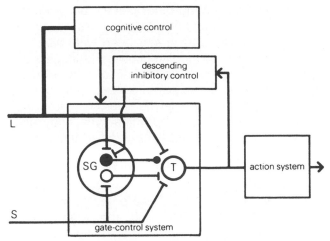

FIGURE V–14 The gate-control theory: Mark II. The new model includes excitatory (white circle) and inhibitory (black circle) links from the substantia gelatinosa (SG) to the transmission (T) cells as well as descending inhibitory control from brain stem systems. The round knob at the end of the inhibitory link implies that its action may be presynaptic, postsynaptic, or both. All connections are excitatory, except the inhibitory link from SG to T cell. (From *The Challenge of Pain* by Ronald Melzack and Patrick D. Wall. Copyright © 1973 by Ronald Melzack. Copyright © 1982 by Ronald Melzack and Patrick D. Wall. Reprinted by permission of Basic Books, Inc., Publishers.)

has been described in detail by Basbaum and Fields,[9] who believe that the system involves structures in the midbrain, medulla, and spinal cord. Activation of cells in the midbrain's periaqueductal gray matter (by electrical stimulation, opiate analgesic drugs, or possibly psychologic factors) in turn stimulates structures in the medulla. These medullary structures then project to and inhibit spinal pain transmission fibers. Pain itself might activate this system, so there is a natural control mechanism limiting the severity of pain experienced.

• **MOLECULAR BASIS OF PAIN TRANSMISSION**

> Some chemical compounds released by injury or inflammation stimulate nociceptors, e.g., *histamine, bradykinin, serotonin,* and *E prostaglandins.* Pain may be reduced by drugs that block these agents, e.g., *steroids aspirin,* and other *nonsteriodal anti-inflammatory drugs (NSAIDs)* that reduce inflammation and block prostaglandins.

Other compounds are associated with pain transmission. Their action occurs at various points in the pain pathways previously described. *Substance P,* a *neuropeptide,* appears to be a pain-specific neurotransmitter that is present in the spinal cord's dorsal horn (at the "gate" in the gate-control model), among other places. Other neuro-peptides undoubtedly *facilitate* pain transmission.

Other peptides are associated with *inhibiting pain.* A group of naturally occurring (endogenous) peptides have properties similar to those of morphine and other narcotic analgesics. The central nervous system has specific neuroreceptors that bind (or make use of) morphine. The body also manufactures substances that bind to these sites and have analgesic properties. These naturally occurring, opium-like compounds are called *endogenous opioids,* or *endorphins.* "Endorphin" has become a generic term for these peptides, which include both β-endorphin and the enkephalins. Electrical stimulation of brain-stem centers activates a profound analgesic effect, which appears to relate to endorphin release.[3,8,9]

Other neurotransmitters are involved in the downward inhibition of pain. It is interesting that serotonin, which *facilitates* pain in nociceptors, also acts as one of the transmitters in the descending pain *inhibition* system. The background level of many of these neurotransmitters fluctuates throughout the day, which may explain the following:

> Pain sensitivity is higher (lower pain threshold) in the afternoon than in the morning. Also, an individual's analgesic requirement may differ at different times of the day. There is increasing evidence that people who experience chronic, high levels of pain may be deficient in some of these neurotransmitters.

• CENTRAL CONTROL OF PAIN

> Pain perception does not depend solely on the degree of physical damage. It is also determined by anxiety, past experience, attention, expectation, and the meaning of the situation in which injury occurs. Brain activities, e.g., distraction or anxiety, may affect the severity and quality of the pain experienced.

• SUMMARY

Directions. In the space provided, rewrite the above selection in your own words, focusing on the main ideas and major details.

• COMPREHENSION QUESTIONS

Directions.   Below are 10 multiple-choice questions. Circle the letter of the best answer from the four choices.

1 The gate-control is a model of:
    a how thoughts affect the experience of pain
    b how emotions affect the experience of pain
    c how to eliminate pain
    d how neural units interact during the experience of pain

2 The gate-control theory was first presented in:
    a 1965
    b 1695
    c 1956
    d 1984

3 According to Figure V–13, the pain-modulating network ranges from the brain stem to the:
    a midbrain
    b spinal cord
    c medulla
    d dorsolateral funiculus

4 Another name for the spinal cord transmission cell is the:
    a SG
    b DFL
    c T cell
    d PAG cell

5 The newer model of the gate-control theory is called:
    a Mark II
    b Marc 2
    c Basbaum and Fields
    d Pain inhibition

6 The newer model of the gate-control theory emphasizes the probability that:
    a a system exists within the brain stem
    b a system within the brain stem inhibits pain transmission
    c a system within the brain stem prevents pain
    d there is a gate that prevents all pain within the brain

7 The severity of pain is limited by a:
    a control of the midbrain structure
    b circuit in the medulla
    c transfer of pain from the spinal cord
    d natural control mechanism

8 Figure V–14 indicates that the inhibitory link from SG to T cell is:
  a causing excitatory connections
  b causing pain to increase
  c excitatory
  d not excitatory

9 In Figure V–14 the white circle is:
  a inhibitory
  b excitatory
  c the new model
  d a descending control of pain

10 Figure V–14 presents:
  a Basbaum and Fields
  b Melzack and Wall
  c Mark II
  d the first gate-control theory

Comprehending? Yes ____ No ____

• Reading Selection 15 •

• PREVIEW QUESTION

What does Figure V–15 describe?

• VOCABULARY

Underline any medical terminology or general vocabulary words you may need to learn in order to understand the ideas in this reading selection.

• INTERVENTION FOR INCREASED INTRACRANIAL PRESSURE

The treatment of increased ICP includes intervention previously discussed for people with altered states of consciousness. Specific treatment to reduce ICP pressure includes:
- Surgical removal of the cause
- Nonsurgical treatment, e.g., osmotic diuretics, steroids, mechanical ventilation

• Surgical Intervention

Various *surgical techniques* are used to treat people with increased ICP. Optimally, the cause is located and removed. Other techniques include (a) surgical placement of a shunt to allow drainage if CSF is blocked and (b) decompressive surgery. The latter is done by removing some brain tissue, e.g., part of the temporal lobe, to give the remaining structures room to expand. If compliance is low at surgery, the bone flap removed to gain access to the brain is not replaced or the dura may not be closed. Subsequent surgery is then required to repair the defect.

• Nonsurgical Intervention

OSMOTIC DIURETICS

The most commonly used *diuretic* is mannitol, which removes fluid from the *normal* brain tissue and not from edematous tissue. Side effects of large doses of mannitol include (a) production of hyperosmolar states, (b) decreased effectiveness

with repeated use, and (c) aggravation of edema in some people.

STEROIDS

Steroids, such as dexamethasone, may be used. The mechanisms by which steroids work are unknown, but some physicians believe they are useful in decreasing brain swelling. Their use is controversial. Antacids or cimetidine are usually also prescribed because of the risk of gastrointestinal hemorrhage.

MECHANICAL VENTILATION

Hyperventilation, induced by a ventilator or by "bagging" a person, is used. It induces *hypocapnia,* which reduces cerebral blood volume and ICP. This intervention may be life-saving while preparing a person for other treatments. Manual hyperventilation is sometimes done during ICP elevations or when sudden clinical signs of deterioration appear. Continuous controlled hyperventilation is a mainstay in the treatment of ICP.

NURSING INTERVENTION

Whether or not hyperventilation is used, pay meticulous attention to maintaining respiratory function. Assess an intubated person often. Frequent arterial blood gases are drawn. Acid-base imbalances are corrected by physician prescription to ensure adequate oxygenation.

Maintain a patent airway by suctioning to prevent build-up of carbon dioxide and elevation of ICP. Adequately oxygenate intubated people before each passage of a suction catheter. Since hy-

---

From Luckmann and Sorensen, pp. 419–420.

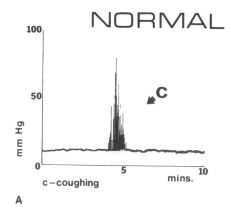

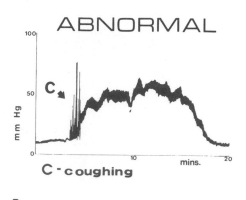

FIGURE V–15 Two examples of what happens when intracranial volume is increased by coughing, vomiting, suctioning, straining, etc. *A* demonstrates a sudden momentary rise in ICP. However, because compliance is normal, the increased intracranial pressure dissipates rapidly. *B* demonstrates what happens during coughing when compliance is low. (From Hanlon, K.: Intracranial compliance interpretation and clinical application. *Journal of Neurosurgical Nursing* 9:35, March 1977.)

perinflation as well as the addition of positive end-expiratory pressure (PEEP) raises ICP, keep the passage of a suction catheter as brief as possible. *Never exceed 15 seconds.* Do not suction via the nose as drainage may indicate CSF leak and it is important to be able to observe it.

It is also important to prevent venous obstruction. Raise the head of the bed 30°. Avoid turning the person's head sharply to either side, and keep the head in alignment with the rest of the body. Maintain a regular bowel program since excessive strain can cause a Valsalva maneuver, which can result in venous back-up and increased ICP.

Fluid administration for people with increased ICP is controversial. Administer fluid exactly as prescribed. Currently the tendency is to use a slightly hypertonic solution, e.g., dextrose 5% ½-normal saline. Such fluid remains in the vascular space and therefore contributes less to cerebral edema. Balanced salt solutions are generally used, but other solutions may be required if complications occur that render the person hemodynamically unstable.

It is important to avoid the use of fluid (e.g., dextrose 5% in water) that moves rapidly into the brain to cause edema. Remember to document the fluid administered with medications and in keeping monitoring devices open, e.g., indwelling arterial catheter lines. A large amount of fluid can be administered by these routes. The *type* and *amount* of such fluids must be taken into account.

> Carefully monitor fluid to ensure it is not infused too rapidly.

The actual amount of fluid infused per hour is determined by various factors. *Never infuse more than the prescribed amount.* If fluid therapy falls behind, consult the physician. This is especially important for a person with low intracranial compliance. Also remember that mechanical ventilation causes a person to retain fluid.

Increased temperature in people with increased ICP raises the metabolic rate and aggravates ICP further. Therefore, hyperthermia requires vigorous treatment with cooling measures and prescribed medication.

Seizures also cause a marked increase in ICP. People with irritative lesions are particularly prone to seizures.

THERAPEUTIC COMA

When other methods of controlling increased ICP have failed, *barbiturate-induced coma* may be used to protect the brain from further injury and reduce metabolic demands on the brain. The person requires full ventilatory support in a critical care unit, along with careful monitoring of cardiac output, blood pressure, pulmonary artery wedge pressure, and arterial blood gases. Hemodynamic parameters are monitored closely because of the cardiac depressant properties of barbiturates. Such depression may be compensated for by low-dose dopamine to provide inotropic support to the heart and maintain arterial systolic blood pressure greater than 90 mm Hg. A person in a therapeutic coma is unresponsive and without protective reflexes (skin, cornea, and airway). Intense nursing care is therefore required.

• SUMMARY

Directions. In the space provided, rewrite the above selection in your own words, focusing on the main ideas and major details.

• COMPREHENSION QUESTIONS

Directions. Below are 10 multiple-choice questions. Circle the letter of the best answer from the four choices.

1 An example of brain tissue is:
 a hypocapnia
 b dexamethasone
 c hyperventilation
 d part of the temporal lobe

2 Mannitol is a:
 a fluid
 b diuretic
 c brain tissue
 d edematous tissue

3   A controversial method for decreasing brain swelling is the use of:
   a diuretics
   b antacids
   c steroids
   d carbon dioxide

4   Figure V–15 indicates what happens when ICP volume is:
   a increased
   b decreased
   c surgically removed
   d untreated

5   Example *B* in Figure V–15 demonstrates:
   a what happens during coughing
   b rapid dissipation of ICP
   c what happens during coughing when compliance is normal
   d what happens during coughing when compliance is low

6   A mainstay in the treatment of ICP is:
   a sporadic ventilation
   b continuous controlled hyperventilation
   c building up carbon dioxide
   d elevating ICP

7   Edema may be caused by:
   a any amount of fluid
   b dehydration
   c fluid moving rapidly into the brain
   d increasing body temperature

8   People with irritative lesions are particularly prone to:
   a fluid retention
   b hyperthermia
   c raised body temperature
   d seizures

9   Barbituate-induced coma may be used to:
   a protect the brain
   b prevent seizures
   c cure edema
   d avoid hyperthermia

10   A patient in a therapeutic coma requires:
   a some nursing care
   b home supervision
   c intense nursing care
   d big intake of barbituates

Comprehending?   Yes ____   No ____

• References •

Arnold, E., and Boggs, K.: Interpersonal relationships: professional communications skills for nurses, Philadelphia, 1989, W.B. Saunders.

Brunner, L.S., and Suddarth, D.S.: Textbook of medical surgical nursing, Philadelphia, 1988, J.B. Lippincott.

Crosby, L.J., et al.: Pharmacology for nursing care, Philadelphia, 1990, W.B. Saunders.

Ignatavicius, D.D., and Bayne, M.V.: Medical-surgical nursing: a nursing process approach, Philadelphia, 1991, W.B. Saunders.

Iyer, P.W., et al.: Nursing process and nursing diagnosis, ed. 2, Philadelphia, 1991, W.B. Saunders.

Kozier, B., and Erb: Concepts and issues in nursing practice, 1988, Addison-Wesley.

Kozier, B., et al.: Introduction to nursing, Reading, Mass., 1989, Addison-Wesley.

Ladewig, P.A., et al.: Essentials of maternal newborn nursing, Reading, Mass., 1990, Addison-Wesley.

Lewis, N. (ed.): Roget's new pocket thesaurus in dictionary form, New York, 1968, Washington Square Press.

Lindberg, J.B., Hunter, M.L., and Kruszewski, A.Z.: Introduction to nursing—concepts, issues, and opportunities, Philadelphia, 1990, J.B. Lippincott.

Luckmann, J., and Sorensen, K.C.: Medical-surgical nursing: a psychophysiological approach, ed. 3, Philadelphia, 1987, W.B. Saunders.

Matteson, M.A., and McConnell, E.S.: Gerontological nursing, concepts and practice, Philadelphia, 1988, W.B. Saunders.

Miller, B.F., and Keane, C.B.: Encyclopedia and dictionary of medicine, nursing, and allied health, ed. 4, Philadelphia, 1987, W.B. Saunders.

Mish, F.C,. et al. (eds.): Webster's ninth new collegiate dictionary, Springfield, Mass., 1985, Merriam-Webster.

Potter, P.A., and Perry, A.G.: Fundamentals of nursing, St. Louis, 1990, Mosby.

Shafler, M., and Marieb, E.N.: The nurse, pharmacology, and drug therapy, 1989, Addison-Wesley.

Sorensen, K.C., and Luckmann, J.: Basic nursing: a psychopharmacological approach, ed. 3, Philadelphia, 1987, W.B. Saunders.

Varcarolis, E.M.: Foundations of psychiatric mental health nursing, Philadelphia, 1990, W.B. Saunders.

Ulrich, S., et al.: Nursing care planning guides, a nursing diagnosis approach, Philadelphia, 1990, W.B. Saunders.

• Glossary •

abbreviation(s) A shortened form of a written word or phase used in place of the whole.

abuse Improper use or treatment.

adaptation Adjustment to environmental conditions.

affect The external expression of emotion attached to ideas or mental representations of objects.

afferent Toward a center or specific site of reference.

affixes One or more sounds or letters occurring as a bound form attached to the beginning or end of a word, base, or phrase or inserted within a word or base and serving to produce a derivative word or an inflectional form.

afterbirth The placental and fetal membranes expelled from the uterus after childbirth.

agoraphobia Fear of open and public spaces.

align To bring into line or alignment.

allegation(s) A statement by a party to a legal action of what he undertakes to prove.

alter(ed) To make different without changing into something else.

Alzheimer's disease Irreversible senile dementia characterized by intellectual deterioration, disorganization of the personality, and functional disabilities in carrying out the tasks of daily living.

ambulatory care Care of patients who are not confined to bed.

analgesia Absence of sensibility to pain.

anatomy The science dealing with the form and structure of living organisms.

anestheticlike A drug or agent used to abolish the sensation of pain.

angina Spasmodic choking or suffocative pain.

anonymity The quality or state of being anonymous.

anonymous Not named or identified.

anorexia Lack or loss of appetite for food.

antigen Any substance that is capable, under appropriate conditions, of inducing a specific immune response and of reacting with that response.

anti-inflammatory Effective against a response provoked by physical, chemical and biologic agents.

antonyms Words of opposite meaning.

anxiety Painful or apprehensive uneasiness of mind over an impending or anticipated ill.

appendicitis Inflammation of the vermiform appendix.

applicable Relevant.

approximate To come close.

arbitrary Based on or determined by individual preference.

arthritis Inflammation of a joint.

assert To state or declare positively and often forcefully or aggressively.

assumption The supposition that something is true.

asthma Condition caused by spasmodic constriction of bronchi.

auscultation Listening for sounds produced within the body.

autonomy Self-directing freedom.

avoidance An act or practice of avoiding or withdrawing from something.

basophils Any structure, cells, or histologic elements staining readily with basic dyes.

benign Not malignant.

biologic Pertaining to the scientific study of living organisms.

biomechanics The application of mechanical laws to living structures.

block To hinder progress.

blood pressure The pressure of blood within the arteries.

bulimia An eating disorder characterized by episodic binge eating followed by purging behavior such as self-induced vomiting and laxative abuse.

cal/day Calories per day.

caption(s) The explanatory comment or designation accompanying a pictorial illustration.

cardiovascular Pertaining to the heart and blood vessels.

care plan A nurse's systematic strategies for taking care of patients.

charting The keeping of a clinical record of the important facts about a patient and the progress of his or her illness.

chronic Persisting for a long time.

chronological order Of, relating to, or arranged in or according to the order of time.

clarify To make understandable.

clotting The formation of a jellylike substance over the ends or within the walls of a blood vessel, with resultant stoppage of the blood flow.

coagulability The state of being capable of forming or being formed into clots.

cognitive Having to do with that operation of the mind process by which we become aware of objects of thought and perception, including all aspects of perceiving, thinking, and remembering.

colleagues Associates in a profession or in a civil or ecclesiastical office.

collegiate Designed for or characteristic of college students.

concept Something conceived in the mind; thought, notion.

concise Marked by brevity of expression or statement; free from all elaboration and superfluous detail.

concrete To make actual or real.

consistency Firmness of constitution or character; persistency.

controversial Of, relating to, or arousing controversy.

controversy A discussion marked especially by the expression of opposing views; dispute.

conversely Reversed in order, relation, or action.

coping The process of contending with life difficulties in an effort to overcome or work through them.

core Central and often foundational part.

corticosteroids Hormones produced by the adrenal cortex; also, their synthetic equivalents.

credence Something believed to be true.

cyst A closed epithelium; live sac or capsule containing a liquid or semisolid substance.

decipher(ed) To make out the meaning of despite indistinctness or obscurity.

deficits Lack or impairment in a functional capacity.

delegate To appoint.

deposit To place, especially for safekeeping (or as a pledge).

detrimental Obviously harmful.

development Process of growth and differentiation.

deviation Noticeable or marked departure from accepted norms of behavior.

diabetes A general term referring to a variety of disorders characterized by excessive urination.

diacritical mark An accent near or through an orthographic or phonetic character or combination of characters indicating a phonetic value different from that given the unmarked or otherwise marked element.

diagnosed To have identified or recognized a disease.

diaphoresis Perspiration.

dilemma A difficult or persistent problem.

discs (disks) Circular or rounded flat plates.

DNA Deoxyribonucleic acid.

document To support with written information.

dressing Materials used for protecting a wound.

dynamic Marked by energy.

edema An abnormal accumulation of fluid in the intercellular spaces of the body.

elaborate To expand on something in detail.

endocrine Pertaining to internal secretions; hormonal.

endogenous opiate A sedative narcotic produced within the organism.

enhance(s) To add or contribute to.

enzyme Any protein that acts as a catalyst, increasing the rate at which a chemical reaction takes place.

epidermis The outermost and nonvascular layer of the skin.

episode An event that is distinctive and separate, although part of a larger series.

etymology The history of a linguistic form (as a word) shown by tracing its development since its earliest recorded occurrence in the language where it was found.

euphoria A feeling of well-being or elation.

exacerbate(ion) To make more violent, bitter, or severe.

excessive Exceeding the usual, proper, or normal.

excitatory An act of irritation or stimulation.

exocrine Secreting externally via a duct.

exogenous Originating outside the organism.

exotic Strikingly or excitingly different or unusual.

expedient Faster and easier.

external Of, or relating to, or connected with the outside or an outer part.

extracurricular Lying outside one's regular duties or routines.

extraneous Unrelated.

feedback The return to a point of evaluative or corrective information about an action or process.

fibrocartilage Cartilage made up of parallel, thick compact collagenous bundles, separated by narrow clefts, containing the typical cartilage cells (chondrocytes).

flexibility Characterized by a ready capability to adapt to new, different, or changing requirements.

footnotes A note of reference, explanation, or comment usually placed below the text on a printed page.

former First mentioned in order of two things mentioned or understood.

friction The rubbing of one body against another.

fulcrum The support about which a lever turns.

gastrointestinal Pertaining to the stomach and intestines.

generativity Pertaining to reproduction.

gestures The use of motions of the limbs or body as a means of expression.

glossary A collection of textual glosses or specialized terms with their meanings.

glucose A simple sugar, a monosaccharide in certain foodstuffs, especially fruit, and in normal blood; the chief source of energy in living organisms.

gout A hereditary form of arthritis in which uric acid appears in excessive quantities in the blood and may be deposited in the joints and other tissues.

graphic Pertaining to a visual representation.

gravity The quality of having weight.

gynecology The branch of medicine dealing with diseases of the genital tract in women.

habitual Resorted to on a regular basis.

hallucinations Sensory impressions that have no basis in external stimulations.

haphazard Marked by lack of plan, order, or direction.

hematoma A localized collection of clotted blood in an organ.

hemoglobin An allosteric protein found in erythrocytes that transports molecular oxygen (O_2) in the blood.

hemorrhage The escape of blood from a ruptured vessel.

hindrance Impediment.

hypertension Persistently high blood pressure.

hyponatremia Deficiency of sodium in the blood; salt depletion.

hypotension Lowered blood pressure.

hysterectomy Surgical removal of the uterus.

idiom The language peculiar to people or to a district, community, or class.

immobility Incapable of being moved.

immune system The body's ability to recognize and dispose of substances it interprets as foreign and harmful to its well-being.

impairments Injury.

impending About to occur.

imperative Not to be avoided or evaded.

impression A telling image impressed in the sense or the mind.

incision A cut or wound made by a sharp instrument.

incorporated To unite or work into something al-

ready existing so as to form an indistinguishable whole.

inflammatory Pertaining to a response elicited by injury or destruction of tissues.

ingrained Forming a part of the essence or innermost being.

inguinal hernia Hernia occurring in the groin, or inguine where the abdominal folds of flesh meet the thighs.

inherent Innate.

initial Of or relating to the beginning.

internal Situated near the inside of the body.

interventions Interference in the affairs of another to accomplish a goal.

intractable Not easily relieved or cured.

intricate Having many complexly interrelating parts or elements.

irrigate To wash a body cavity or wound by a stream of water or fluid.

kinship The quality or state of being kin; relationship.

legend An explanatory list of the symbols on a map or chart.

leverage The action of a lever or the mechanical advantage gained by it.

life-style A way of living.

limitation Restraint.

locus A point.

major Greater in importance.

maladaptive Marked by poor or inadequate adaptation.

malnutrition Poor nourishment resulting from improper diet or from some defect in metabolism that prevents the body from using its food properly.

mandates Requires.

mandatory Containing a command.

maximize To make the most of.

medulla The central or inner portion of an organ.

melanin A dark, sulfur-containing pigment normally found in the hair, skin, ciliary body, choroid of the eye, pigment layer of the retina, and nerve cells.

metabolic Having to do with the disposition of the nutrients absorbed into the blood following digestion.

minor Inferior in importance.

miscommunication Failure to communicate clearly.

mobility The ability to move in one's environment with ease and without restriction.

modification The making of a limited change in something.

momentum A property of a moving body that determines the length of time required to bring it to rest when under the action of a constant force or movement.

monitoring To watch, observe, or check, especially for a special purpose.

moral Of or relating to principles of right and wrong in behavior.

motivated To have provided a reason or cause for action.

multitude A great number.

mutations Permanent, transmissible changes in the genetic material.

mysoline Trademark for preparation of primidone, an anticonvulsant.

myths An unfounded or false notion.

myxorrhea A flow of mucus.

naloxone A narcotic antagonist structurally related to oxymorphone used as an antidote to narcotic overdosing and as an antagonist for pentazocine overdose.

neoplasia The formation of a neoplasm, a tumor.

network An interconnected or interrelated chain, group, or system.

neuron Nerve cell.

nitroglycerin A chemical well known as an explosive, but also having medical uses.

nonbiologic Not pertaining to living organisms.

nutrition The sum of the processes involved in taking in nutriments and assimilating and utilizing them.

obesity Excessive accumulation of fat in the body; increase in weight beyond that considered desirable with regard to age, height, and bone structure.

objective Free from bias.

obstacle Something that impedes progress or achievement.

obstructive To block or close up by an obstacle.

ombudsmen People who investigate complaints.

optimal Most desirable or satisfactory.

ostomy Formation of artificial opening.

overwhelmed Upset.

pallor Paleness, as of skin.

palpitation A heartbeat that is unusually rapid, strong, or irregular enough to make a person aware of it.

pancreas A large, elongated, racemose gland located transversely behind the stomach, between the spleen and duodenum.

paralysis Loss or impairment of motor function in part caused by a lesion of the neural or muscular mechanism.

passive Existing or occurring without being active.

pathogen Any disease-producing agent or microorganism.

pelvic pertaining to the pelvis, the lower portion of the trunk of the body.

percussion In medical diagnosis, striking a part of the body with short, sharp blows of the fingers in order to determine the size, position, and density of the underlying parts by the sound obtained.

physiology The science that treats the functions of the living organism and its parts and of the physical and chemical factors and processes involved.

plasma The fluid portion of the blood in which corpuscles are suspended.

portable Capable of being carried or moved about.

postoperative After a surgical operation.

posture An attitude of the body.

potential Something that can develop or become actual.

preceding That immediately precedes in time or place.

precise Exactly or sharply defined or stated.

prefix An affix attached to the beginning of a word or an inflectional form.

pregnant Containing unborn young within the body.

prematurity Underdevelopment; the condition of a premature infant.

pressure The burden of physical or mental distress.

priority Taking precedence (as in importance).

procrastination To put off intentionally the doing of something that should be done.

pronunciation To present in printed characters the spoken counterpart of.

protocol A system of fixed rules for behavior.

psychosocial Pertaining to or involving both psychic and social aspects.

psychotherapy Any number of related techniques for treating mental illness by psychological methods.

pulmonary Pertaining to the lungs, or to the pulmonary artery.

pulse The beat of the heart as felt through the walls of the arteries.

purification To clear from material defilement or imperfection.

quiescent Marked by inactivity or repose; tranquilly at rest.

receptive Fit to receive and transmit stimuli.

regardless Despite everything.

regimen Regulated activity designed to achieve certain ends.

reinforce To strengthen by additional assistance.

remission A diminution or abatement of symptoms of a disease.

repertoire A list or supply of capabilities.

resuscitate Restoring life or consciousness of one apparently dead, or whose respirations have ceased.

retirement Withdrawal from work.

revisions Alterations.

root The main part of the word.

sabotage An act or process tending to hamper or hurt.

sanitary Promoting or pertaining to health.

schema A mental code of experience that includes a particular organized way of perceiving cognitively.

sclerosis Hardening of a body part.

scoliosis Lateral deviation in the normally vertical line of the spine.

self-concept The way a person feels, thinks or views himself or herself.

sensory Pertaining to sensations or to any response of the senses (hearing, sight, touch, etc.) to incoming stimuli.

shrugging Gesturing with the shoulder.

socialism A system of society or group living in which there is no private property.

sociologic Having to do with the study of social relationships and phenomena.

somatic Pertaining to or characteristic of the body.

spasmodic The nature of a spasm, a sudden involuntary contraction of a muscle or group of muscles.

specialized Designed or fitted for one particular purpose or occupation.

spinal cord That part of the central nervous system lodged in the spinal canal, extending from the foramen magnum to the upper part of the lumbar region.

spiritual Pertaining to the spirit.

stability The strength to stand or endure; firmness.

stable Not changing or fluctuating.

statistics A branch of mathematics dealing with the collection, analysis, interpretation, and presentation of masses of numerical data.

statute A law enacted by the legislative branch of the government.

sterile Free from living microorganisms.

streamlined Stripped of nonessentials.

subjective Arising out of or identified by means of one's perception of one's own state or processes.

suffix An affix occurring at the end of a word, base, or phrase.

summarize Covering the main points succinctly.

superego In psychoanalytic theory, a part of the psyche derived from both the id and the ego, which acts, largely unconsciously, as a monitor.

supplemented Something that completes or makes an addition.

support To provide with substantiation.

supreme Highest in rank or authority.

synonym One of two or more words or expressions of the same language that have the same or nearly the same meaning in some or all senses.

synonymous Having the same or similar meaning.

synthesis The production of a substance by the union of chemical elements, groups, or similar compounds.

systematic Methodical in procedure or plan.

taxonomy The study of the general principles of scientific classification.

thesaurus A book of words and their synonyms.

thrombus An aggregation of blood factors frequently causing vascular obstruction.

tonsillectomy Excision of tonsils.

transmit To send or convey from one person to another.

trauma A wound or injury, especially produced by extreme force.

unabridged Complete; being the most complete of its class.

unilateral Done or undertaken by one person or party.

validation State of being confirmed.

variety The quality or state of having different forms or types.

verify To establish the truth, accuracy, or reality of.

vertebrae The separate segments composing the spine.

visualize To form a mental image.

vital signs The signs of life, namely pulse, respiration, and temperature.

zygote The cell resulting from a union of a male and female gamete; the fertilized ovum.

• Answer Key •

• CHAPTER 1 •

Vocabulary Check

1 d
2 a
3 c
4 d
5 a
6 c
7 b
8 b
9 a
10 c

• CHAPTER 2 •

Five Prereading Strategies

1 Prereading Strategies
2 Using prereading strategies for active reading. The five prereading strategies are: read the title, introduction and summary, boldface headings, key words, and look at graphic aids.
3 Prereading Strategies
Key words
Questions to think about before readings
Five prereading strategies
Vocabulary
Summary
4 Answers will vary
5 Yes

Exercise 2–1

1 Several different types of care plans in use
2 Individually Constructed
Advantages
Disadvantages
Standardized
Advantages
Disadvantages
Computerized
Medical Diagnosis
Nursing Diagnosis
Individually Constructed
Advantages
Disadvantages
Summary

3 extraneous
protocol
inflammatory
trauma
regimen
analgesia
impending
document
credence
4 Yes: Table 6–1 Acute Pain; Figure 6–2 Computerized Care Plan
5 This selection is about the following care plans: individualized, standardized, or computerized.

Vocabulary Check

1 b
2 d
3 a
4 d
5 c
6 b
7 b
8 a
9 c
10 d

• CHAPTER 3 •

Exercise 3–1

Answers will vary

Exercise 3–2

Answers will vary

Exercise 3–3

Answers will vary

Exercise 3–4

Answers will vary

Exercise 3–5

1 Nursing journal
2 General nursing journal

3 Encyclopedia or general nursing textbook

4 General nursing text

5 Nursing journal

6 Encyclopedia

Exercise 3–6

Answers will vary

Vocabulary Check

1 c

2 d

3 c

4 a

5 d

6 b

7 a

8 c

9 a

10 d

• CHAPTER 4 •

Exercise 4–1

TABLE 4–1 Prefixes, Roots, Suffixes

		DEFINITION	EXAMPLE	DEFINITION OF EXAMPLE	YOUR EXAMPLE
Prefix					
1	anti	Against	Anti-inflammatory	An agent that acts against inflammation	Answers will vary
2	*dys	Bad, difficult	Dysfunction	Functioning badly	Answers will vary
3	*endo	Within	Endocrine	Secreting from within	Answers will vary
4	ex	Out	Exhale	To breathe out	Answers will vary
5	fore	Before, in front of	Foresight	To know beforehand	Answers will vary
6	*hem hemato	Relating to the blood	Hemoglobin	A red matter in the blood	Answers will vary
7	*hydra hydro	Relating to water	Hydrocephalus	Water on the brain	Answers will vary
8	*hyper	Over, above, beyond	Hyperactive	Overactive	Answers will vary
9	*hypo	Under	Hypodermic	Injected under the skin	Answers will vary
10	*idio	Relating to the individual organ, distinct	Idiomuscular	Relating to an individual muscle	Answers will vary
11	inter	Between	Interstate	Between states	Answers will vary
12	mal	Poor, bad	Malpractice	Poor practice	Answers will vary
13	*micro	Small	Microscope	An instrument used to see small objects	Answers will vary
14	*neuro	Nerve	Neurobiology	Biology of the nervous system	Answers will vary
15	non	No	Nonviable	Not capable of developing into a living thing	Answers will vary

TABLE 4–1 Prefixes, Roots, Suffixes *Continued*

		DEFINITION	EXAMPLE	DEFINITION OF EXAMPLE	YOUR EXAMPLE
Prefixes cont'd					
16	*ortho	Straight, normal	Orthodontia	The practice of straightening teeth	Answers will vary
17	retro	Backward	Retroactive	Back, toward the past	Answers will vary
18	semi	Half	Semicircle	Half circle	Answers will vary
19	sub	Under	Subconscious	Beneath conscious knowledge	Answers will vary
20	tele	Distant, for	Television	Broadcasting images over a distance	Answers will vary
21	Answers will vary	Answers will vary	Answers will vary	Answers will vary	Answers will vary
22	Answers will vary	Answers will vary	Answers will vary	Answers will vary	Answers will vary
23	Answers will vary	Answers will vary	Answers will vary	Answers will vary	Answers will vary
24	Answers will vary	Answers will vary	Answers will vary	Answers will vary	Answers will vary
25	Answers will vary	Answers will vary	Answers will vary	Answers will vary	Answers will vary
Roots					
1	*arteri arterio	Artery	Arteriosclerosis	Thickening of the walls of the arteries	Answers will vary
2	*arthro arthr	Joint	Arthritis	Disease involving pain and stiffening of the joint	Answers will vary
3	*cardi cardio	Heart	Cardiovascular	Pertaining to the heart and blood vessels	Answers will vary
4	dem, demo	People	Democracy	Government of the people	Answers will vary
5	*derm dermo	Skin	Dermatologist	Skin doctor	Answers will vary
6	fac, fact	Make, do	Factory	Place where things are made	Answers will vary
7	geo	Earth	Geology	Study of the earth	Answers will vary
8	*gyne	Woman	Gynecology	Branch of medicine, dealing with women's diseases	Answers will vary
9	later	Side	Unilateral	One-sided	Answers will vary
10	mit, miss	Send	Transmit	To send across	Answers will vary
11	*nephro nephr	Kidney	Nephritis	Inflammation of the kidney	Answers will vary

Continued.

TABLE 4–1 Prefixes, Roots, Suffixes *Continued*

		DEFINITION	EXAMPLE	DEFINITION OF EXAMPLE	YOUR EXAMPLE
Roots cont'd					
12	nil	Nothing	Nillify	To make into nothing	Answers will vary
13	*oste osteo	Bone	Osteoporosis	Disease of the bones	Answers will vary
14	*path	Disease	Pathology	Study of disease	Answers will vary
15	port	Carry	Transport	To carry across	Answers will vary
16	*psych	Mind	Psychology	Study of the mind	Answers will vary
17	*soma	Body	Somatic	Referring to the body	Answers will vary
18	spec spect	To look at	Spectator	One who watches	Answers will vary
19	ven veno	Vein	Venous	Pertaining to veins	Answers will vary
20	vers	Turn	Reversible	Able to be turned	Answers will vary
21	Answers will vary	Answers will vary	Answers will vary	Answers will vary	Answers will vary
22	Answers will vary	Answers will vary	Answers will vary	Answers will vary	Answers will vary
23	Answers will vary	Answers will vary	Answers will vary	Answers will vary	Answers will vary
24	Answers will vary	Answers will vary	Answers will vary	Answers will vary	Answers will vary
25	Answers will vary	Answers will vary	Answers will vary	Answers will vary	Answers will vary
Suffixes					
1	able, ible	Capable of	Reachable	Capable of being reached	Answers will vary
2	ation	Act of	Purification	The act of making pure	Answers will vary
3	*cide	Causing death	Pesticide	Capable of killing pests	Answers will vary
4	*cyte	Cell	Blastocyte	Undifferentiated embryonic cell	Answers will vary
5	*ectomy	Excision	Tonsillectomy	The removal of the tonsils	Answers will vary
6	er, or, ant	Person who	Actor	One who acts	Answers will vary

TABLE 4–1   Prefixes, Roots, Suffixes *Continued*

		DEFINITION	EXAMPLE	DEFINITION OF EXAMPLE	YOUR EXAMPLE
Suffixes cont'd					
7	ful	Full of	Dreadful	Full of dread	Answers will vary
8	graph	Picture or record	Phonograph	Record player	Answers will vary
9	gram	Instrument that records	Cardiogram	Records heart function	Answers will vary
10	ism	Doctrine	Socialism	Doctrine of public ownership	Answers will vary
11	itis	Inflammation of	Appendicitis	Inflammation of the appendix	Answers will vary
12	*meter	Measure of	Centimeter	Measure of metric length	Answers will vary
13	ology	Study of	Biology	Study of living things	Answers will vary
14	*oplasty	Plastic surgery	Rhinoplasty	Plastic surgery of the nose	Answers will vary
15	*osis	Condition of	Psychosis	Pathological condition of the mind	Answers will vary
16	*ostomy	Opening	Colostomy	An artificial opening created in the large intestine	Answers will vary
17	*phobia	Fear	Agoraphobia	Fear of open space	Answers will vary
18	rupt	Break, burst	Interrupt	To break in	Answers will vary
19	scope	See	Telescope	Instrument for seeing far	Answers will vary
20	*tomy	Cutting	Hysterectomy	Removal of the uterus	Answers will vary
21	Answers will vary	Answers will vary	Answers will vary	Answers will vary	Answers will vary
22	Answers will vary	Answers will vary	Answers will vary	Answers will vary	Answers will vary
23	Answers will vary	Answers will vary	Answers will vary	Answers will vary	Answers will vary
24	Answers will vary	Answers will vary	Answers will vary	Answers will vary	Answers will vary
25	Answers will vary	Answers will vary	Answers will vary	Answers will vary	Answers will vary

Exercise 4–2

Answers will vary

Exercise 4–3

Answers will vary

Exercise 4–4

after injury

Postinjury Phase. Ideally, accidental injuries should be prevented, but in some instances this simply is not possible. Therefore nurses should attend to optimizing postinjury <u>prevention</u> efforts, to minimize the long-range effects of an injury. Many communities have emergency call systems, such as "Lifeline," that allow older people at risk of falling ready access to <u>postfall</u> assistance. The systems work by activating a central emergency call board (such as in an emergency room) when the client pushes a button. These buttons are generally small and may be worn on light clothing. Other alternatives include daily checking systems, in which neighbors, friends, or family phone the older person each day.

the state of preventing

after a fall

An example of a fall-related injury prevention protocol developed for a nursing home is shown on this page. It includes both <u>preinjury</u> and postinjury interventions to reduce injury.

before injury

Evaluation

Criteria for evaluation of nursing care for those with potential for injury are:
1. What is the incidence of injury in the target client population? How does it compare with national averages?
2. What is the incidence of <u>functional</u> impairment <u>attributable</u> to injury in the client population?
3. Are the patients assessed for potential for specific injuries: fall-related injury, other trauma, burns, poisoning?
4. Are steps taken to reduce the at-risk individual's likelihood of sustaining injury?
5. Is the client's lifestyle adversely affected by the injury prevention program?
6. What is the cost of the injury prevention program to the individual, family, and facility or agency?

able to function

able to attribute

NONCOMPLIANCE   *not following advise*
Definition and Scope of Problem

Noncompliance is a term with many definitions and connotations. Even leading experts on nursing diagnosis offer quite different definitions. Carpenito defines noncompliance as "personal behavior that deviates from health-related advice given by health care professionals." Gordon defines it as "failure to participate in carrying out the plan of care *after indicating initial intention to comply.*" The North American Nursing Diagnosis Association has developed yet another definition: "A person's informed decision not to adhere to a <u>therapeutic</u> recommendation."

the condition of intending

act of deciding

that which provides therapy

Compliance is a concern of nurses because the goal of compliance is improved health status. Despite inconsistencies <u>in definition, there is</u> widespread agreement that achieving compliance is problematic in many different categories of patients. Research on compliance shows that noncompliance is found in patients of all ages, social classes, and ethnic groups; it is found in all types of health care delivery systems and in patients whose symptoms vary from <u>nonexistent</u> to life-threatening.

differences

not living

Noncompliance is most often seen in the community setting, where patients have greater control over their daily routines and are more likely to have competing demands on their time. In institutional settings there are fewer opportunities for noncompliance, because many self-care activities are either closely supervised or done for the patient.

The extent of noncompliance by the elderly is thought to be high by some <u>observers</u>, with medication noncompliance rates averaging about 50 per cent. However, variations in the definition of noncompliance used in studies and measurement difficulties make accurate estimates of the extent of this problem among the elderly difficult to obtain.

those who observe

Most of the compliance literature focuses on younger adults. Sackett and Snow's review of 31 compliance studies shows that one third of the studies specifically exclude the elderly, and only 2 of 31 are specific to this population. Much of what we know about compliance in the elderly has been extrapolated from studies of age-heterogeneous groups with specific chronic diseases, such as diabetes and hypertension. The literature that considers the elderly as a discrete group calls attention to sensory deficits and memory impairment as two important contributors to noncompliance.

different kinds

high blood pressure

Vocabulary Check

1 d
2 a
3 c
4 d
5 b
6 a
7 c
8 d
9 a
10 c

• CHAPTER 5 •

Exercise 5–1

1 An abnormal contraction
2 An involuntary trembling of a limb or body part
3 Fear of sexual activity leading to avoidance
4 A replacement for a missing part of the body
5 A thinking function that combines knowledge with comprehension and application

Exercise 5–2

1 Anxiety
2 Unconcerned
3 Impaired
4 Relationship
5 Angry

Exercise 5–3

1 Without attraction
2 Functional
3 Strengths and assets
4 Rejection, devaluation
5 Bed rest

Exercise 5–4

1 Hyperpigmentation, hypopigmentation
2 Specialty, oncology
3 Zygote
4 Margin of safety
5 Epinephrine and norepinephrine

Exercise 5–5

1 Water in the form of vapor
2 An instrument used to measure blood pressure
3 A diseased heart
4 A disorder of the deep veins in the legs
5 Solid substance found in the ground

Exercise 5–6

1 A technique to change behavior
   Pain that won't go away
2 Radioactive tracers
   Dynamic change
3 A goal-directed systematic practice of nursing data
4 The geometric arrangement of body parts in relation to each other
   Best
   Badly
5 The periodic cessation of breathing during sleep
   Evaluated
   The number of times that something happens in a given period

Exercise 5-7

Chart

Word	Definition	Context	Glossary	Dictionary	Medical Dictionary
1. Classification	Sorting information into specific catagories	√			
2. Component	Part			√	
3. Norms	Standards	√			
4. Cue	A piece of information	√			
5. Perception	A sharp understanding			√	
6. Subjective	Affected by feelings	√			
7. Objective	Real	√			
8. Symptoms	Signs or indications	√			
9. Inference	Judgement	√			
10. Clusters	Group of cues	√			
11. Clinical	Pertaining to the clinic				√
12. Concrete	To make actual or real		√		
13. Postoperative	After a surgical operation		√		
14. Appendectomy	The excision of the appendix				√
15. Postpartum	Occurring after childbirth				√

Vocabulary Check

1 a
2 c
3 b
4 d
5 a
6 d
7 a
8 b
9 d
10 a

• CHAPTER 6 •

1 Two
2 \in-sizh-n\
3 Noun
4 Fifteenth century
5 Three
First definition

Exercise 6–1

1 Carcinogen
2 Cardiac

3 Hematoma
4 Hemophilia
5 Menopause
6 Nematodes
7 Perioperative
8 Peripheral
9 Peritonitis
10 Sinusitis

Exercise 6–2

1 _____8_____ Scoliosis
2 _____7_____ Cyst
3 _____1_____ Myotomy
4 _____9_____ Pathogen
5 _____2_____ Glomerulitis
6 _____10_____ Scoliosis
7 _____5_____ Myxorrhea
8 _____3_____ Bulimia
9 _____6_____ Afterbirth
10 _____4_____ Distillation

Exercise 6–3

1 Aorta
2 Chorea

3 Diuretic

4 Hypogastric

5 Phosphate

6 Spina bifida

7 Technologist

8 Convolution

9 Disgraphia

10 Mercury

Exercise 6–4

1 2

2 4

3 2

4 1c

5 1a

6 2

7 1a

8 1

9 3

10 1

Exercise 6–5

1 F

2 T

3 F

4 T

5 T

Thesaurus Entry

<u>Noun</u>

Exercise 6–6

The nurse drew out her notebook from the desk in the
                                              jot down
station. She wanted to <u>note</u> some of the happenings
          observed   *attendant*
she <u>noticed</u> during her shift. In particular the <u>nurse</u>
                          distasteful
wanted to object to some of the <u>objectionable</u> occur-

rences on the floor. However, she wanted to be
impartial   *end*
objective, so the <u>objective</u> of her observation would not
        protest
be to <u>object</u> against the other nurse, but to get him to
          impressions   *care for*
change his <u>notions</u> on what it is to <u>nurse</u> a patient.

Vocabulary Check

1 b

2 d

3 a

4 b

5 d

6 a

7 a

8 c

9 a

10 a

• **CHAPTER 7** •

Exercise 7–1

Answers will vary

Vocabulary Check

1 d

2 a

3 c

4 b

5 b

6 d

7 d

8 c

9 b

10 a

• **CHAPTER 8** •

Exercise 8–1

1 Gestures

2 Examination

3 Systems

4 Texture

5 Description

Exercise 8–2

1	a	Too narrow	4	a	Correct
	b	Correct		b	Too narrow
	c	Not mentioned		c	Too broad
	d	Too broad		d	Not mentioned
2	a	Too broad	5	a	Correct
	b	Not mentioned		b	Too narrow
	c	Correct		c	Not mentioned
	d	Too narrow		d	Too broad
3	a	Too broad			
	b	Not mentioned			
	c	Correct			
	d	Too narrow			

Exercise 8–3

1 Assessing Clients through the Classification Process
2 Validation of Data Interpretation
3 Factors Which Interface with Nurse's Ability to Collect Data
4 Language Barriers Between Nurse and Client
5 Accountability of Nurses for Legal Actions

Exercise 8–4

Answers will vary

Exercise 8–5

Types of Data Collected by Nurse During Assessment

1 Topic: Various Types of Angina Pectoris
   Main Idea: There are several types of angina pectoris.
2 Topic: Reasons for Mental Illness
   Main Idea: Other reasons for mental illness are considered physical or physiological.
3 Topic: Religious Institutions and the Elderly
   Main Idea: Churches and other religious institutions serve the elderly in many ways.
4 Topic: Hospitalization and Patients' Identity Crisis
   Main Idea: In many ways hospitalization creates an identity crisis for the client.
5 Topic: How Antisocial Clients Affect the Nurse
   Main Idea: Clients with antisocial personality disorders, when hospitalized, evoke strong emotions in nurses.

Exercise 8–6

1 Topic: Hospital's Responsibility for Negligence
   Stated Main Idea: Under this theory, the employer will be held liable for negligent acts of its employees performed within the scope of their employment.
2 Topic: Silence in Communication
   Stated Main Idea: Silence also can be used to accent an important point in a verbal communication, a brief silence following an important verbal message.
3 Topic: Allergic Rhinitis
   Unstated Main Idea: Most common allergies like hay fever run in families, occur before a person is 30, and diminish with age.
4 Topic: Social Stresses of the Ill Child
   Stated Main Idea: The social realities the child has to contend with are forces that compel the nurse to consider the child's illness from a broad interpersonal perspective.
5 Topic: Symptoms of Depression
   Unstated Main Ideas: There are many indications of depression.

Exercise 8–7

Topic: Ethical Theories
Main Idea Paragraph 1: Ethical theories describe approaches for resolving dilemmas commonly faced by nurses.
Main Idea Paragraph 2: There are two major ethical theories used to help nurses resolve health care dilemmas: deontology and utilitarianism.
Main Idea Paragraph 3: One of the flaws with this approach is that most situations have extenuating circumstances.
Main Idea Paragraph 4: The utilitarian approach states that actions are right or wrong on the basis of the consequences of the actions. Utilitarians focus on the results of actions rather than on their motivations. This view is quite different from the deontological position, which would maintain that the nurse must tell the truth without exception.
Main Idea of the Entire Passage: There are two ethical theories that nurses use to resolve dilemmas: deontology and utilitarianism; however, both these theories have limitations.

Vocabulary Check

1 d
2 b
3 b
4 a
5 b
6 c
7 c
8 a
9 a
10 b

• CHAPTER 9 •

Exercise 9–1

Three types of MS are seen
↑
Classic picture of exacerbation followed by remission   ←— Benign
                                                         ←— Mild
                                                         ←— Moderate
↑
Progressive MS characterized by absence of periods of remission   Progressive
                                                                  ←— Deterioration occurs over several years
↑
Combined—begins with classic presentation of MS and converts to a progressive course

Exercise 9–2

1 The term depression is used loosely for a wide range of conditions. It may be used to denote normal, everyday mood variations, mild but pathological depressive disorders, or severe psychotic depression. All have very different etiological natures and varying clinical implications (Varcarolis, pp. 70–71). __example__

2 Research has identified three body types or configurations and the personality traits most often associated with them. These types are endomorph—heavyset, sociable, friendly, relaxed; mesomorph—sturdy well-developed bone and muscle, vigorous, energetic, assertive; ectomorph—thin, slender, inhibited, private (Ignatavicius and Bayne, p. 159). __example__

3 There are people who are not able to resolve a particular loss. Between 10% and 20% of newly bereaved persons have serious emotional problems (Ignatavicius and Bayne, p. 202). __data__

4 The nurse assesses muscle strength by having the client (1) squeeze the nurse's hands, (2) attempt to keep the arms flexed while the nurse pulls downward on the lower arms, and (3) push both feet against a flat surface (a box or a board) while the nurse applies resistance (Ignatavicius and Bayne, p. 283). __procedure__

5 Hyponatremia has little direct effect on cardiac muscle contractibility; however, alterations in cardiac output are associated with hyponatremia. In some instances, cardia pathologic changes (such as profound congestive heart failure with generalized edema formation) actually cause the hyponatremia. Ignatavicius and Bayne, p. 283). cause

6 Proceeding from a level at age 2 or 3 which all animals with four legs are horses or some other type of one-dimensional animal, the child is unable to distinguish fantasy from reality, to consider another's view-point or to accept the possibility of alternate options in the pre school years (Arnold and Boggs, p. 419). __description__

7 Don't ask irrelevant questions. Respond to the client in brief concise sentences and don't introduce a lot of explanation. Let the client tell you what he or she is experiencing (Ignatavicius Bayne, p. 460). __procedure__

8 Chronic disease is America's primary health problem. Approximately 50% of the population (110 million people) have one or more chronic illnesses, and nearly 32.4 million people have limitations in performing selfcare activities (Ignatavicius and Bayne, pp. 490–491). __data__

9 Intellect does not decline solely as a result of aging. However, a decrease in intellectual level may be caused by insufficient oxygen supply to the CNS (Ignatavicius and Bayne, p. 847). __cause__

10 Generally, clients with swallowing problems are able to tolerate or swallow soft or semisoft foods and fluids (mechanically soft or dental diet, junior baby foods) better than thin liquids (water, juice, or broth) or a regular meal (Ignatavicius and Bayne, p. 890). __description__

Exercise 9–3

• **EXERCISE 9–3** •   *Unstated Main Idea. Iron deficiency anemia is seen in all countries and populations*

Below is a passage from a nursing textbook. In each paragraph, underline the stated main idea. If the main idea is unstated, create your own in the margin. Underline twice the major details that support the main idea.

The adult body contains about 50 mg of iron per 100 mL of blood. Total body iron ranges between 2 and 6 g, depending on the size of the individual and the amount of hemoglobin the client's cells contain. Approximately two-thirds of this iron is contained in hemoglobin; the other third is stored in the bone marrow, the spleen, the liver, and muscle. If an individual has an iron deficiency, the iron stores are depleted first, followed by a reduction in hemoglobin. As a result, RBCs are small in size (microcytic) and diminished in number to the extent that the client has relatively mild manifestations of anemia, including weakness and pallor.

Iron deficiency anemia is the most common type of anemia. It can result from blood loss, increased internal demands (e.g., with pregnancy, adolescence, infection, and high-metabolism states), malabsorption (e.g., in celiac sprue and after partial or total gastrectomy), or dietary inadequacy (e.g., as a result of chronic alcoholism or poverty). In this anemia, the basic problem is a decreased supply of iron for the developing RBC.

Iron deficiency anemia is seen frequently in underdeveloped countries, as well as in technologically advanced societies, such as in the United States. It can occur at any age, but is more frequently noted in women, children, the elderly, and those with restricted diets (e.g., as a result of low income) or unbalanced diets.

The primary treatment of iron deficiency anemia is an increase in the oral intake of iron. Iron is obtained from food. Important sources are red meats, organ meats, kidney beans, whole-wheat products, spinach, egg yolks, carrots, and raisins. An adequate diet supplies the body with about 12 to 15 mg of iron per day, of which only 5% to 10% is absorbed. The amount of iron normally absorbed daily from the diet is sufficient to meet the needs of healthy men and healthy women after the childbearing age, but is not sufficient to supply the greater needs of menstruating women and adolescents during growth spurts. Fortunately, if iron intake is inadequate or if bleeding or pregnancy occurs, the gastrointestinal (GI) tract is capable of increasing the absorption of iron to about 20% to 30% of the total daily intake. When iron deficiency anemia develops in nonmenstruating women or adult men, other possible sources of insidious blood loss should be explored (such as GI lesions) (Ignatavicius and Bayne, p. 2254).

Vocabulary Check

1 b
2 c
3 a
4 d
5 b
6 d
7 a
8 b
9 c
10 c

• CHAPTER 10 •

Example 10–1
second, next, then, next, final

Example 10–2
thus

Example 10–3
on the other hand

Example 10–4
also

Exercise 10–1

1 Simple listing
2 Comparison-contrast
3 Cause-effect
4 Cause-effect
5 Chronological (time order)

Exercise 10–2

1	Organizational pattern	Simple listing
	Topic	Three layers of skin
	Main idea	Skin is the largest body organ and has three layers.
	Major details	Epidermis
		Dermis
		Subcutaneous tissue
2	Organizational pattern	Simple listing
	Topic	Reasons for bathing
	Main idea	People bathe for reasons other than hygiene.
	Major details	Relax
		Time alone
		Stimulant

3	Organizational pattern	Cause and effect
	Topic	Supreme power of the U.S. Constitution
	Main idea	The U.S. Constitution is the supreme law of the land.
	Major details	Gives court power
		Restricts rights of Congress and states
		Comes before any statute
4	Organizational pattern	Compare and contrast
	Topic	Similarities and differences between nursing diagnosis and medical diagnosis
	Main idea	Nursing diagnoses are not medical diagnoses although there are similarities between the two.

Major details

Similarities	**Differences**
Obtaining person's history	Focus
	Specific goals and objectives
Performing physical exam	Medical diagnosis to learn source of symptoms
Organizing data base	Nursing diagnosis describes combination of signs and symptoms

Analyzing data obtained
Use of:
  Physical skills
  Intellectual skills
  Assessment skills
  Observational skills
Purpose of diagnosis: to identify problem and plan solution

5 Organizational pattern — Chronological (time order)

Topic — Development of infant posture and locomotion

Main idea — The infant gradually progresses in skill of locomotion and walks alone at about 12 to 14 months.

Major details

Birth: legs tucked up
2-3 months: legs extended
5-6 months: sits with support
6½-7½ months: sits without support
8-9 months: creeps
9-11 months: pulls up on furniture
11-12 months: stands alone walks with help
12-14 months: walks alone

Exercise 10–3

1 c
2 c
3 b
4 a
5 d
6 b
7 d
8 a
9 c
10 d

Vocabulary Check

1 c
2 b
3 a
4 b
5 c
6 d
7 b
8 d
9 a
10 c

• CHAPTER 11 •

Exercise 11–1

1 Medical-Surgical Nursing—A Psychophysiologic Approach, Third Edition.
2 Joan Luckmann and Karen Creason Sorensen
3 W.B. Saunders Company
4 No

Exercise 11–2

1 Section 1—Unifying Concepts of Advanced Nursing Care
Section 2—Specific Problems in Medical Surgical Nursing
Section 3—A Summation of Holistic Health Assessment
2 1—empathy
2—therapeutic communication
3—advocacy

Exercise 11–3

1 Four
2 Nursing People Experiencing Cardiovascular Disorders
3 Section Two
4 1836

Exercise 11–4

Answers will vary

Exercise 11–5

1 Clinical Skills: A System of Clinical Examination
2 Nursing

Exercise 11–6

1 Body Systems Assessment Criteria
2 Five

Exercise 11–7

1 743
2 1328

Exercise 11–8

Answers will vary

Exercise 11–9

Answers will vary

Exercise 11–10

1 Sociologic Assessment
2 _____
3 _____
4 c
5 Answers will vary

Exercise 11–11

Answers will vary

Vocabulary Check

1 b
2 a
3 c
4 b
5 b
6 c
7 b
8 c
9 a
10 b

• CHAPTER 12 •

Exercise 12–1

1 Intensive Care Unit
2 Two
3 Patient and health care worker
4 Person is in need of service (help).
5 The picture visually depicts the complexity of all the equipment required to treat the seriously ill.

Exercise 12–2

1 Summary of Normal Play-Age Growth and Development
2 3, 4, 5
3 4
4 5
5 Physical competency
Intellectual competency
Emotional competency
Nutrition
Play
Safety

Exercise 12–3

1 Problem list
2 Six
3 1963
4 Four
5 Two

Exercise 12–4

1 Some major complications of immobility
2 Pressure sores
Pneumonia
Urinary tract
3 Depression
Insomnia
Sensory deprivation

4 Leg
5 Discomfort
6 Urinary tract infections
Pneumonia
Pressure sores
Constipation
Stiff joints
Thrombus
Foot drop
Depression
Insomnia
Sensory deprivation

Exercise 12–5

1 The Nursing Process
2 Data gathering
Problem identification
Intervention planning
Care plan implementation
Intervention evaluation
3 Nursing assessment
4 1—data gathering
5 It gives an overview of the text.

Exercise 12–6

Answers will vary

Vocabulary Check

1 d
2 d
3 b
4 d
5 b
6 a
7 b
8 c
9 c
10 a

• CHAPTER 13 •

Exercise 13–1

Answers will vary

Exercise 13–2

a Answers will vary
b Answers will vary

Vocabulary Check

1 b
2 c
3 c

4 b

5 b

6 c

7 d

8 d

9 b

10 c

Sebaceous glands' function diminishes with age
  In men decrease is minimal
  More so in women after menopause
Sweat glands change with age
  Decrease in size
  Decrease in number
  Decrease in function
    Older people have difficulty sweating
    Impairs older people's ability to maintain body temperature

• CHAPTER 14 •

Exercise 14–1

—Free radicals are "highly reactive cellular components derived from atoms or molecules in which an electron pair has been transiently separated into two electrons that exhibit independence of motion."

—Lipofuscin is a pigmented material rich in lipids and proteins that accumulates in many organs with aging.

—Lipofuscin appears to have some relationship to free radicals and the process of aging because the substance is associated with oxidation of unsaturated lipids.

Exercise 14–2

Answers will vary

Exercise 14–3

Answers will vary

Exercise 14–4

Answers will vary

Exercise 14–5

1 %

2 ?

3 '

4 "

5 →

6 ←

7 @

8 5

9 ×

10 $

Exercise 14–6

Two major types of skin glands
  Sebaceous glands
    Originate in dermis
    Secrete sebum
  Sweat glands
    Eccrine
      Promotes body cooling
    Apocrine
      Responsible for body odor

Exercise 14–7

Answers will vary

Exercise 14–8

Answers will vary

Exercise 14–9

Answers will vary

Exercise 14–10

Answers will vary

Exercise 14–11

Answers will vary

Vocabulary Check

1 a

2 d

3 c

4 b

5 d

6 b

7 c

8 d

9 a

10 d

• CHAPTER 15 •

Exercise 15–1

1 d

2 c

3 a

4 c

5 d

Exercise 15–2

1 b

2 b

3 b

4 c

5 a

Exercise 15–3

1 d
2 c
3 b
4 a
5 c

Exercise 15–4

1 b
2 b
3 b
4 c
5 a

Exercise 15–5

Part I
1 third
2 the legal system
3 governor
4 state
5 American Nurses Association

Part II
1 e
2 d
3 a
4 c
5 b

Part III
1 b
2 d
3 c
4 b
5 c
6 a
7 d
8 b
9 a
10 a

Part IV
1 F
2 T
3 T
4 F
5 T

Exercise 15–6

Answers will vary

Exercise 15–7

Answers will vary

Exercise 15–8

Answers will vary

Vocabulary Check

1 d
2 d
3 a
4 d
5 c
6 b
7 b
8 b
9 b
10 a

• READING SELECTION 1 •

Preview Question

Answers will vary

Vocabulary

Answers will vary

Summary

Answers will vary

Comprehension Questions

1 c
2 a
3 d
4 b
5 d
6 a
7 c
8 a
9 d
10 b

• READING SELECTION 2 •

Preview Question

Answers will vary

Vocabulary

Answers will vary

Summary

Answers will vary

Comprehension Questions

1 d
2 a
3 b
4 d
5 c
6 b
7 d
8 b
9 a
10 d

• READING SELECTION 3 •

Preview Question

Stage 1—vascular stage
Stage 2—cellular exudate stage
Stage 3—tissue repair and replacement stage

Vocabulary

Answers will vary

Summary

Answers will vary

Comprehension Questions

1 a
2 b
3 d
4 d
5 a
6 d
7 c
8 a
9 b
10 a

• READING SELECTION 4 •

Preview Question

Head and neck
Vertebral spine
Upper and lower extremities

Vocabulary

Answers will vary

Summary

Answers will vary

Comprehension Questions

1 b
2 d
3 b
4 b
5 a
6 c
7 d
8 b
9 a
10 d

• READING SELECTION 5 •

Preview Question

To determine the normal functioning of the nervous system, both motor and sensory

Vocabulary

Answers will vary

Summary

Answers will vary

Comprehension Questions

1 b
2 c
3 d
4 a
5 d
6 c
7 a
8 d
9 b
10 c

• READING SELECTION 6 •

Preview Question

Answers will vary

Vocabulary

Answers will vary

Summary

Answers will vary

Comprehension Questions

1 a
2 b

3 d

4 c

5 b

6 b

7 a

8 c

9 d

10 a

5 a

6 d

7 b

8 b

9 a

10 c

• READING SELECTION 7 •

Preview Question

(a) Anatomy and physiology of the external, middle, and inner ear

(b) Answers will vary

Vocabulary

Answers will vary

Summary

Answers will vary

Comprehension Questions

1 a

2 d

3 b

4 c

5 a

6 d

7 b

8 c

9 a

10 d

• READING SELECTION 8 •

Preview Question

How the Blood Flows Through the Heart

Vocabulary

Answers will vary

Summary

Answers will vary

Comprehension Questions

1 c

2 d

3 a

4 b

• READING SELECTION 9 •

Preview Question

The scalp, skull or brain

Vocabulary

Answers will vary

Summary

Answers will vary

Comprehension Questions

1 b

2 c

3 c

4 d

5 a

6 d

7 b

8 c

9 c

10 d

• READING SELECTION 10 •

Preview Question

(a) No

(b) They are pathologic

Vocabulary

Answers will vary

Summary

Answers will vary

Comprehension Questions

1 b

2 b

3 a

4 c

5 d

6 a

7 b

8 a
9 c
10 b

• READING SELECTION 11 •

Preview Question

It allows the surgeon to directly visualize the heart during the operation.

Vocabulary

Answers will vary

Summary

Answers will vary

Comprehension Questions

1 d
2 b
3 c
4 b
5 a
6 d
7 b
8 a
9 d
10 a

• READING SELECTION 12 •

Preview Question

Elderly women with osteoporosis

Vocabulary

Answers will vary

Summary

Answers will vary

Comprehension Questions

1 b
2 c
3 d
4 b
5 c
6 b
7 d
8 a
9 c
10 b

• READING SELECTION 13 •

Preview Question

Respiratory depression
Circulating depression
Nausea and vomiting
Paresthesia
Physical dependence
Tolerance

Vocabulary

Answers will vary

Summary

Answers will vary

Comprehension Questions

1 b
2 a
3 c
4 a
5 c
6 b
7 a
8 d
9 a
10 c

• READING SELECTION 14 •

Preview Question

It explains many aspects of pain and how pain may be controlled by thoughts, emotion and action.

Vocabulary

Answers will vary

Summary

Answers will vary

Comprehension Questions

1 d
2 a
3 b
4 c
5 a
6 b
7 d
8 d
9 b
10 c

• READING SELECTION 15 •

Preview Question

Two examples of what happens when intracranial volume is increased by coughing, vomiting, suctioning, straining, etc.

Vocabulary

Answers will vary

Summary

Answers will vary

Comprehension Questions

1 d
2 b
3 c
4 a
5 d
6 b
7 c
8 d
9 a

Index

Note: Page numbers in *italics* refer to illustrations; page numbers followed by t refer to tables.

A

Abbreviations, in note taking, 186
Abducens nerve, assessment of, 238
Acceptance, 221
Acoustic nerve, assessment of, 238–239
Active listening, 173–178
  benefits of, 176
  exercises in, 175–176
  function of, 174
  key words related to, 173
  problems in, 174–175
  strategies for, 175–176
  vs. hearing, 178
Addiction, to analgesics, 275
Adie's pupil, 237–238
Affect, person's, 98
Affixes, 37–44
  examples of, 38–39
  exercise with, 42
  introduction to, 38
  misapplication of, 39
  types of, 38–39
Alignment, correct, *150*
  defined, 150
Alphabetical order, review of, 65
Alzheimer's disease, 259–262
  assessment findings in, 259–260
  factors predisposing to, 259
  nursing diagnoses in, 260–262
  nursing intervention in, 260, 261t
Amnesia, post-traumatic, 255
Analgesics, side effects of, 274–277
Anger, about dying, 221
Annulus, 247
Anorexia, 203
Antonym(s), 50–51
  defined, 50
  dictionary guide to, 63
  examples of, 50–51
Anxiety, about test taking, 215
  from prolonged incapacitation, 271
  relieving, 4
Apnea, sleep, defined, 55
Appendix, exercise related to, 140–141
  function of, 140
Appositive, 51–52
  examples of, 51–52

Arthritis, 203
  gouty, *160*, 160–161
Assessment, sociologic, 146–147
Assumptions, 121–122
Auditory screening, 246
Auscultation, 116
Aversion, sexual, defined, 48
Avoidance, 9

B

Battle's sign, 255
Behavior modification, 54
Bibliography, exercise related to, 138–139
  function of, 138
Biomechanics, defined, 149
Blood flow, cardiac, 251–253
Body alignment, correct, *150*
  defined, 150
Body movement, effective, 150–151
Brain, injuries to, 255–256
Brain stem, contusions of, 256

C

Calendars, daily, 8, *9*
  monthly, *6*
  use of, 5–6
  weekly, *7*
Cancer, cells in, 109
  in elderly, 107
Cardiac blood flow, 251–253
Care plans, nursing, 185
  computerized, 18–20, *19*
  standardized, 17–18
Carotid artery, occlusion of, from head injury, 257
Cerebrospinal fluid, leakage of, 255
Charting, 194
Chronological order, 182
Circulation, cardiovascular, 251–253
Circulatory depression, intervention for, 274
Classification, process of, 56–57
Clusters, 57
Cochlea, 248
Coma, therapeutic, for increased intracranial pressure, 284–285
Communication, confidentiality of, 216

Communication (*Continued*)
  role relationships in, 31–32
  strategies for, 31–32
Comparison, defined, 115
Complement, defined, 47
Compliance, defined, 48
  goal of, 42
  of elderly, 43
Comprehension, reading. See *Reading comprehension.*
Computers, nursing care planning with, 18–20, *19*
Concentration, improving, 1–11
  by finding main idea, 86
  by finding topic, 86, 91–92
  by monitoring comprehension, 24–34
  by prereading strategies, 12–23
  by time management, 3–11
  graphic aids in, 155
Concussion, defined, 255
Conscience, defined, 29
Consciousness, level of, 256
Consistency, 5–6, 10
Constipation, from analgesics, 274–275
Consultation, defined, 48
Contents, table of, example of, 134–137
    function of, 132
Context clues, 45–60
  antonyms as, 50–51
  appositives as, 51–55
  defined, 46–47
  direct definition as, 47–48
  student use of, 55–56
  synonyms as, 48–50
  testing based on, 206
  types of, 47–51
Contrast, defined, 115
Control, locus of, 16
Contusion, brain stem, 256
  cerebral, 256
  findings in, 256
Conversely, defined, 183
Corneal reflex, assessment of, 238
Corticosteroid, 29
Cranial nerve, assessment of, 237–239
  damage to, 255
  eighth, 248
Cues, examples of, 57
  for note taking, 191–192
Cyclitis, defined, 242

D

Data, defined, 107
  objective, 57, 91–92
  subjective, 57, 91–92
Daydreaming, 174
Death, conceptualizations of, 221–222
Deficits, 200
Definition, direct, as context clues, 47–48
  shades of meaning for, 65

Delusional thinking, 201
Dementia, 259–263
  findings in, 259
Dependence, on analgesics, 275
Depression, 29, 221
  circulatory, from analgesics, 274
  respiratory, from analgesics, 274
    intervention for, 274
Dermis, 117
Details, 102–112
  cause, 107
  description, 108–109
  examples as, 108
  function of, 103
  in examinations, 202–203
  in main idea, 103–104
  in note taking, 184–189
  key words related to, 102–103
  listening for, 175
  major, exercise for identifying, 110–111
    in note taking, 189
    vs. minor, 104–105
  minor, in note taking, 189
  procedure, 108
  types of, 107–108
    exercise for identifying, 109–110
Diagnosis(es), nursing, 119–120
Diagrams, example of, *162*
  exercise for reading, 168, *169*, 170, *170*
  function of, 161
Dictionary, 63–71
  collegiate, 63
  guide words in, 66
  locating entries in, 65
  medical, 63
  pronunciation key of, 66
  purpose of, 63
  reading entries in, 64–65
  selection from, 67
  unabridged, 63
Distractions, external, 28
  giving in to, 175
  internal, 28
  types of, 10
Diuretics, osmotic, for increased intracranial pressure, 283
Dying, conceptualizations of, 221–222

E

Ear(s), anatomy and physiology of, 246–250
  external structures of, *246*
  inner, 248
  internal structures of, *247*
  middle, 247, *247*, 248, *248*
Edema, from head injury, 257
Education, client level of, 15
Elderly, abuse of, 107
  cancer in, 107

Elderly *(Continued)*
  noncompliance of, 43
Elimination patterns, alteration in, in Alzheimer's disease, 261
Endolymph, 248
Endorphins, 280
Enkephalins, 280
Epidermis, 117
Epitympanum, 247
Equilibrium, assessment of, 239
Etymology, 63
  abbreviations related to, 64
Examinations. See *Test-taking strategies.*
Extracorporeal membrane oxygenator, 265
Extremities, assessment of, 233–234
Eye(s), assessment of, 237

F

Facial nerve, assessment of, 238
Facts. See *Details.*
Family(ies), synonyms for, 147
Family coping, ineffective, in Alzheimer's disease, 262
Fasciculation, defined, 48
Femur, fracture of, 268–273, *269*
  assessment of, 268
  complications of, 269, 270
  extracapsular, 268
  internal fixation of, 268–269, *269*
  intervention in, 268–269
  intracapsular, 268
  nursing diagnoses related to, 270–272
  postoperative care for, 270
  normal, *269*
5 W's, 145
  exercise related to, 145
Flashcards, creating, 70–80
Former, defined, 184
Fracture, learning/teaching guide about, 271
  of hip. See *Femur, fracture of.*
  of skull, 254–255
Friction, defined, 149
Fulcrum, defined, 149

G

Glands, skin, types of, 190
Glossary, 70, 72
  example of, 73
  exercise related to, 138
  function of, 138
Glossopharyngeal nerve, 239
Glucose, 29
Goals, self-monitoring of, 7–8
  setting and prioritizing, 4–5, 5t
Gout, defined, 160
Gouty arthritis, *160*, 160–161
Graph, exercise for reading, 164
Graphic aids, 154–172

Graphic aids *(Continued)*
  examination of, 15
  key words related to, 154–155
  purpose of, 155
  reading, 161, 163
  relationship of, to written text, 155–157, 159
  types of, 159–161
Graphs, characteristics of, 159, *159*
  example of, *163*
Gravity, center of, 150
  defined, 149
  line of, 150, *150*
Gunn's pupil sign, 237

H

Habitual, defined, 118
Hallucinations, defined, 200–201
Handwriting, streamlined, 185–186
Head, assessment of, 233
Head injuries, 254–257
  health care facility required for, 255t
  primary, 254–256
  secondary, 257
Headings, in note taking, 193–194
  textbook, 144
  use of, 14
Hearing loss, assessment of, 238
Heart, blood flow in, 251–253
Heart-lung machine, *265*
  purposes of, 264–265
  risks of, 265
Hematoma, from head injury, 257
Hemorrhage, 119
Hip fracture. See *Femur, fracture of.*
Hyperbaric, defined, 53
Hypertension, 122
Hyperuricemia, defined, 160
Hypobaric, defined, 53
Hypocapnia, induced, 283
Hypoglossal nerve, assessment of, 239
Hypothermia, in open heart surgery, 264

I

Idea, main. See *Main idea.*
Illusions, defined, 201
Illustrations. See *Graphic aids; Pictures.*
Immobility, complications of, 269
Impairments, 203
Incontinence, in Alzheimer's disease, 260
Index, example of, 143
  exercise related to, 142
  function of, 142
Infant, posture and locomotion of, development of, *120*
Inference, defined, 57
Inflammatory responses, 229–232
  cellular exudate stage of, 230

Inflammatory responses (*Continued*)
  tissue repair and replacement stage of, 230
  vascular stage of, 229–230
Ingrained, defined, 200
Interpretation, process of, 57
Interventions, planning, 15
Intimacy, defined, 146
Intracranial pressure, increased, 283–286
    effects of, *284*
      nonsurgical intervention for, 283–285
      surgical intervention for, 283
Iridocyclitis, defined, 242
Iritis, defined, 242

J

Joints, assessment of, 234, *234*

K

Key words, examples of, 16
  use of, 14–15
Knee joint, goniometric measurement of, *234*
Kübler-Ross, Elisabeth, 221

L

Learning, assumptions about, 121–122
  factors influencing, 15
  readiness for, 121–122
Lectures, note taking for. See *Note taking*.
Level of consciousness, 256
Leverage, defined, 149
Lifestyle, client, 32
  effect of, on client's ability to learn, 16
Listening, active. See *Active listening*.
Lists, to-do, 8, 8t
Living-dying, patterns of, 221–222, 222t
Locomotion, development of, *120*
Locus of control, 16

M

Main idea. See also *Topic*.
  details in, 103–104
  examples of, 92–93
  listening for, 175
  locating, 95–96
  of reading selection, 92–98
  unstated, 96–98
Malleus, 247
Malnutrition, 203
Mannitol, for increased intracranial pressure, 283
Mechanical ventilation, for increased intracranial pressure, 283
Melanin, 117
Membrane(s), Reissner's, 248
  tympanic, 247
Mental patients, rights of, 93

Mobility, 202
  impaired, from femur fracture, 270–271
Momentum, defined, 149
Moral codes, 29
Motivation, client, 15
Movement, body, effective, 150–151
Multiple sclerosis, types of, 106
Myths, 200

N

Narcotics, side effects of, 274–275
Nausea, from analgesics, 274
Neck, assessment of, 233
Nerve(s). See specific nerves.
Network, social, assessment of, 147
Neuritic plaque, defined, 48
Neuropeptides, in pain transmission, 279–280
Noncompliance, definition of, 42
  scope of, 42–43
Non-rapid eye movement sleep, 116
Note taking, 179–196
  abbreviations in, 186
  by taping, 192
  checklist for, 180–181
  cues in, 191–192
  detail in, 184–185
  determining important points for, 191–192
  formulating questions from, 193–194
  headings in, 193
  indicating major and minor points in, 189–190
  key words related to, 180
  organizational factors in, 182–183, *183*
  quantity of, 183–184
  relationship of, to active listening, 176
  reviewing, 192
  rote, 174
  shorthand in, 187–188
  streamlined handwriting in, 185–186
  studying, 192, 194–195
  symbols in, 188–189
  verbal tips for, 191
Nursing care plans, computerized, 18–20, *19*
  standardized, 17–18
Nursing diagnosis(es), 119–120
Nursing process, characteristics of, 55
  diagram of, *170*
Nutrition, in Alzheimer's disease, 260–261
Nystagmus, 238

O

Obesity, 203
Oculomotor nerve, assessment of, 237–238
Olfactory nerve, assessment of, 237
Ombudsmen, 93
Open heart surgery, 264–267
Opioids, endogenous, 280
  side effects of, 274–275

Optic nerve, assessment of, 237
Optimal, defined, 116
Osmotic diuretics, for increased intracranial pressure, 283
Ostomy, learning outcomes related to, 16

P

Pain, gate-control theory of, 278–282, *279*
  intractable, defined, 54
  nursing care plan in, 18
  perception of, 280
  physiology of, 278
  theories of, 104–105
  transmission of, facilitation of, 280
   inhibition of, 280
   molecular basis of, 279–280
Pain threshold, 280
Palpation, 116
Pancreas, endocrine functions of, 47
  exocrine functions of, 47
Paragraph, finding topic of, 88–92
  main idea in, 95–96
  organization of, by cause and effect, 115
   by comparison-contrast, 115
   by simple listing, 115–116
   chronological, 114–115
   exercises for identifying, 116–123
   improving reading comprehension with, 113–125
   key words related to, 113–114
   recognizing, 114
Paralysis, facial, 255
Paraphrasing, 175
Paresthesia, from analgesics, 275
Pars flaccida, 247
Parts of speech, 64
Passive, defined, 174
Percussion, 116
Perilymph, 248
Pictures. See also *Graphic aids.*
  exercise for, 164
  purpose of, 160
Pinna, 246
Positive end-expiratory pressure, 284
Postphlebitic syndrome, characteristics of, 54
Posture, correct, *150*
  defined, 150
  development of, *120*
Powerlessness, from prolonged incapacitation, 271–272
Preceding, defined, 174
Preface, example of, 133
  purpose of, 132
Prefixes, definitions of, 38, 40t
  examples of, 40t
Prereading strategies, 12–23
  example of, 15–16
  exercises for, 17–30
Prevention, protocol for, 42–43
Priorities, setting, 4–5

Procrastination, anxiety caused by, 4, 9
Pronunciation, dictionary guide to, 63, 64
Pronunciation key, 66
Prosthesis, defined, 48
Protocol, 17
Psychotherapy, defined, 193
Pupils, assessment of, 237
  with head injuries, 256

Q

Questions, detail, in examinations, 202–203
  essay, 212–216
  examples of, 148
  formulating, 144
   from notes, 193–194
  inference, in examinations, 204
  main idea, 199
  objective test, 207–213

R

Rapid eye movement sleep, 116
Reading, purpose in, 98–99
  study skills related to, 129–153
Reading comprehension, 83–125
  improving, details in, 102–112. See also *Details.*
   graphic aids in, 155
   paragraph organization in, 113–125
  monitoring, 24–34
   by defining new words, 27–28
   by questions, 32
   by rereading, 25–26
   by research, 30
   by summarizing, 26–27
   by visualization, 28–29
   in longer passages, 30–32
   strategies for, 25–30
  of topic, 86–97
Reflex(es), corneal, assessment of, 238
Reissner's membrane, 248
REM sleep, 116
Rereading, 25–26
Research, as monitoring strategy, 30
Respiration, assessment of, with head injuries, 256
Respiratory depression, from analgesics, 274
  intervention for, 274
Retention, improvement of, graphic aids in, 155
Revisions, 213
Rinne test, 239
Roots, word, definitions of, 38, 40t–41t
  examples of, 40t–41t

S

Sabotage, 186
Scalp, injuries to, 254
Schema, defined, 30
Scoliosis, defined, 203

Seizures, from increased intracranial pressure, 284
Self-care deficit, in Alzheimer's disease, 260
Self-concept, 194
Semicircular canals, 248
Sexual aversion, defined, 48
Shorthand, note taking with, 187–188
Significant others, 147
Skeletal system, assessment of, 233–236
    deformities of, 234
Skin glands, types of, 190
Skin integrity, impaired, nursing process in, 225–228
Skull, injuries to, 254–255
Sleep, REM versus non-REM, 116
Sleep apnea, defined, 55
Social network, assessment of, 147
Social status, in therapeutic relationship, 31–32
Sociologic assessment, 146–147
Speech, parts of, 64
Spelling, dictionary guide to, 63
Spinal accessory nerve, assessment of, 239
Spinal cord transmission cell, 278
Spine, assessment of, 233
Stability, defined, 149
Steroids, for increased intracranial pressure, 283
Study guide, preparation of, 146
Study skills, 127–218
    active listening as, 173–178
    graphic aids as, 154–172
    in textbook reading, 129–153
    note taking as, 179–196
    test-taking strategies as, 197–218
Substance P, in pain transmission, 279–280
Substantia gelatinosa, 278
Suffixes, definitions and examples of, 41t
Summarizing, 26–27, 148
    in note taking, 184–189
    of textbook selections, 145
    with graphic aids, 157
Superego, subsystems of, 29
Support systems, 147
Sutures, 226
    classification of, 225–226
Syllabication, dictionary guide to, 63
Symbols, note taking with, 188–189
Symptoms, defined, 57
Synonym(s), 48–50
    defined, 48
    dictionary guide to, 63
Synonymous, defined, 174

T

Table of contents, example of, 134–137
    function of, 132
Tables, example of, 158t, 162t
    exercise for reading, 165, 168
    function of, 161
Taping, note taking with, 192
Taste, assessment of, 239

Taxonomy, defined, 119
Test-taking strategies, 197–218
    exercise for, 211–212
    for avoiding anxiety, 216
    for essay tests, 212–216
    for matching tests, 207
    for multiple-choice tests, 199–213
        with detail questions, 202–203
        with inference questions, 204–206
        with main idea questions, 199–201
        with vocabulary in context questions, 206–207
    for objective tests, 198–199, 208–210
    for short answer tests, 207
    for true-false tests, 207
    key words related to, 197–198
    practice tests as, 216
    preparation in, 198
Text, relationship of, to graphic aids, 155–157, 159
Textbook, formulating questions about, 144
    exercise related to, 148
    graphic aids in. See *Graphic aids.*
    headings in, 144
    main ideas and details of, 5 W's for determining, 145
    preparing study guide for, 146
        exercise related to, 148
    previewing, 144
        exercise related to, 147
    reading strategies for, 144–151
    study skills for reading, 129–153
        exercise using, 149–151
    studying, 146
    summarizing selections from, 145
        exercise related to, 148
    surveying, 130–138
    typographical clues in, 144
    underlining in, 146
        exercise related to, 148
Therapeutic index, 52
Thesaurus, 72–75
    defined, 72
    example of, 75
    purpose of, 72
    use of, 74
Thinking, delusional, 201
Thought processes, alteration in, in Alzheimer's disease, 260
Time management, 3–11
    calendars in, 5–6
    goal setting in, 4–5
    organizing skills in, 4
Title page, exercise related to, 130–131
    information contained on, 130
Tolerance, of analgesics, 275
Topic, 86–92. See also *Main idea.*
    defined, 86
    finding, 86–88
        as aid to concentration, 91–92
    in paragraphs, 88–92
Tremor, defined, 48

Trigeminal nerve, assessment of, 238
Trochlear nerve, assessment of, 238
Tympanic membrane, 247

U

Underlining, 146, 148
Understanding, defined, 48
Uveitis, 242–243
   management of, 243
   overview of, 242

V

Vagus nerve, assessment of, 239
Ventilation, mechanical, for increased intracranial pressure, 283
Ventricular fibrillation, from induced hypothermia, 264
Vestibulocochlear nerve, assessment of, 238–239
Vision, impairment of, 243, 255
   peripheral, testing of, 237
Visual aids. See *Graphic aids.*
Visualization, as comprehension strategy, 28–29
Vocabulary. See also *Words.*
   development of, 35–82
     with affixes, 37–44
     with context clues, 45–60

Vocabulary (*Continued*)
     with dictionaries, 63–71
     with glossaries, 70, 72
     with thesaurus, 72–75
Vomiting, from analgesics, 274

W

Word bank, 78–82
   advantages of, 79–81
   creating, 79–81
Words. See also *Vocabulary.*
   components of, 38–39. See also *Affixes.*
   definitions of, approximate, 46
     as comprehension strategy, 27–28
     precise, 47
     sources for, 62–75
   guide, 66
   remembering, 79
   roots of, 38, 40t–41t
   unknown, encountering, 79
     indicating, 79
Wound(s), closure of, 225–226

Z

Zygote, 52

LEARNING CENTRE